BARRON'S

PCAT*

Pharmacy College Admission Test

7TH EDITION

Marie A. Chisholm-Burns, Pharm.D., MPH, MBA, FCCP, FASHP, FAST

Dean and Professor
University of Tennessee College of Pharmacy
Memphis, Knoxville, and Nashville, Tennessee

Contributing Authors:

Alan Wolfgang, Ph.D.
Assistant Dean for Student Affairs
The University of Georgia College of Pharmacy
Athens, Georgia

Mark A. McCombs, M.S.
Senior Lecturer, Department of Mathematics
University of North Carolina at Chapel Hill
Chapel Hill, North Carolina

Suzanne Carpenter, M.S.
Associate Professor of Chemistry
Armstrong State University
College of Science and Technology
Savannah, Georgia

Christina Spivey, Ph.D.
Assistant Professor
Department of Clinical Pharmacy
University of Tennessee College of Pharmacy
Memphis, Tennessee

Sara Gremillion, Ph.D.
Associate Professor, Department of Biology
Armstrong State University
College of Science and Technology
Savannah, Georgia

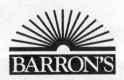

BARRON'S

*PCAT is a registered trademark of Pearson, which does not endorse this book.

All inquiries should be addressed to:
Barron's Educational Series, Inc.
250 Wireless Boulevard
Hauppauge, NY 11788
www.barronseduc.com

ISBN: 978-1-4380-0866-0

Library of Congress Catalog Card No.: 2017930893

PRINTED IN THE UNITED STATES OF AMERICA
9 8 7 6 5 4 3 2 1

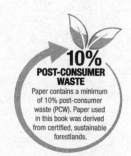

10%
POST-CONSUMER
WASTE
Paper contains a minimum
of 10% post-consumer
waste (PCW). Paper used
in this book was derived
from certified, sustainable
forestlands.

Contents

Introduction

━━━

Grades achieved in pre-pharmacy courses and Pharmacy College Admission Test (PCAT) scores are often the most important criteria used to evaluate students for admission to colleges and schools of pharmacy. Therefore, it is crucial for you to perform your very best on the PCAT. The PCAT was developed to provide college admission committees with comparable information about the academic abilities of applicants in designated areas.

This study guide can be very useful in preparing you for the PCAT, and for pharmacy education in general. When used properly and in combination with other materials, such as those offered on the official PCAT website (*www.pcatweb.info*), this guide will enhance your chances in the applicant pool of a college or school of pharmacy. All chapters are written by practicing pharmacists and/or educators (professors or instructors) with extensive experience in the admission procedures of U.S. pharmacy schools. In addition, each of the chapter authors has special expertise in the designated subject; this will further help you do your best on the PCAT.

This guide should help focus your review by outlining and reviewing subjects that are currently included on the PCAT. In addition, this guide can be very useful in the early stages of your pre-pharmacy education by pointing out the areas that will be covered on the PCAT. Thus, you will be able to prioritize topics for studying, a step that will aid you in achieving your desired score.

Remember, your pre-pharmacy courses are designed to serve as the foundation for your pharmacy education. The PCAT is intended to determine your grasp of this material and your ability to apply it during your continued education. To be successful on the PCAT, it is important that you not only understand the material in a particular course, but that you can also apply it in your future program of higher education. If you take your pre-pharmacy courses with this in mind, the PCAT should be less difficult.

Use this and any other study guide as just that—a guide to what and how to study. The chance that the same exact questions contained in this text will be on the exam you take is remote; however, the likelihood that the same material will be covered is great. When reviewing a particular question, do not just look for the sentence or phrase that "answers the question"; study the topic and refresh your understanding of the material. Pay particular attention to facts that are related but differ in a "testable" way. For example, do you remember the terms *mitosis* and *meiosis*? You may remember these words and perhaps know that they have something to do with cell propagation, but that is not enough. If the multiple-choice answers to a question on the PCAT include descriptions of both mitosis and meiosis, you must be able to distinguish between the terms to select the correct answer, or risk receiving no more credit than someone who never took a biology course.

This book reviews all the sections of the PCAT (as of 2017) and therefore serves as a good focal point to begin studying for the exam. Please keep in mind, however, that this is a guide; its purpose is not to review all required pre-pharmacy courses, but rather to aid you in studying for the PCAT. For optimal performance, it is strongly suggested that you use this guide along with your pre-pharmacy coursework to prepare for the PCAT.

FORMAT AND USE OF THIS BOOK

The format of this book is user-friendly. Chapter 1 covers general information about the pharmacy profession, pharmacy school admissions, and pharmacy education. In Chapters 2 and 3, general information on the current PCAT and specific test-taking strategies and tactics are presented, respectively. Five chapters addressing biological processes, chemical processes, quantitative reasoning, critical reading, and writing follow. Also, each chapter (with the exception of the writing chapter) has a set of questions with full explanatory answers to test, review, and enhance your knowledge of the various subjects. The chapter on writing your PCAT essay contains helpful tips for writing effectively. Finally, so you can practice taking the exam and evaluating your skills, two sample PCATs with full explanatory answers are provided in Chapters 9 and 10.

Planning for a Career in Pharmacy

1

A CAREER IN PHARMACY

Over the last few decades, pharmacy practice has undergone significant changes. Since the 1960s, the pharmacy profession has branched out in many directions other than traditional pharmacy settings (community and hospital). Once you have graduated from pharmacy school and have successfully passed a pharmacy state board licensure examination, career opportunities in pharmacy are great. These opportunities include, but are not limited to, community pharmacy (chain and independent), hospital pharmacy, pharmaceutical industry, government agencies, geriatric pharmacy, clinical pharmacy, pharmacy services, managed care pharmacy, pharmaceutical research, pharmacy and medical education, nuclear pharmacy, and other specialty areas.

Job opportunities are diverse for a person who earns a degree in pharmacy. In addition, postgraduate training or graduate education provides an excellent opportunity for continuing your pharmacy education, thereby enhancing your career opportunities in this field. Although career counseling is best done in a pharmacy program, the purpose of this section is to familiarize you with several pharmacy careers (see the list that follows). Once accepted into a pharmacy school, you should inquire further about career opportunities in pharmacy.

Examples of Career Opportunities in Pharmacy

Academia
- Administration
- Biological Science
- Clinical Pharmacy
- Continuing Education
- Experiential Education
- Medicinal Chemistry
- Pharmaceutics
- Pharmacy Administration
- Pharmacy Practice

Administration
- Continuing Education
- Professional Relations

Business
- Administration
- Management
- Marketing
- Sales

Clinical
- Adult Medicine
- Ambulatory Care
- Clinical Coordinator
- Clinical Manager
- Critical Care
- Drug Information
- Family Medicine
- Geriatrics
- Infectious Disease
- Internal Medicine
- Nutrition
- Oncology
- Pain Management

Pediatrics
Pharmacokinetics
Poison Control
Psychiatry
Surgery
Transplantation

Community
Apothecary
Compounding Pharmacy
Franchise
Home Health Care
Long-term Care
Specialty Pharmacy

Computer Technology Consultant
Clinical Pharmacy
Home Health Care
Long-term Care

Drug Information

Federal
Alcohol, Drug Abuse, and
  Mental Health
Armed Services
Clinical Pharmacy
Drug Enforcement Administration
Food and Drug Administration
Health Administration
Health Care Financing
Indian Health Services
Medicare

Hospital
Administration
Clinical Pharmacy
Inventory Control
Staff

Independent
Apothecary
Clinical Pharmacy
Franchise
Home Health Care
Long-term Care
Specialty Pharmacy

Industry
Regulatory Affairs
Medical Communication
Medication Safety

Mail-Order Pharmacy

Managed Care Pharmacy

Nuclear Pharmacy

Pharmacy Associations

Research and Development
Biological Sciences
Clinical Outcomes
Cosmetics/Formulation
Informatics
Medicinal Chemistry
Pharmaceutical Research
Pharmaceutics
Pharmacogenomics
Pharmacognosy
Pharmacology
Pharmacy Administration
Pharmacy Practice

State
Board of Pharmacy
Clinical Outcomes
Department of Consumer Affairs
Department of Health
Medicaid

Technical/Scientific
Drug Information
Manufacturing
Postmarketing Surveillance
Product Control

Veterans Administration Facilities

Veterinary Pharmacy

IMPORTANT CONSIDERATIONS WHEN PLANNING YOUR PHARMACY EDUCATION

On the following page is a flowchart that displays some general guidelines to help you when planning your pharmacy education and completing the admission process at a U.S. college/school of pharmacy. For additional information, refer to the pre-pharmacy advisor at the institution where you are taking your pre-pharmacy required courses and the college/school of pharmacy you wish to attend. The information given in this chapter should not replace or supersede information obtained from your pre-pharmacy advisor or the college/school of pharmacy in which you would like to continue your education.

Pre-Pharmacy Curricula

You should be familiar with the requirements of each of the institutions to which you plan to apply. Many students who apply to pharmacy school have more than the minimum pre-pharmacy course requirements and/or have attended college for more than two years. You may be able to complete the required pre-pharmacy coursework within two years (of course, this depends on the individual requirements of the pharmacy school); however, there are some schools that require more than two years of coursework. Obviously, the pre-pharmacy curricula at each school may vary, but there are typically some similarities that will give you an idea of the type of courses required. Below is an outline detailing the subject areas covered by many pre-pharmacy curricula. Please note: additional coursework may be required and the courses listed below may or may not be required at many schools of pharmacy; therefore, it is imperative to check with the school of pharmacy for its exact pre-pharmacy requirements.

REMEMBER

The information provided in this book regarding the PCAT is current at the time of the book's writing; for the most recent PCAT updates and information, please refer to the official PCAT website at *www.pcatweb.info.*

PRE-PHARMACY CURRICULUM OUTLINE

- Humanities and Fine Arts Courses

  - English—two courses or one year.
  - Literature—one course.
  - Communication/Speech—one course.

- Social Science Courses

  - History—one or more courses.
  - Political Science—one course. This may be covered with an additional History course.
  - Economics—one course.
  - Other Social Science elective—one course (e.g., Sociology, Psychology, Anthropology, or additional History courses).

- Math and Science Courses

  - Pre-Calculus—one course. Some programs may only require Calculus courses, but prerequisites may be required of some post-secondary applicants.
  - Calculus/Analytical Geometry—one or two courses.
  - Statistics—one course.
  - Biological Sciences—two courses or one year with labs. Some programs may require Anatomy and Physiology and/or Microbiology as pre-pharmacy courses.
  - Chemistry—four courses or two years. These courses include General Chemistry and Organic Chemistry with labs. Some programs may require Biochemistry.
  - Physics—up to two courses or one year. Physics is not required by some programs.

Pharmacy School Applicant Guidelines

Identify pharmacy school(s) of interest.
Important considerations that may help you
in the identification process include:
- school's geographical location;
- your program preference;
- cost and scholarship availability;
- school's reputation; and
- academic requirements for admission.

Identify what pre-pharmacy courses are required.
- This information will vary between different
  pharmacy schools.
- Since many pre-pharmacy courses are sequential,
  it is important to focus on the scheduling of courses.
- As soon as possible, make an appointment
  to consult with the pre-pharmacy advisor
  at your school.

Take pre-pharmacy courses.
- It is important to make the best grades and
  get the best background possible in these
  courses. Keep materials from courses as they
  may be helpful to study for the PCAT.

**Apply to pharmacy school(s) and/or
PharmCAS (www.PharmCAS.org).**
Check with your pre-pharmacy advisor
concerning the most appropriate
time to apply.
- Apply as early as possible and when
  appropriate, considering when you will
  be finished with pre-pharmacy requirements.
- If faculty or personal references are
  required, select professors and others who
  know you well, will provide a good
  reference, and will send it in *on time*.
- If the school utilizes PharmCAS, check to
  see if supplemental forms are required.

**Is the PCAT required by
the pharmacy school(s)
to which you are applying?**

YES

NO

Register to take the PCAT.
Allow yourself the opportunity to take
the PCAT more than once; check with
your pre-pharmacy advisor and the
PCAT website (*www.pcatweb.info*)
for scheduling and registration.
Check with the pharmacy school(s)
concerning their policy on taking the
PCAT more than once and how
multiple PCAT scores are considered
in the admission process.

**Complete the application
process and await status letter.**
Make sure you follow up if you
are offered admission. You will
need to confirm and may have
to provide a tuition deposit and/or
complete a background check.

**Check with each pharmacy
school/college about interview.**

Each institution's program will have its own pre-pharmacy course requirements; you should obtain this information directly from the desired school. Many colleges and universities offer pre-professional advising programs to assist students in course selection. Utilize these advisors and the recruitment and admission staff of your desired pharmacy program as important resources. Since many programs only accept students once a year, if you do not complete the pre-pharmacy curriculum by the designated time, it may delay acceptance by an entire academic year. If you have previously completed coursework for which you expect to receive credit, in lieu of some specific pre-pharmacy prerequisites, verify whether the course will satisfy requirements early in your application process.

Doctorate of Pharmacy Degree Curricula

DOCTORATE OF PHARMACY DEGREE ("2 + 4," "3 + 4," AND "4 + 4" PROGRAMS)

Each school or college of pharmacy has a list of courses that are considered prerequisites to the pharmacy professional program. For many schools, the pre-pharmacy prerequisites can take two years or longer to complete. A two-year pre-pharmacy curriculum, along with the four-year professional curriculum, comprises what is called a "2 + 4" professional doctor of pharmacy degree program. There are a few pharmacy programs in which students take courses year round (i.e., they attend classes in the summer), and thereby complete the equivalent of a standard four-year curriculum in three calendar years. Some programs require three years of pre-pharmacy coursework ("3 + 4" program). Some programs require eighty or more hours of pre-pharmacy coursework, and may even require applicants to have earned a bachelor's degree (such programs are referred to as "4 + 4" programs); thus, it could take considerably longer than two years to complete the pre-pharmacy requirements for many schools.

DOCTORATE OF PHARMACY DEGREE ("0 + 6" PROGRAM)

Another variation of the "2 + 4" program is the "0 + 6" program. This program allows students to be accepted directly into the school or college of pharmacy where they will complete the pre-pharmacy core as part of a six-year academic program. Most of these programs also consider applicants to the professional program; however, if the student is accepted, he or she will enter at the beginning of the third year of the program.

PharmCAS

The Pharmacy College Application Service (PharmCAS) is a centralized application service designed to assemble, process, and distribute applicants' information. Most pharmacy programs utilize this service to gather admission data from applicants, advisors, and other sources. The system is similar to those used by other professional programs such as medical schools, law schools, and veterinary medicine programs. The information presented here is current as of the preparation of this edition of this book.

PharmCAS is designed to be a comprehensive application system that provides a mechanism to distribute information about an applicant to one or more participating pharmacy schools. According to the information detailed on the PharmCAS website, the system operates to benefit applicants, participating pharmacy schools, and advisors of pre-pharmacy

TIP

Familiarize yourself
with PharmCAS
by obtaining
information from
their website,
www.PharmCAS.org.

students. Information for each participating school is provided on the PharmCAS website. Listed below are some examples of the information that is provided:

1. application deadlines
2. transcript submission requirements
3. pre-pharmacy requirements
4. recommendation submission procedures
5. any special or additional requirements for specific schools

Non-participating schools—those NOT participating in PharmCAS—are listed and links to various school websites are provided. Be aware that PharmCAS participating schools may still require that supplemental application data be submitted directly to the school to which the student is applying.

As of 2017, the application fee for an individual to submit an application to a single participating school is $175. There is a graduated fee scale to apply for more than one school. For example, to apply for a second school, an additional $55 is required. The PharmCAS website contains the most current information.

The PharmCAS website lists several sources of instructions. Applicants are encouraged to familiarize themselves with the "Step-by-Step" checklist, PharmCAS Application Instructions, and Applicant Code of Conduct. Visit the PharmCAS website at *www.PharmCAS.org.*

In addition to various supplemental materials that may be required by schools participating in PharmCAS, applicants must submit transcript request forms to the registrar of each U.S. and Canadian college or university they have attended. A requirement as of 2017 is the provision for letters of reference to be submitted via PharmCAS. You may enter the names of up to four reference writers on your PharmCAS application. Evaluators will be sent an email from PharmCAS with information on how to submit an electronic letter of reference to PharmCAS; hard copy letters of recommendation will not be accepted. PharmCAS will forward these references to designated schools when your file is complete. PharmCAS does not forward references to schools which require that reference letters be submitted to them directly. Again, the applicant should consult the PharmCAS website for specific instructions for the program or programs in which he or she is interested.

Some participating pharmacy programs offer an "early decision" process via the PharmCAS system. As of the 2016–2017 application cycle, the early decision application deadline is September 6. The PharmCAS website indicates that an applicant must contact the schools offering early decision to obtain information regarding early decision guidelines. Additionally, if you are offered admission as an early decision application participant, you are obligated to accept that offer AND you will not be permitted to apply to another PharmCAS institution. PharmCAS institutions that participate in the early decision process will announce those choices by a date selected annually.

Part of the application process for PharmCAS requires that the applicant enter all coursework and grades using personal transcripts or grade reports. These entries are verified by PharmCAS upon receipt of official copies of your transcripts. Additional copies of your official transcripts may be required by the institution(s).

Students who have completed college-level work at foreign institutions must contact the schools to which they are applying, or get specific information from the school's website. Usually, foreign transcripts must be submitted to a service that specializes in this type of evaluation. Individual schools vary in their procedures for accepting credit toward the completion of pre-pharmacy coursework from non-U.S. accredited programs.

Applicants who submitted and paid for an application to PharmCAS in the previous cycle are eligible to have their application information carried over to the new cycle. Please refer to the application instructions on the PharmCAS website for further details.

The PharmCAS system offers a mechanism for an applicant to pursue a number of pharmacy programs while possibly reducing the amount of repeated materials that must be submitted. Currently, the majority of all pharmacy programs utilize PharmCAS. Applicants should contact each pharmacy school of interest to obtain admission requirements.

For current information on PharmCAS, please visit *www.PharmCAS.org*, as information in this section may change.

TIP

Make sure that you check to see if any additional materials are required, even if a school uses PharmCAS.

U.S. Colleges and Schools of Pharmacy Admission Requirements

Applications for admission to schools and colleges of pharmacy have increased significantly in the twenty-first century. For example, the American Association of Colleges of Pharmacy (AACP) reported an average application-to-enrollment ratio of approximately 3:1 for U.S. schools of pharmacy in 1990; however, in 2015 the average applicant-to-enrollment ratio was about 5.4:1. The increased number of applicants can be interpreted in many ways in terms of pharmacy practice and education. You should prepare yourself to be the most competitive.

As of 2017, there were approximately 140 schools of pharmacy with accreditation or preaccreditation status in the U.S. The listing of schools can be found through the Accreditation Council for Pharmacy Education website (*www.acpe-accredit.org*) or through the AACP website (*www.aacp.org*). All schools of pharmacy utilize the college pre-pharmacy grade point average (GPA) when evaluating candidates for admission. In addition to the GPA, the PCAT is utilized by most pharmacy schools when selecting students. Therefore, the two main academic performance selection criteria for admission are the PCAT scores and the pre-pharmacy GPA. Schools also conduct interviews to evaluate students for acceptance; however, whether a candidate is selected for an interview is often dependent on his or her GPA and PCAT performance.

Since acceptance into pharmacy school is very competitive, it is extremely important for you to do your best in both.

U.S. Colleges and Schools of Pharmacy

The following information represents the U.S. colleges and schools of pharmacy as reported by the Accreditation Council for Pharmacy Education (ACPE). More than 95% of the schools listed here have been accredited by ACPE. To obtain the most current information and accreditation status, contact the specific college or school of pharmacy in which you are interested.

Albany College of Pharmacy

Appalachian College of Pharmacy

Auburn University

Belmont University

Butler University

California Health Sciences University

California Northstate University

Campbell University

Cedarville University

Chapman University

Chicago State University

Concordia University

Creighton University

Drake University

Duquesne University

D'Youville College

East Tennessee State University

Fairleigh Dickinson University

Ferris State University

Florida A&M University

Hampton University

Harding University

High Point University

Howard University

Husson University

Idaho State University

Keck Graduate Institute

Ketchum University

Lake Erie College of Osteopathic
   Medicine

Larkin Health Sciences Institute

Lipscomb University

Loma Linda University

Long Island University

Manchester University

Marshall University

Massachusetts College of Pharmacy
   and Health Sciences (MCPHS)
      University—Boston

MCPHS University—Worcester

Medical University of South Carolina

Mercer University

Midwestern University—Chicago

Midwestern University—Glendale

North Dakota State University

Northeast Ohio Medical University

Northeastern University

Notre Dame of Maryland University

Nova Southeastern University

Ohio Northern University

Ohio State University

Oregon State University

Pacific University

Palm Beach Atlantic University

Philadelphia College

Presbyterian College

Purdue University

Regis University

Roosevelt University

Rosalind Franklin University

Roseman University of Health Sciences

Rutgers University

Samford University

Shenandoah University

South College

South Dakota State University

South University

Southern Illinois University—Edwardsville

Southwestern Oklahoma State University

St. John Fisher College

St. John's University

St. Louis College of Pharmacy

Sullivan University

Temple University

Texas A&M University—Kingsville

Texas Southern University

Texas Tech University

Thomas Jefferson University

Touro College
Touro University
Union University
University of Arizona
University of Arkansas
University at Buffalo—State University
   of New York
University of California—San Diego
University of California—San Francisco
University of Charleston
University of Cincinnati
University of Colorado
University of Connecticut
University of Findlay
University of Florida
University of Georgia
University of Hawaii
University of Houston
University of Illinois
University of the Incarnate Word
University of Iowa
University of Kansas
University of Kentucky
University of Louisiana
University of Maryland
University of Maryland Eastern Shore
University of Michigan
University of Minnesota
University of Minnesota—Duluth
University of Mississippi
University of Missouri
University of Montana
University of Nebraska

University of New England
University of New Mexico
University of North Carolina
University of North Texas
University of Oklahoma
University of the Pacific
University of Pittsburgh
University of Puerto Rico
University of Rhode Island
University of Saint Joseph
University of the Sciences in Philadelphia
University of South Carolina
University of South Florida
University of Southern California
University of Tennessee Health Science
   Center
University of Texas at Austin
University of Texas at Tyler
University of Toledo
University of Utah
University of Washington
University of Wisconsin
University of Wyoming
Virginia Commonwealth University
Washington State University
Wayne State University
West Coast University
West Virginia University
Western New England University
Western University of Health Sciences
Wilkes University
Wingate University
Xavier University of Louisiana

Directory of U.S. Colleges and Schools of Pharmacy (by State)

ALABAMA

Harrison School of Pharmacy
Auburn University
2316 Walker Building
Auburn University, Alabama 36849-5501
(334) 844-8348
pharmacy.auburn.edu/
Branch Campus: Mobile, Alabama
Professional Degree Offered: Doctor of Pharmacy

McWhorter School of Pharmacy
Samford University
800 Lakeshore Drive
Birmingham, Alabama 35229
(205) 726-2982
www.samford.edu/pharmacy
Professional Degree Offered: Doctor of Pharmacy

ARIZONA

College of Pharmacy—Glendale
Midwestern University
19555 North 59th Avenue
Glendale, Arizona 85308
(623) 572-3215
www.midwestern.edu/programs-and-admission/
    az-pharmacy.html
Professional Degree Offered: Doctor of Pharmacy

College of Pharmacy
University of Arizona
1295 N. Martin Avenue
P.O. Box 210202
Tucson, Arizona 85721
(520) 626-1427
www.pharmacy.arizona.edu/
Branch Campus: Phoenix, Arizona
Professional Degree Offered: Doctor of Pharmacy

ARKANSAS

College of Pharmacy
Harding University
915 East Market Avenue
Searcy, Arkansas 72149
(501) 279-5528
www.harding.edu/pharmacy
Professional Degree Offered: Doctor of Pharmacy

College of Pharmacy
University of Arkansas for Medical Sciences
4301 West Markham Street, Slot 522
Little Rock, Arkansas 72205
(501) 686-8889
pharmcollege.uams.edu
Branch Campus: Fayetteville, Arkansas
Professional Degree Offered: Doctor of Pharmacy

CALIFORNIA

College of Pharmacy
California Health Sciences University
120 N. Clovis Avenue
Clovis, California 93612
(559) 325-3600
chsu.org
Professional Degree Offered: Doctor of Pharmacy

College of Pharmacy
California Northstate University
9700 West Taron Drive
Elk Grove, California 95757
(916) 631-8108
pharmacy.cnsu.edu/
Professional Degree Offered: Doctor of Pharmacy

School of Pharmacy
Chapman University
9401 Jeronimo Road
Suite 212
Irvine, California 92618
(714) 516-5600
www.chapman.edu/pharmacy
Professional Degree Offered: Doctor of Pharmacy

School of Pharmacy
Keck Graduate Institute
535 Watson Drive
Claremont, California 91711
(909) 607-9145
www.kgi.edu/pharmacy
Professional Degree Offered: Doctor of Pharmacy

School of Pharmacy
Loma Linda University
Shryock Hall
24745 Stewart Street
Loma Linda, California 92350
(909) 558-1300
pharmacy.llu.edu
Professional Degree Offered: Doctor of Pharmacy

College of Pharmacy
Marshall B. Ketchum University
2575 Yorba Linda Boulevard
Fullerton, California 92831
(714) 872-5698
www.ketchum.edu/index.php/academics/ph
Professional Degree Offered: Doctor of Pharmacy

College of Pharmacy
Touro University—California
1310 Club Drive, Mare Island
Vallejo, California 94592
(707) 638-5200
cop.tu.edu/
Professional Degree Offered: Doctor of Pharmacy

Skaggs School of Pharmacy and Pharmaceutical
    Sciences
University of California—San Diego
9500 Gilman Drive
La Jolla, California 92093
(858) 822-4900
pharmacy.ucsd.edu/
Professional Degree Offered: Doctor of Pharmacy

School of Pharmacy
University of California at San Francisco
513 Parnassus Avenue
UCSF Box 0150, Room S-960
San Francisco, California 94143
(415) 476-2733
pharmacy.ucsf.edu/
Professional Degree Offered: Doctor of Pharmacy

Thomas J. Long School of Pharmacy
    and Health Sciences
University of the Pacific
3601 Pacific Avenue
Stockton, California 95211
(209) 946-2211
www.pacific.edu/Academics/Schools-and-Colleges/
    Thomas-J-Long-School-of-Pharmacy-and-
    Health-Sciences.html
Professional Degree Offered: Doctor of Pharmacy

School of Pharmacy
University of Southern California
1985 Zonal Avenue
Los Angeles, California 90089-9121
(323) 442-1369
pharmacyschool.usc.edu/
Professional Degree Offered: Doctor of Pharmacy

School of Pharmacy
West Coast University
590 N. Vermont Avenue
Los Angeles, California 90004
(866) 424-7476
pharmacy.westcoastuniversity.edu
Professional Degree Offered: Doctor of Pharmacy

College of Pharmacy
Western University of Health Sciences
309 E. Second Street
Pomona, California 91766
(909) 469-5335
www.westernu.edu/pharmacy
Professional Degree Offered: Doctor of Pharmacy

COLORADO

School of Pharmacy
Regis University
3333 Regis Boulevard
Denver, Colorado 80221-1099
(303) 458-4344 or (800) 388-2366 (ext. 4344)
*www.regis.edu/RHCHP/Schools/School-of-
Pharmacy.aspx*
Professional Degree Offered: Doctor of Pharmacy

Skaggs School of Pharmacy and Pharmaceutical
Sciences
University of Colorado Anschutz Medical
Campus
Pharmacy and Pharmaceutical Sciences Building
12850 East Montview Boulevard
Aurora, Colorado 80045
(303) 724-2882
www.ucdenver.edu/pharmacy
Professional Degree Offered: Doctor of Pharmacy

CONNECTICUT

School of Pharmacy
The University of Connecticut
69 North Eagleville Road
Storrs, Connecticut 06269
(860) 486-2216
pharmacy.uconn.edu/
Professional Degree Offered: Doctor of Pharmacy

School of Pharmacy
University of St. Joseph
229 Trumbull Street
Hartford, Connecticut 06103-0501
(860) 231-5858
*www.usj.edu/academics/schools/school-of-
pharmacy*
Professional Degree Offered: Doctor of Pharmacy

DISTRICT OF COLUMBIA

College of Pharmacy
Howard University
2300 Fourth Street, Northwest
Washington, DC 20059
(202) 806-6530
*healthsciences.howard.edu/education/colleges/
pharmacy*
Professional Degree Offered: Doctor of Pharmacy

FLORIDA

College of Pharmacy and Pharmaceutical
Sciences
Florida Agricultural and Mechanical University
1415 South Martin Luthur King, Jr. Boulevard
Tallahassee, Florida 32307
(850) 599-3301
pharmacy.famu.edu/
Branch Campus: Crestview, Florida
Professional Degree Offered: Doctor of Pharmacy

College of Pharmacy
Larkin Health Sciences Institute
18301 North Miami Avenue, Suite 1
Miami, Florida 33169
(305) 760-7500
www.ularkin.org/pharmacy
Professional Degree Offered: Doctor of Pharmacy

College of Pharmacy
Nova Southeastern University
3200 South University Drive
Fort Lauderdale, Florida 33328
(954) 262-1300
pharmacy.nova.edu
Branch Campuses: Palm Beach Gardens and
Miami, Florida; San Juan, Puerto Rico
Professional Degree Offered: Doctor of Pharmacy

Lloyd L. Gregory School of Pharmacy
Palm Beach Atlantic University
901 South Flagler Drive
West Palm Beach, Florida 33401
(561) 803-2750
www.pba.edu/school-of-pharmacy
Professional Degree Offered: Doctor of Pharmacy

College of Pharmacy
University of Florida
1225 Center Drive
Gainesville, Florida 32611
(352) 273-6217
pharmacy.ufl.edu/
Branch Campuses: Jacksonville, Orlando,
and St. Petersburg, Florida
Professional Degree Offered: Doctor of Pharmacy

College of Pharmacy
University of South Florida
12901 Bruce B. Downs Boulevard
Tampa, Florida 33612
(813) 974-5699
health.usf.edu/pharmacy/index.htm
Professional Degree Offered: Doctor of Pharmacy

GEORGIA

College of Pharmacy and Health Sciences
Mercer University
3001 Mercer University Drive
Atlanta, Georgia 30341
(678) 547-6232
pharmacy.mercer.edu
Professional Degree Offered: Doctor of Pharmacy

School of Pharmacy
Philadelphia College of Osteopathic Medicine
625 Old Peachtree Road, NW
Suwanee, Georgia 30024
(868) 282-4544
*www.pcom.edu/academics/programs-and-degrees/
doctor-of-pharmacy*
Professional Degree Offered: Doctor of Pharmacy

School of Pharmacy
South University
709 Mall Boulevard
Savannah, Georgia 31406
(912) 201-8120
www.southuniversity.edu/
Branch Campus: Columbia, South Carolina
Professional Degree Offered: Doctor of Pharmacy

College of Pharmacy
The University of Georgia
250 W. Green Street
Athens, Georgia 30602-2351
(706) 542-1911
www.rx.uga.edu/
Branch Campuses: Albany, Augusta, and
Savannah, Georgia
Professional Degree Offered: Doctor of Pharmacy

HAWAII

Daniel K. Inouye College of Pharmacy
The University of Hawaii at Hilo
200 West Kawili Street
Hilo, Hawaii 96720-4091
(808) 933-2909
pharmacy.uhh.hawaii.edu
Professional Degree Offered: Doctor of Pharmacy

IDAHO

College of Pharmacy
Idaho State University
970 South 5th Street, Stop 8288
Pocatello, Idaho 83209-8288
(208) 282-3475
pharmacy.isu.edu/live/
Branch Campuses: Meridian, Idaho; Anchorage,
Alaska
Professional Degree Offered: Doctor of Pharmacy

ILLINOIS

College of Pharmacy
Chicago State University
9501 South King Drive
206 Douglas Hall
Chicago, Illinois 60628-1598
(773) 821-2500
www.csu.edu/collegeofpharmacy/
Professional Degree Offered: Doctor of Pharmacy

Chicago College of Pharmacy
Midwestern University
555 31st Street
Downers Grove, Illinois 60515
(630) 515-7200
*www.midwestern.edu/programs-and-admission/
il-pharmacy.html*
Professional Degree Offered: Doctor of Pharmacy

College of Pharmacy
Roosevelt University
1400 N. Roosevelt Boulevard
Schaumburg, Illinois 60173
(847) 619-7300
www.roosevelt.edu/Pharmacy.aspx
Professional Degree Offered: Doctor of Pharmacy

College of Pharmacy
Rosalind Franklin University of Medicine and
    Science
3333 Green Bay Road
North Chicago, Illinois 60064
(847) 578-3204
*www.rosalindfranklin.edu/academics/college-of-
pharmacy*
Professional Degree Offered: Doctor of Pharmacy

School of Pharmacy
Southern Illinois University, Edwardsville
Campus Box 2000
Edwardsville, Illinois 62026-2000
(618) 650-5150
www.siue.edu/pharmacy/
Professional Degree Offered: Doctor of Pharmacy

College of Pharmacy
University of Illinois at Chicago
833 South Wood Street
Chicago, Illinois 60612
(312) 996-7240
www.uic.edu/pharmacy/
Branch Campus: Rockford, Illinois
Professional Degree Offered: Doctor of Pharmacy

INDIANA

College of Pharmacy and Health Sciences
Butler University
Pharmacy Building 107
4600 Sunset Avenue
Indianapolis, Indiana 46208
(317) 940-9322
www.butler.edu/cophs/
Professional Degree Offered: Doctor of Pharmacy

College of Pharmacy
Manchester University
10627 Diebold Road
Fort Wayne, Indiana 46845
(260) 470-2700
www.manchester.edu/pharmacy
Professional Degree Offered: Doctor of Pharmacy

School of Pharmacy and Pharmaceutical Sciences
Purdue University
575 Stadium Mall Drive
West Lafayette, Indiana 47907
(765) 494-1361
www.pharmacy.purdue.edu/
Professional Degree Offered: Doctor of Pharmacy

IOWA

College of Pharmacy and Health Sciences
Drake University
Cline 106
2507 University Avenue
Des Moines, Iowa 50311-4505
(515) 271-3018 or 1-800-44-DRAKE (ext. 3018)
www.drake.edu/pharmacy
Professional Degree Offered: Doctor of Pharmacy

College of Pharmacy
The University of Iowa
115 South Grand Avenue
Iowa City, Iowa 52242
(319) 335-8795
pharmacy.uiowa.edu/
Professional Degree Offered: Doctor of Pharmacy

KANSAS

School of Pharmacy
University of Kansas
2010 Becker Drive
Lawrence, Kansas 66047-1620
(785) 864-3591
pharmacy.ku.edu/
Branch Campus: Wichita, Kansas
Professional Degree Offered: Doctor of Pharmacy

KENTUCKY

College of Pharmacy
Sullivan University
2100 Gardiner Lane
Louisville, Kentucky 40205
(502) 413-8640
pages.sullivan.edu/pharmacy
Professional Degree Offered: Doctor of Pharmacy

College of Pharmacy
University of Kentucky
789 South Limestone
Lexington, Kentucky 40536-0596
(859) 323-2755
pharmacy.uky.edu
Professional Degree Offered: Doctor of Pharmacy

LOUISIANA

College of Health and Pharmaceutical Sciences
School of Pharmacy
The University of Louisiana at Monroe
1800 Bienville Drive (physical address)
700 University Avenue (mailing address)
Monroe, Louisiana 71201
(318) 342-3800
rxweb.ulm.edu/pharmacy/
Professional Degree Offered: Doctor of Pharmacy

College of Pharmacy
Xavier University of Louisiana
1 Drexel Drive
New Orleans, Louisiana 70125
(504) 520-5397
www.xula.edu/cop/
Professional Degree Offered: Doctor of Pharmacy

MAINE

School of Pharmacy
Husson University
One College Circle
Bangor, Maine 04401
(207) 404-5660
www.husson.edu/pharmacy
Professional Degree Offered: Doctor of Pharmacy

College of Pharmacy
University of New England
716 Stevens Avenue
Portland, Maine 04103
(207) 221-4225
www.une.edu/pharmacy
Professional Degree Offered: Doctor of Pharmacy

MARYLAND

School of Pharmacy
Notre Dame of Maryland University
4701 North Charles Street
Baltimore, Maryland 21210
(410) 532-5551
www.ndm.edu/academics/school-of-pharmacy
Professional Degree Offered: Doctor of Pharmacy

School of Pharmacy
University of Maryland
20 North Pine Street
Baltimore, Maryland 21201
(410) 706-7650
www.pharmacy.umaryland.edu/
Branch Campus: Rockville (Shady Grove),
    Maryland
Professional Degree Offered: Doctor of Pharmacy

School of Pharmacy and Health Professions
University of Maryland Eastern Shore
116 Somerset Hall
1 Backbone Road
Princess Anne, Maryland 21853
(410) 621-2292
www.umes.edu/pharmacy
Professional Degree Offered: Doctor of Pharmacy

MASSACHUSETTS

School of Pharmacy—Boston
MCPHS University
179 Longwood Avenue
Boston, Massachusetts 02115
(617) 732-2800
www.mcphs.edu/en/mcphs-life
Professional Degree Offered: Doctor of Pharmacy

School of Pharmacy—Worcester
MCPHS University
19 Foster Street
Worcester, Massachusetts 01608
(508) 890-8855
www.mcphs.edu/en/mcphs-life
Branch Campus: Manchester, New Hampshire
Professional Degree Offered: Doctor of Pharmacy

Bouvé College of Health Sciences—School of
    Pharmacy
Northeastern University
360 Huntington Avenue
Mailstop R218TF
Boston, Massachusetts 02115
(617) 373-7000
www.northeastern.edu/bouve/pharmacy
Professional Degree Offered: Doctor of Pharmacy

School of Pharmacy
Western New England University
1215 Wilbraham Road
Springfield, Massachusetts 01119
(413) 796-2113
www1.wne.edu/pharmacy/index.cfm
Professional Degree Offered: Doctor of Pharmacy

MICHIGAN

College of Pharmacy
Ferris State University
220 Ferris Drive, PHR 105
Big Rapids, Michigan 49307
(231) 591-3780
www.ferris.edu/colleges/pharmacy/
Branch Campus: Grand Rapids, Michigan
Professional Degree Offered: Doctor of Pharmacy

College of Pharmacy
The University of Michigan
428 Church Street
Ann Arbor, Michigan 48109-1065
(734) 764-7312
pharmacy.umich.edu
Professional Degree Offered: Doctor of Pharmacy

Eugene Applebaum College of Pharmacy
    and Health Sciences
Wayne State University
259 Mack Avenue
Detroit, Michigan 48201
(313) 577-1716
www.cphs.wayne.edu
Professional Degree Offered: Doctor of Pharmacy

MINNESOTA

College of Pharmacy
University of Minnesota
5-130 Weaver-Densford Hall
308 Harvard Street, SE
Minneapolis, Minnesota 55455
(612) 624-1900
www.pharmacy.umn.edu
Professional Degree Offered: Doctor of Pharmacy

College of Pharmacy, Duluth
University of Minnesota
232 Life Science
1110 Kirby Drive
Duluth, Minnesota 55812
(218) 726-6000
www.pharmacy.umn.edu/duluth
Professional Degree Offered: Doctor of Pharmacy

MISSISSIPPI

School of Pharmacy
The University of Mississippi
P.O. Box 1848
University, Mississippi 38677-1848
(662) 915-7265
pharmacy.olemiss.edu/
Branch Campus: Jackson, Mississippi
Professional Degree Offered: Doctor of Pharmacy

MISSOURI

St. Louis College of Pharmacy
4588 Parkview Place
St. Louis, Missouri 63110
(314) 367-8700
www.stlcop.edu
Professional Degree Offered: Doctor of Pharmacy

School of Pharmacy
University of Missouri—Kansas City
UMKC Health Sciences Building
2464 Charlotte Street
Kansas City, Missouri 64108
(816) 235-2833
pharmacy.umkc.edu
Branch Campuses: Columbia and Springfield,
Missouri
Professional Degree Offered: Doctor of Pharmacy

MONTANA

College of Health Professions and Biomedical
Sciences
Skaggs School of Pharmacy
The University of Montana
341 Skaggs Building
Missoula, Montana 59812-1512
(406) 243-4656
health.umt.edu/pharmacy
Professional Degree Offered: Doctor of Pharmacy

NEBRASKA

School of Pharmacy and Health Professions
Creighton University Medical Center
2500 California Plaza
Omaha, Nebraska 68178
(402) 280-2950
spahp.creighton.edu
Professional Degree Offered: Doctor of Pharmacy

College of Pharmacy
University of Nebraska Medical Center
986000 Nebraska Medical Center
Omaha, Nebraska 68198-6000
(402) 559-4333
www.unmc.edu/pharmacy/
Professional Degree Offered: Doctor of Pharmacy

NEVADA

College of Pharmacy
Roseman University of Health Sciences
11 Sunset Way
Henderson, Nevada 89014
(702) 940-2007
*www.roseman.edu/explore-our-colleges/college-of-
pharmacy*
Branch Campus: South Jordan, Utah
Professional Degree Offered: Doctor of Pharmacy

NEW JERSEY

School of Pharmacy
Fairleigh Dickinson University
Mailstop M-SP1-01
230 Park Avenue
Florham Park, New Jersey 07932
(973) 443-8401
www.fdu.edu/academic/pharmacy
Professional Degree Offered: Doctor of Pharmacy

Ernest Mario School of Pharmacy
Rutgers, the State University of New Jersey
160 Frelinghuysen Road
Piscataway, New Jersey 08854
(848) 445-2675
pharmacy.rutgers.edu/
Professional Degree Offered: Doctor of Pharmacy

NEW MEXICO

College of Pharmacy
University of New Mexico
MSC 09 5360
1 University of New Mexico
Albuquerque, New Mexico 87131-0001
(505) 272-3241
pharmacy.unm.edu/
Professional Degree Offered: Doctor of Pharmacy

NEW YORK

Albany College of Pharmacy and Health Sciences
106 New Scotland Avenue
Albany, New York 12208
(518) 694-7200
www.acphs.edu
Branch Campus: Colchester (Burlington),
    Vermont
Professional Degree Offered: Doctor of Pharmacy

School of Pharmacy
D'Youville College
320 Porter Avenue
Buffalo, New York 14202
(716) 829-8440
*www.dyc.edu/academics/schools-and-
    departments/pharmacy*
Professional Degree Offered: Doctor of Pharmacy

Arnold and Marie Schwartz College of Pharmacy
    and Health Sciences
Long Island University
75 Dekalb Avenue
Brooklyn, New York 11201
(718) 488-1234
www.liu.edu/pharmacy/
Professional Degree Offered: Doctor of Pharmacy

Wegmans School of Pharmacy
St. John Fisher College
3690 East Avenue
Rochester, New York 14618
(585) 385-8430
www.sjfc.edu/schools/school-of-pharmacy
Professional Degree Offered: Doctor of Pharmacy

College of Pharmacy and Health Sciences
St. John's University
8000 Utopia Parkway
Queens, New York 11439
(718) 990-6275
*www.stjohns.edu/academics/schools-and-colleges/
    college-pharmacy-and-health-sciences*
Professional Degree Offered: Doctor of Pharmacy

Touro College of Pharmacy—New York
230 West 125th Street
New York, New York 10027
(646) 981-4700
tcop.touro.edu
Professional Degree Offered: Doctor of Pharmacy

School of Pharmacy and Pharmaceutical Sciences
University at Buffalo—The State University
    of New York
285 Kapoor Hall
Buffalo, New York 14214-8033
(716) 645-2825
www.pharmacy.buffalo.edu/
Professional Degree Offered: Doctor of Pharmacy

NORTH CAROLINA

College of Pharmacy and Health Sciences
Campbell University
P.O. Box 1090
Buies Creek, North Carolina 27506
(800) 760-9734 or (910) 893-1690
www.campbell.edu/cphs
Professional Degree Offered: Doctor of Pharmacy

Fred Wilson School of Pharmacy
High Point University
One University Parkway
High Point, North Carolina 27268
(336) 841-9198
www.highpoint.edu/pharmacy
Professional Degree Offered: Doctor of Pharmacy

Eshelman School of Pharmacy
University of North Carolina at Chapel Hill
301 Pharmacy Lane, CB 7355
Chapel Hill, North Carolina 27599-7355
(919) 966-9429
www.pharmacy.unc.edu/
Branch Campus: Asheville, North Carolina
Professional Degree Offered: Doctor of Pharmacy

School of Pharmacy
Wingate University
515 N. Main Street
Levine College of Health Sciences
Wingate, North Carolina 28174
(704) 233-8633
pharmacy.wingate.edu/
Branch Campus: Hendersonville, North Carolina
Professional Degree Offered: Doctor of Pharmacy

NORTH DAKOTA

College of Health Professions
School of Pharmacy
North Dakota State University
NDSU Dept. 2650
123 Sudro Hall
P.O. Box 6050
Fargo, North Dakota 58108-6050
(701) 231-7456
www.ndsu.nodak.edu/pharmacy/
Professional Degree Offered: Doctor of Pharmacy

OHIO

School of Pharmacy
Cedarville University
251 N. Main Street
Cedarville, Ohio 45314
(937) 766-7480
www.cedarville.edu/Academics/Pharmacy.aspx
Professional Degree Offered: Doctor of Pharmacy

College of Pharmacy
Northeast Ohio Medical University
4209 State Route 44
P.O. Box 95
Rootstown, Ohio 44272
(800) 686-2511
www.neomed.edu
Professional Degree Offered: Doctor of Pharmacy

Raabe College of Pharmacy
Ohio Northern University
525 S. Main Street
Ada, Ohio 45810
(419) 772-2275
www.onu.edu/pharmacy
Professional Degree Offered: Doctor of Pharmacy

College of Pharmacy
The Ohio State University
217 Lloyd M. Parks Hall
500 West 12th Avenue
Columbus, Ohio 43210
(614) 292-2266
pharmacy.osu.edu
Professional Degree Offered: Doctor of Pharmacy

James L. Winkle College of Pharmacy
University of Cincinnati
3225 Eden Avenue
Kowalewski Hall, Suite 136
Cincinnati, Ohio 45267-0004
(513) 558-3784
pharmacy.uc.edu/
Professional Degree Offered: Doctor of Pharmacy

College of Pharmacy
University of Findlay
300 Davis Street
Findlay, Ohio 45840
(419) 434-5327
www.findlay.edu/pharmacy
Professional Degree Offered: Doctor of Pharmacy

College of Pharmacy and Pharmaceutical
  Sciences
The University of Toledo
3000 Arlington Avenue, MS 1014
Toledo, Ohio 43614
(419) 383-1904
www.utoledo.edu/pharmacy
Professional Degree Offered: Doctor of Pharmacy

OKLAHOMA

College of Pharmacy
Southwestern Oklahoma State University
100 Campus Drive
Weatherford, Oklahoma 73096
(580) 774-3105
www.swosu.edu/pharmacy/
Professional Degree Offered: Doctor of Pharmacy

College of Pharmacy
University of Oklahoma
P.O. Box 26901
Oklahoma City, Oklahoma 73126-0901
(405) 271-6484
pharmacy.ouhsc.edu
Professional Degree Offered: Doctor of Pharmacy

OREGON

College of Pharmacy
Oregon State University
203 Pharmacy Building
Corvallis, Oregon 97331
(541) 737-3424
pharmacy.oregonstate.edu/
Branch Campus: Portland, Oregon
Professional Degree Offered: Doctor of Pharmacy

School of Pharmacy
Pacific University
222 Southeast 8th Avenue, Suite 451
Hillsboro, Oregon 97123
(503) 352-7271
www.pacificu.edu/future-graduate-professional/
  colleges/college-health-professions/school-
  pharmacy
Professional Degree Offered: Doctor of Pharmacy

PENNSYLVANIA

Mylan School of Pharmacy
Duquesne University
600 Forbes Avenue
Pittsburgh, Pennsylvania 15282
(412) 396-6393
www.duq.edu/academics/schools/pharmacy
Professional Degree Offered: Doctor of Pharmacy

School of Pharmacy
Lake Erie College of Osteopathic Medicine
1858 West Grandview Boulevard
Erie, Pennsylvania 16509
(814) 866-8409
www.lecom.edu/academics/school-of-pharmacy
Branch Campus: Bradenton, Florida
Professional Degree Offered: Doctor of Pharmacy

School of Pharmacy
Temple University
3307 North Broad Street
Philadelphia, Pennsylvania 19140
(215) 707-4900
pharmacy.temple.edu/
Professional Degree Offered: Doctor of Pharmacy

Jefferson College of Pharmacy
Thomas Jefferson University
901 Walnut Street
Health Professions Academic Building
Philadelphia, Pennsylvania 19107
(877) 533-3247 or (215) 503-8890
www.jefferson.edu/university/pharmacy.html
Professional Degree Offered: Doctor of Pharmacy

School of Pharmacy
University of Pittsburgh
Student Services
1104 Salk Hall
3501 Terrace Street
Pittsburgh, Pennsylvania 15261
(412) 624-5240
www.pharmacy.pitt.edu/
Professional Degree Offered: Doctor of Pharmacy

Philadelphia College of Pharmacy
University of the Sciences
600 South 43rd Street
Philadelphia, Pennsylvania 19104
(215) 596-8805
www.usciences.edu/philadelphia-college-of-
  pharmacy/index.html
Professional Degree Offered: Doctor of Pharmacy

Nesbitt School of Pharmacy
Wilkes University
Stark Learning Center
84 West South Street
Wilkes-Barre, Pennsylvania 18766
(570) 408-4280
*www.wilkes.edu/academics/colleges/nesbitt-
college-of-pharmacy/index.aspx*
Professional Degree Offered: Doctor of Pharmacy

PUERTO RICO

School of Pharmacy
University of Puerto Rico
Medical Sciences Campus
School of Pharmacy Building
Office 248
P.O. Box 365067
San Juan, Puerto Rico 00936
(787) 758-2525 ext. 5422
farmacia.rcm.upr.edu/
Professional Degree Offered: Doctor of Pharmacy

RHODE ISLAND

College of Pharmacy
University of Rhode Island
Pharmacy Building
7 Greenhouse Road
Kingston, Rhode Island 02881
(401) 874-5842
web.uri.edu/pharmacy/
Professional Degree Offered: Doctor of Pharmacy

SOUTH CAROLINA

College of Pharmacy
Medical University of South Carolina
280 Calhoun Street
MSC 141
Charleston, South Carolina 29425
(843) 792-3115
academicdepartments.musc.edu/cop
Professional Degree Offered: Doctor of Pharmacy

School of Pharmacy
Presbyterian College
307 North Broad Street
Clinton, South Carolina 29325
(864) 938-3900
pharmacy.presby.edu
Professional Degree Offered: Doctor of Pharmacy

College of Pharmacy
University of South Carolina
715 Sumter Street
Columbia, South Carolina 29208
(803) 777-4151
sc.edu/study/colleges_schools/pharmacy/index.php
Branch Campus: Greenville, South Carolina
Professional Degree Offered: Doctor of Pharmacy

SOUTH DAKOTA

College of Pharmacy
South Dakota State University
Avera Health and Science Center 133
Box 2202C
Brookings, South Dakota 57007
(605) 688-6197
www.sdstate.edu/pha/index.cfm
Professional Degree Offered: Doctor of Pharmacy

TENNESSEE

School of Pharmacy
Belmont University
1900 Belmont Boulevard
Nashville, Tennessee 37212
(615) 460-8122
www.belmont.edu/pharmacy
Professional Degree Offered: Doctor of Pharmacy

Bill Gatton College of Pharmacy
East Tennessee State University
P.O. Box 70414
Johnson City, Tennessee 37614-1704
(423) 439-6338
www.etsu.edu/pharmacy
Professional Degree Offered: Doctor of Pharmacy

College of Pharmacy and Health Sciences
Lipscomb University
One University Park Drive
Nashville, Tennessee 37204
(615) 966-7181
www.lipscomb.edu/pharmacy
Professional Degree Offered: Doctor of Pharmacy

School of Pharmacy
South College
3904 Lonas Drive
Knoxville, Tennessee 37909
(865) 251-1800
www.southcollegetn.edu
Professional Degree Offered: Doctor of Pharmacy

School of Pharmacy
Union University
1050 Union University Drive
Jackson, Tennessee 38305
(731) 661-5910
www.uu.edu/academics/sop
Professional Degree Offered: Doctor of Pharmacy

College of Pharmacy
University of Tennessee Health Science Center
881 Madison Avenue, Suite 226
Memphis, Tennessee 38163
(901) 448-6036
www.uthsc.edu/pharmacy
Branch Campuses: Knoxville and Nashville,
    Tennessee
Professional Degree Offered: Doctor of Pharmacy

TEXAS

Irma Lerma Rangel College of Pharmacy
Texas A&M University Health Science Center
1010 West Avenue B
Kingsville, Texas 78363
(361) 221-0604
pharmacy.tamhsc.edu
Branch Campus: College Station, Texas
Professional Degree Offered: Doctor of Pharmacy

College of Pharmacy and Health Sciences
Texas Southern University
3100 Cleburne Street
Houston, Texas 77004
(713) 313-6700
*tsu.edu/academics/colleges-and-schools/college-of-
    pharmacy-and-health-sciences/*
Professional Degree Offered: Doctor of Pharmacy

School of Pharmacy
Texas Tech University Health Sciences Center
1300 Coutler Avenue
Amarillo, Texas 79106
(806) 414-9393
www.ttuhsc.edu/sop/
Branch Campuses: Abilene, Dallas, and Lubbock,
    Texas
Professional Degree Offered: Doctor of Pharmacy

College of Pharmacy
University of Houston
3455 Cullen Boulevard, Room 141
Houston, Texas 77204-5000
(713) 743-1239
www.uh.edu/pharmacy
Professional Degree Offered: Doctor of Pharmacy

Feik School of Pharmacy
University of the Incarnate Word
4301 Broadway, CPO #99
San Antonio, Texas 78209
(210) 883-1000
www.uiw.edu/pharmacy/
Professional Degree Offered: Doctor of Pharmacy

College of Pharmacy
University of North Texas System
3500 Camp Bowie Boulevard
Fort Worth, Texas 76107
(817) 735-2000
www.unthsc.edu/college-of-pharmacy
Professional Degree Offered: Doctor of Pharmacy

College of Pharmacy
The University of Texas at Austin
2409 University Avenue
Stop: A1900
Austin, Texas 78712-0120
(512) 471-1737
www.utexas.edu/pharmacy/
Branch Campuses: El Paso, Rio Grande Valley,
    and San Antonio, Texas
Professional Degree Offered: Doctor of Pharmacy

Ben and Maytee Fisch College of Pharmacy
University of Texas at Tyler
3900 University Boulevard
Tyler, Texas 75799
(903) 565-5777
www.uttyler.edu/pharmacy
Professional Degree Offered: Doctor of Pharmacy

UTAH

College of Pharmacy
University of Utah
30 South 2000 East
Salt Lake City, Utah 84112
(801) 581-6731
pharmacy.utah.edu/
Professional Degree Offered: Doctor of Pharmacy

VIRGINIA

Appalachian College of Pharmacy
1060 Dragon Road
Oakwood, Virginia 24631
(866) 935-7350
www.acp.edu
Professional Degree Offered: Doctor of Pharmacy

School of Pharmacy
Hampton University
Kittrell Hall
Hampton, Virginia 23668
(757) 727-5071
pharm.hamptonu.edu
Professional Degree Offered: Doctor of Pharmacy

Bernard J. Dunn School of Pharmacy
Shenandoah University
1775 N. Sector Court
Winchester, Virginia 22601
(540) 665-1282 or (888) 420-7877
www.su.edu/pharmacy/
Branch Campus: Ashburn, Virginia
Professional Degree Offered: Doctor of Pharmacy

School of Pharmacy
Virginia Commonwealth University
Medical College of Virginia Campus
P.O. Box 980581
410 North 12th Street, Room 500
Richmond, Virginia 23298-0581
(804) 828-3000
www.pharmacy.vcu.edu/
Branch Campuses: Inova (Falls Church) and
    Charlottesville, Virginia
Professional Degree Offered: Doctor of Pharmacy

WASHINGTON

School of Pharmacy
University of Washington
H364 Health Sciences Building
Seattle, Washington 98195-7631
(206) 543-2030
sop.washington.edu/
Professional Degree Offered: Doctor of Pharmacy

College of Pharmacy
Washington State University
P.O. Box 1495
Spokane, Washington 99210-1495
(509) 368-6605
www.pharmacy.wsu.edu/
Branch Campus: Yakima, Washington
Professional Degree Offered: Doctor of Pharmacy

WEST VIRGINIA

School of Pharmacy
Marshall University
One John Marshall Drive-CEB
Huntington, West Virginia 25755-2950
(304) 696-7302
www.marshall.edu/pharmacy
Professional Degree Offered: Doctor of Pharmacy

School of Pharmacy
University of Charleston
2300 MacCorkle Avenue, Southeast
Charleston, West Virginia 25304
(304) 357-4889
pharmacy.ucwv.edu/pharmacy
Professional Degree Offered: Doctor of Pharmacy

School of Pharmacy
West Virginia University
P.O. Box 9500
Morgantown, West Virginia 26506-9500
(304) 293-5101
pharmacy.hsc.wvu.edu/
Professional Degree Offered: Doctor of Pharmacy

WISCONSIN

School of Pharmacy
Concordia University
12800 North Lake Shore Drive
Mequon, Wisconsin 53097
(262) 243-5700
www.cuw.edu/programs/pharmacy
Professional Degree Offered: Doctor of Pharmacy

School of Pharmacy
University of Wisconsin—Madison
777 Highland Avenue
Madison, Wisconsin 53705-2222
(608) 262-6234
pharmacy.wisc.edu/
Professional Degree Offered: Doctor of Pharmacy

WYOMING

School of Pharmacy
University of Wyoming
Health Sciences Center, Room 292
Department 3375
1000 East University Avenue
Laramie, Wyoming 82071
(307) 766-6120
www.uwyo.edu/pharmacy/
Professional Degree Offered: Doctor of Pharmacy

Admission Committees

The individuals who wrote the "Admission Committees" and "The Interview Process" sections of this book have served on pharmacy school admission committees for several years. Based on their experiences, they have summarized their observations of students who were successful in being accepted into a college/school of pharmacy. The following describes the purpose of the admission committee and provides tips to successfully guide you through the admission process.

The purpose of the admission committee for a pharmacy school is to select the most qualified students to enter the program. The phrase "most qualified student" will have a slightly different interpretation by each committee and may vary slightly within an institution from year to year. As soon as possible, contact the institutions in which you are interested and request materials regarding application requirements. Much of this data may be available on the school's website, and therefore it is important to review materials most schools make available on the Internet. By reviewing these materials, you should be able to determine not only the requirements for the institution, but which factors are utilized to select students for admission.

The committees will use various sources of information and mechanisms to compare students to make selection decisions. You should make sure that the information requested is provided for the committee. If you have a special interest, ability, or experience that you think would be helpful in your application, include a letter or other supporting documentation in the materials you submit to the institution(s) for the committee to consider.

TIP

Provide additional information that you think is important for the committee to understand your interest in pharmacy and their program in particular.

As important as it is for you to do well academically and to take the required courses, the practice of pharmacy requires various skills and talents that you may develop and enhance prior to attending a pharmacy school. Some of these areas include:

- Work Experience
- Verbal and Written Communication Skills
- Community Involvement/Leadership
- Entrepreneurial Ability

Some institutions will request information regarding the activities listed above as part of the application; others may rely on recommendations to provide this information. Schools utilize a personal interview as part of the application process to give the student a chance to present information regarding his or her personal and academic background. You should determine how to best develop and exhibit your skills in these areas, and also how to communicate this information to the pharmacy college(s)/school(s). If your current school has a career center that offers practice interviews, take advantage of that opportunity to optimize your interview skills.

Work experience provides the student with a background about the workplace in general. It also gives students a chance to develop good work habits and communication skills. Work experience in the profession of pharmacy will be an excellent way for you to understand what pharmacy is about and whether your interests and skills are compatible. Also, you will be able to find out more information about the variety of career opportunities that exist in the practice of pharmacy. Work experience in pharmacy is great, but other jobs can also be supportive and provide information about a student's interests and abilities. Work in a doctor's office, a health clinic, or a hospital setting should provide the student with a background in health care issues, contact with patients, and a chance to see various health care professionals in action. Additionally, seemingly unrelated jobs in retail or food services still provide a medium for the student to develop good work skills, communication skills, and the ability to work with people. No matter what work experience you have, try to see what aspects of that job might apply to your activities as a pharmacist or pharmacy student. Make sure to communicate this effectively to the admission committee.

Communication skills are important in all aspects of pharmacy. Students and pharmacists must be able to communicate effectively with a wide range of people. Also, they must be able to communicate about potentially complex subject matter in a manner that is effective for their audience, whether it be a patient, another student, a professor or other health care professionals. Additionally, the ability to listen effectively is just as important as the ability to communicate.

Community involvement is a way for the admission committee to determine more about the character of an applicant. The practice of pharmacy requires that a person be empathetic to the needs of the patient or other professional contacts. This means that a pharmacist can be most effective when he or she can "put him- or herself in the other's shoes." By showing a history of participation in organizations that show compassion by assisting others, you may be more likely to have the desired character to practice effectively and ethically. It is suggested that you show a history of participation in these types of activities, not just recent participation in one or two events to have something to place on an application or state in an interview. Make sure that you can talk about the type of activities or events you have been involved in, not just list organizations or events.

Entrepreneurship is the interest in new opportunities—not only business ventures, but also professional development and new ways of doing things. Pharmacy, like most professions, will go through various changes throughout one's career, and the ability and interest to pursue new avenues of practice assures that one will continue to be competent and competitive. A committee might assess an applicant's entrepreneurial abilities through questions in the interview such as "tell me about a project you instituted or carried out with others." By asking such a question, the committee might be looking for creativity, leadership skills, and motivation.

It is important to consider the composition of the admission committee. Committees may consist of any combination of faculty members, pharmacists, non-pharmacists, alumni members, students, and administrative members. Be sure to think in terms of what that type of individual would want to know about you that will help them realize you will be a good pharmacy student and practitioner.

Not all students will have experience or strong backgrounds in each of the areas mentioned; however, you want to have a good mixture of skills and talents. Do not go out and try to "check-off all the boxes" just to satisfy the committee. It is important that you represent yourself completely and honestly to the committee so that your interest can best be served and the committee can assess not only what you bring to the program, but how the program will benefit your development as a pharmacist.

The Interview Process

Schools require an interview as part of the admission process. The structure and goals of this process will vary between programs. This general information regarding interviews is meant to help you have a better idea of what to expect, and therefore be more effective in communicating your abilities and desires to the interviewers. One of the most positive benefits of preparing yourself for an interview is that it gives you a structured assessment of your strengths, weaknesses, and professional goals. By quantifying these at this critical time in your career, you will be sure of your goals and motivation for your chosen career path.

There are many texts that provide copious information on how interviews are structured and can prepare you for this event. Most of these address the pursuit of a job in your chosen field. This fact makes their recommendations a bit more structured than might be appropriate for an academic interview for a position in a professional program. Overall, the committee or interviewer is not looking for one right person for the job. They look for a wide range of backgrounds and interests that will not only assure student success in a rigorous academic program, but will also provide support for a variety of practice settings. Not everyone will work in a direct patient care environment for his or her whole career. As important as patient empathy is to a health care professional, some are going to be better than others and some will work in an area where this skill is not the most important one required. There is room for diversity in pharmacy programs in every sense of the word. Thus, interviewers may evaluate candidates on a range of criteria including communication skills, critical thinking, maturity, and motivation. Just as interviewees will vary, so will the interviewers. Some will be more skilled than others and some may look at the applicant in terms of their own career choices. It is important for you to try and listen to the interviewer, and determine what is meant by the question being asked and how you should best relate your own feelings while being sensitive to the setting and the audience. Remember that honesty is the best policy. If you feel that you have to compromise your interests to say what the interviewer wants to hear, you should review your choice of this institution or career pursuit.

Overall, the greatest benefit to be gained by the interview is for the committee to see the sincerity of the interest you have in the program and a career in pharmacy. Also, it is important that you receive positive reinforcement of your goals and helpful information from the institution administering the interview.

Based on our experience, here are three of the most common topics discussed during a pharmacy application interview:

- Professional Background
- Academic Background
- Personal Background

The following table lists questions you may want to consider as you prepare for the interview process.

TIP

Get as much information as possible about the program and have some good questions ready (for example, a question about points that were brought up by committee members). This shows that you are "thinking on your feet."

- **What qualities do you possess that you believe are especially suited to the pharmacy profession?**
- **What is the basis for your interest in the pharmacy profession?**
- **What have you done to increase the likelihood of your acceptance into pharmacy school? What sets you apart from other applicants?**
- **What are your plans if you do not gain entry to pharmacy school this year?**
- **Describe a project you worked on that required problem-solving and critical thinking skills.**
- **Describe how you prepare for exams.**
- **What skills and abilities have facilitated your academic success thus far and which will promote your success in pharmacy school?**

- Describe an obstacle you have faced in the past and what you learned about yourself as a result.
- Name five things you are most proud of and why.
- What are the advantages and disadvantages of working with a team on a project?
- Describe a time when you were involved in a conflict during a team activity. How was the conflict resolved?
- Describe your best friend. How would your best friend describe you?
- How do you manage your time between school and other activities?
- What are the most important attributes of a good pharmacist?
- Describe an ethical dilemma you have faced in the past and how you resolved the dilemma.
- Do you have any hobbies? What do you do to have fun and relax?
- What qualities do you possess that make you a good leader?

PROFESSIONAL BACKGROUND

Basically, you have been preparing all of your life for the interview. However, you should spend some significant time before the interview making an "inventory" of your answer to the question "why pharmacy?" Here are some self-assessment questions to help prepare you for this type of discussion.

- Why have you chosen pharmacy as a career path? When did you first consider pharmacy as a career?
- Do you know anyone who is a pharmacist?
- What other careers did you consider?
- What steps have you taken to learn more about pharmacy as a profession?
- Who influenced your choice of career, and how (actively or through example)?
- Who would you consider to be your mentor? Why?
- What type of jobs have you held? What have been your likes and dislikes about those jobs? Have these jobs influenced your decision to pursue pharmacy as a career?
- What other careers or academic pursuits interest you?
- What jobs are available to pharmacists? What type of career in pharmacy interests you most?
- What will you do if you are not admitted into a school or college of pharmacy?
- Have you held any leadership positions such as in an organization or on a sports team?
- What hobbies or extracurricular activities are you involved in?
- What are your opinions on professional and community service?
- How would you describe yourself? What are your strengths and weaknesses?
- What is the most challenging personal situation you have faced? How did you cope?
- Can you provide an example of a situation in which you faced a moral or ethical dilemma? How did you confront or resolve this situation?

Any student can come up with answers to these types of questions. Ideally, there is no right or wrong answer. What the committee should be looking for is the background information that you relate to support your answers. Understand that any answer to the questions, such as the ones on page 30, should include an implicit explanation of why or how you arrived at that decision. This is the best way to relate to the committee the maturity of your decision-making process and career interest. It also helps minimize the problem with a difficult interviewer who may be looking for your answer to match his or her choices. If you have a good explanation of how you arrived at that decision, it validates your answer.

Be aware of the professional questions being posed to you as an applicant. The interviewers have been in their profession a long time and often can only relate to subject matter that they have come to accept as common knowledge. An example of a question being asked about a professional setting scenario is "What would you do if a patient comes in and needs a prescription refill and there are no refills indicated on the prescription?" The possible answers are myriad, and often the question is asked of a student who has retail pharmacy experience and has observed a pharmacist handle this situation many times. If you do not have any experience or any idea of how to answer this question, consider explaining your lack of experience in that area and stating that this is the type of thing you know training in the professional program will provide. Then, try to relate the question to something you are more familiar with. For example, you might respond, "It sounds like this is a question that deals with utilizing appropriate people skills and ethical behavior on the part of the pharmacist; let me tell you about a situation that I dealt with in a job where we had an employee who was involved in stealing . . . ." This allows you to put the question on your own terms and to talk about something with which you are familiar. Follow-up your description with a question as to whether that scenario related sufficiently to the professional question posed by the interviewer(s).

Ideally, you will have some pharmacy or related experiences to utilize in the interview. This not only shows your competency in areas that you have been trained, but also, that you are making your decision regarding a career choice based on personal experience. Pharmacy jobs for pre-pharmacy students can be difficult to obtain, particularly if you are in an area with a high concentration of pharmacy students. Often, students first think of retail or community pharmacy because this practice option is so visible, but do not neglect opportunities in hospitals, clinics, long-term care facilities, and many other areas where pharmacists or other healthcare professionals have the opportunity to work with interested students. Maybe you started working in a related area as early as high school. In doing this, you may have had the opportunity to advance to a position which provides direct contact with the operation of a pharmacy. If you are unable to obtain a job in a pharmacy, you may be able to obtain relevant experience by shadowing pharmacists or volunteering in health care settings that provide pharmacy services.

ACADEMIC BACKGROUND

The nature of academic performance reported to the institution you are applying to is very quantitative. All require that transcripts be provided and often calculate a single grade point average (GPA) for ranking the applicant pool. Some interviews may be conducted "blind" in that the interviewers do not have access to the student's credentials prior to the interview. In this case, you may still bring this information into the process if they refer to your performance or discuss this as part of the interview. If academic success is a strong point in your background, by all means, include it in your discussions. Most interviewers will have had the chance to review a student's admission file before and during the interview. It is important that all available materials, transcripts, and other required information have been provided and that your application is as complete as possible. Also, the committee may ask specific questions regarding courses in which you did especially well or faced challenges. Do not try to ignore bad academic events or specific grades. Address them honestly to the committee and explain any extenuating circumstances which may have adversely affected performance in the short term. In most circumstances, you should avoid blaming the instructor in a course; it is important to take responsibility for your own performance. Point out improvements or trends which show improved effort or understanding of vital material. Talk about additional courses that you may have taken which, even though not required, might provide a benefit during the pharmacy program or in professional practice. Even courses in business, psychology, writing, or education can be very applicable and helpful in one's career pursuit. Usually, high school grades or performance are not an issue, but if you had a particularly good experience in a class or with a teacher who was pivotal in your career choice or academic performance, it would be good to include this in your discussion.

Be aware of the pre-pharmacy requirements for the program and discuss how you plan to complete any remaining courses in time to begin the professional program in the desired term. If you have courses for which you hope to receive credit toward pharmacy prerequisites, check that out with the admission office before the interview. Often the interviewers are faculty who, though familiar with the requirements of the program, are not the ones to make transfer credit decisions. Thus, questions concerning transfer credit should be addressed to the admissions office.

Often you will be asked if you have applied to other pharmacy or academic programs. Again, be honest and discuss other plans you have or pursuits you have considered. Considering other programs or even other academic pursuits, which are based on the interests you have stated in the interview, should be a positive factor and show that you are a serious and mature student. However, if you detect that the interviewers feel some competitiveness toward another pharmacy program which you are considering, tell them that this shows how serious you are about your pursuit of a career in pharmacy. We believe it is a good idea to consider and apply to any program you feel you could attend and get the education that will allow you to pursue your career goals.

PERSONAL BACKGROUND

The interview is a chance to put some "personality" into your application. The process prior to the time of the interview is very quantitative, with GPAs and PCAT scores often being the primary consideration that allowed you an interview. It is your responsibility to make the impression on the interviewers that you will do well in their institution and will be the type of pharmacist they want to represent their institution. Talk not only about the experiences in your background that led you to pharmacy, but also talk about the experiences that helped you to develop a personality that will support you through the academic program and as a pharmacist. Include information about outside activities, sports, and hobbies. Include involvement in organizations in addition to academic pursuits, such as membership in service groups. Membership in honor societies should be mentioned; discuss activities or opportunities that were provided during your membership, not just that you were a member because of your grades or other academic qualities.

The various background areas overlap, each one providing important information on how you got to where you are and what type of student and person you are. Therefore, it is natural that the relationship between academics, professional pursuits, and personality will be extensions of each other.

TIP

Don't just state that you were a member of a particular organization. Discuss what you did in it to show your leadership abilities or interest in providing service to the community.

ON-SITE ESSAY

Some schools may require that you complete an essay during your interview at the school/college. Examples of possible essay topics include:

- You just learned your patient has been nonadherent to his medication. Describe how you would convince this patient to take his medication as prescribed, and the importance of medication adherence.
- What are two messages or themes about responsibility for personal health care and well being that you feel are important to advance to American teenagers today?
- What one or two areas of health maintenance and disease treatment should U.S. scientific research efforts and resources be directed toward during the next 10 years?
- What are some knowledge or skill requirements essential for practitioners in today's community and environment? Why?

The length of the essay and the time allotted for completion of the essay will vary by school/college. Essay evaluation criteria may include use of language, grammar, punctuation, clarity, and cohesiveness. We recommend that you take a few minutes at the beginning of the essay-writing session to prepare an outline to help guide your writing process. We also recommend that you save a few minutes at the end of the essay-writing session to review and edit your essay as necessary. Other general essay-writing tips can be found in Chapter 8.

CONCLUSION OF THE INTERVIEW

At the end of the interview make sure you summarize your interest in the program and "wrap-up" any issues regarding remaining coursework. State your plans for future academic terms, and make sure you know what the next step will be and when you can expect to hear from the committee regarding the results of your application.

TIPS FOR SUCCESSFUL INTERVIEWING

- Arrive on time for the interview. Arriving late may send the message that the interview is not a priority to you.
- Try not to appear nervous. Arriving to the interview early will give you the opportunity to adjust to the environment and may decrease your anxiety.
- Dress professionally.
- Be courteous.
- Be positive and friendly, and smile.
- Answer all questions as completely as possible.
- Speak clearly.
- Make eye contact with the interviewers.
- Don't exhibit unnecessary movements.
- Educate yourself on the institution.
- If you have questions, ask if there is enough time to ask your questions. If so, ask questions.
- If you have any additional materials that you want the committee to review, bring them with you to the interview.
- Listen attentively and learn from the interview. The information exchange should be a two-way process.
- Bring a pen and notebook to the interview. Have a list of questions that you may want to ask and make notes as appropriate.
- Don't limit yourself to one or two word answers.
- Participate in mock interviews.

Graduate Degrees in Pharmacy

Master of Science (M.S.) and Doctor of Philosophy (Ph.D.) degrees are available for pharmacy disciplines including, but not limited to, medicinal chemistry, pharmaceutics, pharmacology, pharmacy care administration, and toxicology. Many colleges of pharmacy also offer dual degree programs which allow students to pursue a graduate degree while enrolled in a PharmD program. Examples of common dual degree programs include the PharmD/Master of Business Administration (MBA), the PharmD/Master of Public Health (MPH), and the PharmD/PhD. For more information regarding graduate programs, you should contact the specific college or school of pharmacy in which you are interested.

Postgraduate Training: Residencies and Fellowships

A graduate of a college or school of pharmacy may decide to pursue postgraduate training in a specific area of pharmacy practice or pharmacy research (see the later section entitled "Residency and Fellowship Programs: Areas of Pharmacy Practice and Research"). Residencies and fellowships are two distinct types of postgraduate training programs. General requirements for an applicant seeking a residency or fellowship include graduating from an accredited college or school of pharmacy and an interest in and aptitude for advanced training in pharmacy. A resident or fellow receives a stipend plus benefits (insurance, vacation, etc.). The amount of the stipend and the specific benefits vary according to the individual program.

RESIDENCIES

A residency is an organized, directed postgraduate training program in a defined area of pharmacy practice. Residencies are typically one year in duration; however, some may be longer. The primary goal of a residency is to train pharmacists in a specific area of pharmacy practice. The objective of a residency is to develop competent practitioners who are able to provide pharmacy services such as clinical pharmacy, drug information, pharmacotherapeutic dosing and monitoring, and administration. Residency training is increasingly a requirement for employment in various pharmacy settings.

A pharmacy practice residency is a general residency in pharmacy practice. In addition to pharmacy practice residencies, a host of specialized residencies exist. A specialized residency focuses on a particular niche of pharmacy practice; pediatric pharmacy, psychiatric pharmacy, and nuclear pharmacy are all examples of specialized residencies. Whether the residency is a pharmacy practice residency or a specialty residency, training typically involves structured rotations within the pharmacy department as well as medical rotations with physicians and other health care professionals. The practice experiences of residents are closely directed and evaluated by qualified practitioner-preceptors who are trained in particular areas of pharmacy practice.

The American Society of Health-System Pharmacists is the accrediting body for residencies. To obtain a list of postgraduate pharmacy practice residency programs, write to or visit:

American Society of Health-System Pharmacists
7272 Wisconsin Avenue
Bethesda, Maryland 20814
www.ashp.org

FELLOWSHIPS

A fellowship is a directed, highly individualized postgraduate program, typically two years in duration, that is designed to prepare the participant to become an independent researcher. The primary goal of a fellowship is to develop competency in scientific pharmacy research. A fellow works under the close direction and instruction of a qualified researcher-preceptor. Many fellowships are affiliated with a college or school of pharmacy. Fellowship training may be required or recommended for employment in certain pharmacy settings. To obtain a list of postgraduate fellowship programs, you can write to or visit:

American College of Clinical Pharmacy
13000 W. 87th St. Parkway
Lenexa, Kansas 66215-4530
www.accp.com

RESIDENCY AND FELLOWSHIP PROGRAMS: AREAS OF PHARMACY PRACTICE AND RESEARCH

Administration
Ambulatory Care
Cardiology
Clinical Informatics
Clinical Pharmaceutical
   Sciences
Clinical Pharmacology
Community Pharmacy
Critical Care
Drug Development
Drug Information
Emergency Medicine
Endocrinology
Family Medicine
Geriatrics
HIV Pharmacy

Hospice
Immunology
Infectious Disease
Internal Medicine
Managed Care
Nephrology
Neurology
Nuclear Pharmacy
Nutrition
Obstetrics-Gynecology
Oncology
Outcomes Research
Pain Management
Patient Safety
Pediatrics
Pharmacoeconomics

Pharmacoepidemiology
Pharmacogenomics
Pharmacokinetics
Pharmacometrics
Pharmacotherapy
Pharmacy Practice
Primary Care
Psychiatric Pharmacy
Pulmonary
Rheumatology
Toxicology
Translational Research
Transplantation
Women's Health

The PCAT

2

WHAT IS THE PCAT?

The Pharmacy College Admission Test (PCAT) is a national examination developed by Pearson Education, Inc. The PCAT was developed to provide admission committees of pharmacy schools with comparable information about the academic abilities of applicants in five topic areas: biological processes, chemical processes, quantitative reasoning, critical reading, and writing.

The computer-based exam consists of 192 multiple-choice questions and 1 writing topic. The stem portion of each multiple-choice question may be presented as a question, partial statement, or problem scenario followed by four possible answers. Only one answer is correct. Often the other choices are distractors, may contain errors, do not apply to the question, or may not be the best answer to the question. Often the distractors are taken from the same content area of study as the correct answer, so it is important to recognize specific facts, not just be familiar with topics. The PCAT score is calculated from the number of correct answers. There is NO penalty for guessing, so candidates should not leave any answers blank.

PCAT Contents

As of July 2016, the following is a description of the PCAT's five scoring sections:

- **BIOLOGICAL PROCESSES.** This section consists of 48 general biology, microbiology, and anatomy and physiology questions. Forty minutes are given to complete this section.
- **CRITICAL READING.** This section consists of six reading passages and 48 questions that test candidates' evaluation, comprehension, and analytical skills. Fifty minutes are given to complete this section.
- **QUANTITATIVE REASONING.** This section consists of 48 basic math, algebra, precalculus, calculus, probability, and statistics questions. A calculator will be provided during the exam. Forty-five minutes are given to complete this section.
- **CHEMICAL PROCESSES.** This section consists of 48 general and organic chemistry and basic biochemistry processes questions. Some may involve calculations; remember, a calculator will be provided. Forty minutes are given to complete this section.
- **WRITING.** The candidate will be requested to compose one problem-solving essay. Thirty minutes will be given to write the essay.

Usually the PCAT exam includes multiple-choice experimental questions being tested for possible use in future exams. There is no way to know which items are experimental, so candidates will want to do their best to answer each question correctly.

The Exam

PCAT Sections	2017-2018 PCAT Section Subtests/% of Item Types	Number of Items in Section	Number of Minutes to Complete PCAT Section
1. Biological Processes	General Biology—50% Microbiology—20% Anatomy and Physiology—30%	48 Items	40 Minutes
2. Critical Reading	Comprehension—30% Evaluation—30% Analysis—40%	6 Reading Passages and 48 Items	50 Minutes
3. Quantitative Reasoning	Basic Math—25% Algebra—25% Probability and Statistics—18% Precalculus—18% Calculus—14%	48 Items	45 Minutes
4. Chemical Processes	General Chemistry— 50% Organic Chemistry—30% Basic Biochemistry Processes—20%	48 Items	40 Minutes
5. Writing	Problem Solving Conventions of Language	1 Topic	30 Minutes

PCAT Scoring

Your score report will include separate scaled scores and percentile scores for each of the four multiple-choice content areas. It will also include a composite scaled score and percentile score for the overall multiple-choice exam. Scaled scores are computed from raw scores for each individual test offering so that results can be compared from one test offering to the next. The scaled scores will range from 200 to 600.

Additionally, a percentile score is computed by distributing your performance in a norm group or pool of candidates. The percentile reported for individual sections and the composite score indicate the percentage of students who scored below you. For example, a 75th percentile score on the biological processes section indicates that you did better than 75% of the students in the norm group. Immediately after taking the PCAT, students receive preliminary scores for each of the four content areas and the overall composite score; these preliminary scores will very closely approximate the official PCAT scores received several weeks after taking the test. Students can use these preliminary scores to assess how well they performed on the PCAT and whether they may need to take the test again to improve their scores.

You will receive a single writing score that is based both on mechanics and on the development and presentation of the composition. The writing score is reported on a scale of 1.0 to 6.0, and a mean score for all individuals who have taken the PCAT within the last 12 months is also shown.

The scores used by numerous pharmacy programs in evaluating candidates vary. Some use scaled scores; others use percentiles. Some have minimum scores required in each of the PCAT sections; some use composite scores. Many will use a candidate's highest score on a single attempt if the candidate has taken the test more than once; however, this might not always be the case.

TIP

Check with the school to ensure that your score is as competitive as possible.

After a candidate has taken the PCAT five times, restrictions may be placed on additional registrations. Candidates may be required to provide documentation explaining the circumstances that necessitate taking the PCAT again. If the requested documentation is not provided, the candidate will not be permitted to register. Further details on this policy and the type of documentation that may be required can be found on the PCAT website.

When Is the PCAT Offered?

The PCAT is administered at Pearson VUE Test Centers on multiple dates. To obtain exact dates, visit the PCAT website at *www.pcatweb.info*. Accommodations may be made for individuals with disabilities. Deadlines for registration for the PCAT are available on the PCAT website—onsite, same-day registration is not available.

Fees

For the most current information, visit the PCAT website at *www.pcatweb.info*. The following is the PCAT fee as of 2017.

Online Registration Fee $210.00

For more information concerning special fees, visit the PCAT website.

PCAT Information

For more information concerning the PCAT, contact Pearson at the following address or phone number or visit the website below.

NCS Pearson, Inc.
PCAT Customer Relations—PCAT
19500 Bulverde Road
San Antonio, Texas 78259
1-800-622-3231
www.pcatweb.info

We strongly recommend reviewing the PCAT candidate information booklet available at *www.pcatweb.info*.

When Should You Take the PCAT?

Many considerations are involved in the decision of when and how often to take the PCAT. Many colleges/schools of pharmacy do not penalize applicants for taking the test more than once and often use the highest scores. This practice differs from institution to institution, so you will need to check with the college/school that you are interested in attending. In addition, it is strongly recommended that you take the PCAT no later than the fall of the year prior to the semester that you want to begin pharmacy school. This strategy will allow you to retake the PCAT in the winter if desired or necessary.

The ultimate decision of when and how often to take the PCAT is an individualized one and depends on many circumstances, such as when you feel most comfortable taking the test (this may depend on the number of pre-pharmacy courses you have taken). Other factors that may affect your decision are the admissions policy of the pharmacy college or school you wish to attend and your previous PCAT scores.

Strategies to Increase Your Score

3

PCAT STRATEGIES

When taking the PCAT, work at a comfortable pace but keep in mind that there is a time limit for each section. Be sure to answer every question. Your total PCAT score and the score you receive on each section of the test (excluding the PCAT essay) reflect the number of correct answers only. Some tests penalize for guessing by subtracting the number of wrong answers from the number of correct answers; with the PCAT, however, this is not the case. Although guesses are not likely to make much difference in your scores, you should not ignore this chance to avoid the total loss of points from unanswered questions.

The PCAT is divided into five sections. Three sections are specifically related to course-work covered in the pre-pharmacy curriculum: biological processes, chemical processes, and quantitative reasoning. One section is more comprehensive in nature and measures skills acquired through lifelong learning: critical reading. Because the critical reading section assesses skills acquired over a long period of time, it tends to be more difficult to study for in advance. The writing section is a combination of comprehensive learning, life experiences, and skills potentially obtained during your pre-pharmacy work.

When you take the practice PCAT tests in this book and the actual PCAT test, make sure to keep track of the time allotted for each test section. Pace yourself and work quickly but calmly through all the questions. Although you may be forced to guess on some questions, there is a chance that some of your guesses will be correct.

In addition to the practice tests in this book, you should also consider utilizing the resources available on the official PCAT website (*www.pcatweb.info*). These resources include computer-based practice tests that you may purchase access to.

REMEMBER

On the PCAT, your score is computed from the number of correct answers only. You are NOT penalized for guessing.

FIFTEEN PRESCRIPTIONS TO INCREASE YOUR SCORE

The first section of this chapter discussed general PCAT strategies. In this section you are given fifteen "prescriptions" to improve your PCAT test scores. Students who have taken the PCAT and employed these test-taking tactics have found them quite useful:

- **Rx 1.** Get an adequate amount of sleep the night before the test.
- **Rx 2.** Allow yourself plenty of time to get to the testing site.
- **Rx 3.** Bring an accurate watch.
- **Rx 4.** Bring two forms of proper identification (e.g., driver's license, passport).
- **Rx 5.** Wear comfortable clothes.
- **Rx 6.** Know what to expect. After studying this preparation manual, you will be familiar with the types of questions that may appear on the PCAT.
- **Rx 7.** Read and memorize the directions for each question type or section.
- **Rx 8.** Pace yourself. Work within the time restriction.
- **Rx 9.** Look at all the possible answers before making your final choice.
- **Rx 10.** Eliminate as many wrong answers as possible.
- **Rx 11.** Answer every question.
- **Rx 12.** In preparing for the writing section, review available online essay-writing resources and tutorials. Also, consider purchasing access to the practice writing tests available on the official PCAT website.
- **Rx 13.** In the critical reading section, when asked to find the main idea, be sure to check the opening and summary sentences of the passage.
- **Rx 14.** Remember, you will be provided with a calculator for use on the biological processes, chemical processes, and quantitative reasoning sections.
- **Rx 15.** Do not bring cell phones and other electronic devices to the PCAT as they are not allowed in the testing area. Your PCAT score will be cancelled if you break this rule.

Biological Processes Review and Practice

4

TIPS FOR THE BIOLOGICAL PROCESSES SECTION

The biological processes section of the PCAT measures your knowledge and understanding of principles and concepts in basic biology (including general biology), microbiology, and human anatomy and physiology. Microbiology, human anatomy, and physiology may not be covered in general pre-pharmacy required biology courses. If you do not feel confident in these areas, you can probably improve your PCAT biological processes score by reviewing these subjects independently or by taking a course in these subjects.

The biological processes section of the real PCAT consists of 48 questions (more have been included in this chapter for review purposes). Some questions will be based on brief passages. You should read through each passage and then answer its associated questions, referring back to the passage as needed. You will have 40 minutes to complete the biological processes section. Be sure to answer all questions.

BIOLOGICAL PROCESSES REVIEW OUTLINE

I. General Biology
  A. Cellular and Molecular Biology
   i. Structure and function of cells
     1. Four classes of biomolecules
     2. Organelles
     3. Membranes and membrane transport
   ii. Gene expression and inheritance
     1. Transcription
     2. Translation
     3. Genetics
        a. Chromosomes
        b. Genes
        c. Traits
        d. Genetic diseases
   iii. Cell division and growth
     1. Mitosis
     2. Meiosis
   iv. Energy transformations
   v. Metabolism
     1. Glycolysis
     2. Cellular respiration
     3. Chemiosmotic phosphorylation (ATP production)

B. Diversity of Life Forms
    i. Phylogenetic tree of life
C. Health
    i. Nutrition
       1. Proteins
       2. Fats
       3. Glucose
       4. Vitamins
    ii. Diseases
    iii. Drugs

II. Microbiology
A. Microorganisms
    i. Viruses
    ii. Bacteria
    iii. Fungi
B. Infectious Diseases and Prevention
C. Microbial Ecology
D. Medical Microbiology
E. Immunity

III. Human Anatomy and Physiology
A. Structure
    i. Cells
    ii. Tissue
    iii. Organs
B. Systems
    i. Skeletal/muscular
       1. Axial skeleton
       2. Appendicular skeleton
       3. Bones
       4. Joints
       5. Skeletal muscles
    ii. Nervous/sensory
       1. Neuron
       2. Central nervous system
       3. Peripheral nervous system
       4. Sensory system
    iii. Circulatory/respiratory
       1. Blood
       2. Circulation
       3. Blood vessels
       4. Heart anatomy
       5. Heart function
       6. Respiratory ventilation
       7. Inspiration and expiration
       8. Gas exchange

iv. Digestive/excretory
    1. Digestive organs
    2. Digestive tract
    3. Digestive enzymes
    4. Digestive hormones
    5. Kidney anatomy
    6. Kidney function
    7. Liver anatomy
    8. Liver function

v. Endocrine
    1. Hormones
    2. Pancreas
    3. Thyroid gland
    4. Pituitary gland
    5. Parathyroid glands
    6. Adrenal glands

vi. Reproductive
    1. Reproductive organs (male and female)
    2. Hormone regulation

vii. Integumentary
    1. Skin
    2. Glands
    3. Hair
    4. Nails

viii. Immune
    1. Immune cell types
    2. Immune cell production

ANSWER SHEET
Biological Processes

1. Ⓐ Ⓑ Ⓒ Ⓓ	26. Ⓐ Ⓑ Ⓒ Ⓓ	51. Ⓐ Ⓑ Ⓒ Ⓓ	76. Ⓐ Ⓑ Ⓒ Ⓓ
2. Ⓐ Ⓑ Ⓒ Ⓓ	27. Ⓐ Ⓑ Ⓒ Ⓓ	52. Ⓐ Ⓑ Ⓒ Ⓓ	77. Ⓐ Ⓑ Ⓒ Ⓓ
3. Ⓐ Ⓑ Ⓒ Ⓓ	28. Ⓐ Ⓑ Ⓒ Ⓓ	53. Ⓐ Ⓑ Ⓒ Ⓓ	78. Ⓐ Ⓑ Ⓒ Ⓓ
4. Ⓐ Ⓑ Ⓒ Ⓓ	29. Ⓐ Ⓑ Ⓒ Ⓓ	54. Ⓐ Ⓑ Ⓒ Ⓓ	79. Ⓐ Ⓑ Ⓒ Ⓓ
5. Ⓐ Ⓑ Ⓒ Ⓓ	30. Ⓐ Ⓑ Ⓒ Ⓓ	55. Ⓐ Ⓑ Ⓒ Ⓓ	80. Ⓐ Ⓑ Ⓒ Ⓓ
6. Ⓐ Ⓑ Ⓒ Ⓓ	31. Ⓐ Ⓑ Ⓒ Ⓓ	56. Ⓐ Ⓑ Ⓒ Ⓓ	81. Ⓐ Ⓑ Ⓒ Ⓓ
7. Ⓐ Ⓑ Ⓒ Ⓓ	32. Ⓐ Ⓑ Ⓒ Ⓓ	57. Ⓐ Ⓑ Ⓒ Ⓓ	82. Ⓐ Ⓑ Ⓒ Ⓓ
8. Ⓐ Ⓑ Ⓒ Ⓓ	33. Ⓐ Ⓑ Ⓒ Ⓓ	58. Ⓐ Ⓑ Ⓒ Ⓓ	83. Ⓐ Ⓑ Ⓒ Ⓓ
9. Ⓐ Ⓑ Ⓒ Ⓓ	34. Ⓐ Ⓑ Ⓒ Ⓓ	59. Ⓐ Ⓑ Ⓒ Ⓓ	84. Ⓐ Ⓑ Ⓒ Ⓓ
10. Ⓐ Ⓑ Ⓒ Ⓓ	35. Ⓐ Ⓑ Ⓒ Ⓓ	60. Ⓐ Ⓑ Ⓒ Ⓓ	85. Ⓐ Ⓑ Ⓒ Ⓓ
11. Ⓐ Ⓑ Ⓒ Ⓓ	36. Ⓐ Ⓑ Ⓒ Ⓓ	61. Ⓐ Ⓑ Ⓒ Ⓓ	86. Ⓐ Ⓑ Ⓒ Ⓓ
12. Ⓐ Ⓑ Ⓒ Ⓓ	37. Ⓐ Ⓑ Ⓒ Ⓓ	62. Ⓐ Ⓑ Ⓒ Ⓓ	87. Ⓐ Ⓑ Ⓒ Ⓓ
13. Ⓐ Ⓑ Ⓒ Ⓓ	38. Ⓐ Ⓑ Ⓒ Ⓓ	63. Ⓐ Ⓑ Ⓒ Ⓓ	88. Ⓐ Ⓑ Ⓒ Ⓓ
14. Ⓐ Ⓑ Ⓒ Ⓓ	39. Ⓐ Ⓑ Ⓒ Ⓓ	64. Ⓐ Ⓑ Ⓒ Ⓓ	89. Ⓐ Ⓑ Ⓒ Ⓓ
15. Ⓐ Ⓑ Ⓒ Ⓓ	40. Ⓐ Ⓑ Ⓒ Ⓓ	65. Ⓐ Ⓑ Ⓒ Ⓓ	90. Ⓐ Ⓑ Ⓒ Ⓓ
16. Ⓐ Ⓑ Ⓒ Ⓓ	41. Ⓐ Ⓑ Ⓒ Ⓓ	66. Ⓐ Ⓑ Ⓒ Ⓓ	91. Ⓐ Ⓑ Ⓒ Ⓓ
17. Ⓐ Ⓑ Ⓒ Ⓓ	42. Ⓐ Ⓑ Ⓒ Ⓓ	67. Ⓐ Ⓑ Ⓒ Ⓓ	92. Ⓐ Ⓑ Ⓒ Ⓓ
18. Ⓐ Ⓑ Ⓒ Ⓓ	43. Ⓐ Ⓑ Ⓒ Ⓓ	68. Ⓐ Ⓑ Ⓒ Ⓓ	93. Ⓐ Ⓑ Ⓒ Ⓓ
19. Ⓐ Ⓑ Ⓒ Ⓓ	44. Ⓐ Ⓑ Ⓒ Ⓓ	69. Ⓐ Ⓑ Ⓒ Ⓓ	94. Ⓐ Ⓑ Ⓒ Ⓓ
20. Ⓐ Ⓑ Ⓒ Ⓓ	45. Ⓐ Ⓑ Ⓒ Ⓓ	70. Ⓐ Ⓑ Ⓒ Ⓓ	95. Ⓐ Ⓑ Ⓒ Ⓓ
21. Ⓐ Ⓑ Ⓒ Ⓓ	46. Ⓐ Ⓑ Ⓒ Ⓓ	71. Ⓐ Ⓑ Ⓒ Ⓓ	96. Ⓐ Ⓑ Ⓒ Ⓓ
22. Ⓐ Ⓑ Ⓒ Ⓓ	47. Ⓐ Ⓑ Ⓒ Ⓓ	72. Ⓐ Ⓑ Ⓒ Ⓓ	97. Ⓐ Ⓑ Ⓒ Ⓓ
23. Ⓐ Ⓑ Ⓒ Ⓓ	48. Ⓐ Ⓑ Ⓒ Ⓓ	73. Ⓐ Ⓑ Ⓒ Ⓓ	98. Ⓐ Ⓑ Ⓒ Ⓓ
24. Ⓐ Ⓑ Ⓒ Ⓓ	49. Ⓐ Ⓑ Ⓒ Ⓓ	74. Ⓐ Ⓑ Ⓒ Ⓓ	99. Ⓐ Ⓑ Ⓒ Ⓓ
25. Ⓐ Ⓑ Ⓒ Ⓓ	50. Ⓐ Ⓑ Ⓒ Ⓓ	75. Ⓐ Ⓑ Ⓒ Ⓓ	100. Ⓐ Ⓑ Ⓒ Ⓓ

100 Questions

> **Directions:** Select the best answer to each of the following questions.

1. Which of the following is the fluid medium of the nucleus?
   (A) Chloroplast
   (B) Golgi complex
   (C) Nucleoplasm
   (D) Nucleolus

2. A newly discovered bacterium is found to infect animals and cause a reduction in muscle contractions. Symptoms include labored breathing, difficulty swallowing, and slowed physical movement. All animals presenting these symptoms tested positive for the presence of this bacterium.

   Further studies reveal that the bacterium secretes a toxin called "Toxin β" while in the host. The toxin enters muscle cells and binds to ATP synthase, blocking the active sites where new ATP is formed. Based on the mode of action of how the toxin works, which of the following choices best describes where the toxin localizes in the muscle cells?

   (A) Mitochondrial matrix
   (B) Outer membrane of the mitochondria
   (C) Golgi apparatus
   (D) Nucleus

3. You are an endocrinologist who is testing a new drug to replace testosterone in males with low testosterone. The results of your trial suggest the drug is effective. Which of the following describes your drug?

   (A) Your drug is binding to signal receptors at the surface of a cell.
   (B) Your drug is binding to the little testosterone present in a cell.
   (C) Your drug forms a hormone receptor complex and moves to the nucleus.
   (D) Your drug locates to the surface of the mitochondria.

4. Newly made proteins are directed to a specific location within a cell. Their subcellular location is determined by

   (A) entry into transport vesicles.
   (B) the addition of ubiquitin tag.
   (C) the addition of a phosphate.
   (D) a localization signal within the protein sequence.

QUESTIONS 5 THROUGH 8 REFER TO THE FOLLOWING PASSAGE:

Proteins are biomolecules that are crucial to the structure and function of all cells. Proteins are made of individual amino acids connected via peptide bonds. The sequence of those amino acids is unique to each protein. Once a protein is formed, it will begin to fold into a three-dimensional structure, oftentimes with the help of chaperone proteins. This shape determines the functionality of the protein.

It is possible that proteins may misfold, creating an irregular shape and a non-functional protein. Fortunately, eukaryotic cells have a mechanism called the Unfolded Protein Response to recognize and refold such proteins. Misfolded proteins that are not detected by this system can cause problems within cells. Diseases such as Mad Cow Disease are caused by misfolded proteins.

5. Protein folding is directly related to protein function. Which of the following involves the unequal sharing of electrons between atoms of amino acids which helps proteins fold?
   (A) Electrostatic interactions
   (B) Hydrophobic interactions
   (C) Van der Waals interactions
   (D) Ionic bonding

6. Which of the following best describes the interaction of two non-polar R-groups of amino acids?
   (A) Hydrophobic interactions
   (B) Cohesion
   (C) Adhesion
   (D) Ionic bonding

7. In regard to protein folding, which of the following best describes the attraction of an oxygen dipole to a nitrogen dipole?
   (A) Electrostatic interactions
   (B) Adhesion
   (C) Hydrophobic interactions
   (D) Van der Waals interactions

8. Which of the following cannot denature or unfold an enzyme?
   (A) High pH levels
   (B) High salinity levels
   (C) High temperatures
   (D) High substrate levels

9. The study of the relationship of microorganisms with one another and with their environment is called

    (A) microbiology.
    (B) phylogenetics.
    (C) microbial ecology.
    (D) prokaryotic genetics.

10. In general, enzymes are used by a cell to

    (A) increase the energy required to start a chemical reaction.
    (B) decrease the energy required to start a chemical reaction.
    (C) disrupt a chemical reaction.
    (D) bypass a chemical reaction.

QUESTIONS 11 THROUGH 14 REFER TO THE FOLLOWING PASSAGE:

Human sexual reproduction is a result of the combination of a haploid male sperm and a haploid female egg to form a diploid zygote. Fertility issues in males have been linked to abnormal pH or sugar levels in seminal fluid of the semen. Quantitative or qualitative characteristics of sperm may also lead to infertility (e.g., swimming ability, abnormal morphology). Fertility issues can also occur in females and can include a lack of egg release, reduced egg viability, or the rejection of the fertilized egg by the body.

   Problems with glands or hormone levels can also lead to infertility. Hormones play a key role in successful egg and sperm production as well as preparation of the female body for pregnancy. Estrogen, follicle stimulating hormone (FSH), progesterone, and gonadotropin-releasing hormone are just a few that are involved. Numerous glands are involved in the production and release of these hormones at specific times during sex cell production.

11. If an infertile male is tested and found to have lower than normal levels of FSH, what gland is likely malfunctioning?

    (A) Thyroid
    (B) Testes
    (C) Parathyroid
    (D) Pituitary gland

12. If a 20-year-old female has stopped ovulating, which hormone is likely no longer being produced?

    (A) Estrogen
    (B) Testosterone
    (C) Luteinizing hormone
    (D) Progesterone

13. An infertile female is examined, and it is discovered that the endometrium is not thickening after ovulation. A lack of which hormone is likely the cause?

(A) Progesterone
(B) Estrogen
(C) Gonadotropin-releasing hormone
(D) Luteinizing hormone

14. An infertile female is examined, and it is discovered that her ovaries did not fully develop during puberty. A lack of which hormone is likely the cause?

(A) Progesterone
(B) Estrogen
(C) Gonadotropin-releasing hormone
(D) Testosterone

---

15. Which part of a cell produces ribonucleoproteins such as ribosomes?

(A) Nuclear envelope
(B) Chromosomes
(C) Nucleoplasm
(D) Nucleolus

16. Which of the following can undergo simple diffusion through a membrane?

(A) Glucose
(B) Amino acids
(C) Ions
(D) Gases

QUESTIONS 17 THROUGH 20 REFER TO THE FOLLOWING PASSAGE:

Blood is composed of a variety of cells that transport gases, fight infections, and clot broken blood vessels. The liquid part of blood is called plasma and contains water, proteins, and dissolved nutrients such as sodium ions.

Human blood falls into one of four blood types: A, B, AB, or O, based on antigens present on the surface of red blood cells (Table 1). An understanding of the different blood types is important. For example, if a person loses blood in an accident, a blood transfusion is an option for treatment. Since not all blood is the same, a transfusion of the wrong blood type will lead to rejection by the body as antibodies will attach to the newly acquired red blood cells and an immune response will be launched.

Table 1

Blood type	Antibodies present in host
A+	B type antibodies
A–	B type antibodies
B+	A type antibodies
B–	A type antibodies
AB+	Neither A nor B type antibodies
AB–	Neither A nor B type antibodies
O+	A and B type antibodies
O–	A and B type antibodies

17. A person with which blood type can receive any blood type via transfusion without rejection?

   (A) Blood type O
   (B) Blood type AB
   (C) Blood type A
   (D) Blood type B

18. Which blood type is considered the universal donor for transfusions?

   (A) Blood type O
   (B) Blood type AB
   (C) Blood type A
   (D) Blood type B

19. The presence or absence of which of the following proteins on the surface of red blood cells indicates a positive or negative blood type, respectively?

   (A) Hemoglobin
   (B) Spectrin
   (C) Aquaporins
   (D) Rh

20. If a mother is AB+ blood type and a father is O blood type, which of the following is a possible blood type of their offspring?

   (A) Blood type O only
   (B) Blood type A only
   (C) Blood type B only
   (D) Blood type A or B

21. The theory of spontaneous generation states that

   (A) microorganisms arise from lifeless matter.
   (B) evolution has taken place in large animals.
   (C) humans have generated from apes.
   (D) viruses are degenerative forms of bacteria.

QUESTIONS 22 THROUGH 25 REFER TO THE FOLLOWING PASSAGE:

In 2014, an outbreak of the Ebola virus caused fever, organ failure, and even death in people of Senegal, West Africa. Recent studies on primates may provide evidence for a new, effective treatment. Researchers injected Ebola-infected monkeys with siRNA, or small interfering RNA. This single stranded nucleotide enters infected cells and binds to the viral mRNA, preventing it from binding to ribosomes. The virus is then unable to replicate and the disease progression stops.

   Ebola is a negative sense, single-stranded RNA, or (–)ssRNA, virus. Not all viruses possess (–)ssRNA. For example, the common human cold virus is a positive sense, single-stranded RNA, or (+)ssRNA, virus. Some viruses, such as the Herpes Simplex Virus, include double-stranded DNA (dsDNA) as their genetic material. These three viral types can all be targeted by siRNA therapies.

22. Based on the research described above, what specific step in the life cycle of the Ebola virus is blocked by the siRNA?

   (A) Viral DNA replication
   (B) Viral RNA replication
   (C) Viral transcription
   (D) Viral translation

23. Which of the following ordered steps best represents how Ebola makes a copy of its capsid proteins when it enters a cell?

   (A) (–)ssRNA $\longrightarrow$ mRNA $\longrightarrow$ viral capsid protein
   (B) (–)ssRNA $\longrightarrow$ DNA $\longrightarrow$ mRNA $\longrightarrow$ viral capsid protein
   (C) (–)ssRNA $\longrightarrow$ (+)ssRNA $\longrightarrow$ mRNA $\longrightarrow$ viral capsid protein
   (D) (–)ssRNA $\longrightarrow$ viral capsid protein

24. Which of the following ordered steps best represents how (+)ssRNA virus makes a copy of its capsid proteins when it enters a cell?

   (A) (+)ssRNA $\longrightarrow$ mRNA $\longrightarrow$ viral capsid protein
   (B) (+)ssRNA $\longrightarrow$ DNA $\longrightarrow$ mRNA $\longrightarrow$ viral capsid protein
   (C) (+)ssRNA $\longrightarrow$ (–)ssRNA $\longrightarrow$ mRNA $\longrightarrow$ viral capsid protein
   (D) (+)ssRNA $\longrightarrow$ viral capsid protein

25. Which of the following ordered steps best represents how a dsDNA virus makes a copy of its capsid proteins when it enters a cell?

    (A) dsDNA → integrate into host dsDNA → mRNA → viral capsid protein
    (B) dsDNA → mRNA → viral capsid protein
    (C) dsDNA → (–)ssRNA → (+)ssRNA → viral capsid protein
    (D) dsDNA → (–)ssRNA → (+)ssRNA → mRNA → viral capsid protein

---

26. In eukaryotes, DNA is

    (A) naked.
    (B) bound by histone proteins to form chromatin.
    (C) transcribed into messenger RNA while in a condensed state.
    (D) may be a single-stranded molecule.

27. What metal ion is responsible for the binding of oxygen gas to hemoglobin?

    (A) Magnesium
    (B) Manganese
    (C) Copper
    (D) Iron

28. UV radiation that damages DNA beyond repair can lead to which of the following?

    (A) Infection
    (B) Cancer
    (C) Reduced immune function
    (D) Blood-borne disease

29. Organic molecules, at the very least, must be composed of

    (A) hydrogen.
    (B) carbon.
    (C) carbon and hydrogen.
    (D) carbon, hydrogen, and oxygen.

30. Crossing over of homologous chromosomes occurs during what phase of meiosis?

    (A) Prophase I
    (B) Metaphase II
    (C) Anaphase I
    (D) Telophase II

31. Progression through the cell cycle is regulated by oscillations in the concentrations of which types of molecules?

    (A) Suppressor proteins
    (B) Cyclin-dependent kinases
    (C) Cyclins
    (D) Tubulin

QUESTIONS 32 THROUGH 35 REFER TO THE FOLLOWING PASSAGE:

Phylogenetic trees are pictorial representations of the evolution and relatedness of living organisms. The length of the arms indicates time and the nodes represent common ancestors. Figure 1 below displays the phylogenetic tree showing the evolution of prokaryotes and eukaryotes.

In the past, phylogenetic trees were drawn based on physical or phenotypic characteristics of organisms. Modern day phylogenetic trees are based on DNA sequences to establish relatedness. The phylogenetic tree in Figure 1 is based on the DNA sequence of the ITS (Internal Transcribed Spacer) region of the organisms listed. This section of DNA varies highly between species; therefore, it is often used to track the evolution of different species.

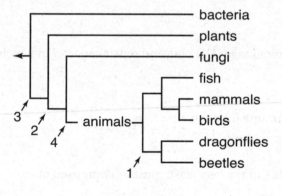

Figure 1

32. Which numbered node represents the most recent common ancestor of fungi and animals?

    (A) Node 1
    (B) Node 2
    (C) Node 3
    (D) Node 4

33. According to the tree, which group is more closely related to birds?

    (A) Fish
    (B) Mammals
    (C) Dragonflies
    (D) Beetles

34. Each node of the phylogenetic tree represents the evolution of a population into two new groups. Which of the following best describes this type of evolution?

    (A) Convergent evolution
    (B) Divergent evolution
    (C) Parallel evolution
    (D) Coevolution

35. The common ancestor of birds and insects did not have the ability to fly. Both of these groups later evolved to have this ability. Which of the following best describes this type of evolution?

    (A) Convergent evolution
    (B) Divergent evolution
    (C) Parallel evolution
    (D) Coevolution

_____

36. The lac operon is usually in the _____ position and is activated by a(n) _____ molecule.

    (A) on; repressor
    (B) off; repressor
    (C) on; inducer
    (D) off; inducer

37. The process of splitting glucose into two molecules of pyruvate while creating ATP is called

    (A) the Krebs cycle (the citric acid cycle).
    (B) the electron transport chain.
    (C) glycolysis.
    (D) fermentation.

38. The stage in cell division marked by chromosome separation is

    (A) anaphase.
    (B) metaphase.
    (C) prophase.
    (D) telophase.

39. The main role of apoptosis is to

    (A) remove damaged or diseased cells from tissue.
    (B) remove old or damaged organelles within a cell.
    (C) repair unfolded or misfolded proteins within a cell.
    (D) repair damaged DNA within a cell.

QUESTIONS 40 THROUGH 43 REFER TO THE FOLLOWING PASSAGE:

Cell signaling is the means by which cells can communicate with their environment. Cells produce and secrete a wide variety of signal molecules. In bacteria, signal molecules are secreted by individuals and later interpreted by other individuals in the colony. This process is called quorum sensing, and it is required if bacterial colonies are to launch pathogenic attacks on a host.

In eukaryotic cells, signals play a role in many processes from mating to immune responses. The chemistry of these molecules is also diverse, ranging from a small gas to a large nucleotide. Table 2 below includes categories and examples of eukaryotic signal molecules.

Table 2

Category of signal molecule	Example
Gas	Nitric Oxide
Sterol	Testosterone
Neurotransmitter	Acetylcholine
Protein	Insulin
Nucleotide	ATP

40. Which cell membrane protein is responsible for binding a signal molecule and initiating cell signaling?

    (A) Enzyme
    (B) Receptor
    (C) Transcription regulator
    (D) Transporter

41. Once cell signaling has begun, which type of protein will interpret the signal and cause a change in gene expression?

    (A) Enzymes
    (B) Receptors
    (C) Transcription regulators
    (D) Transporters

42. Of the types of signal molecules listed in Table 2, which molecule may diffuse through the cell plasma membrane to find its intracellular receptor?

(A) Sterol
(B) Protein
(C) Nucleotide
(D) Neurotransmitter

43. Of the types of signal molecules listed in Table 2, which molecule signals the relaxation of smooth muscles associated with blood vessels?

(A) Nitric oxide
(B) Acetylcholine
(C) Testosterone
(D) Insulin

---

44. Myosin is considered to be which of the following types of cellular proteins?

(A) Motor proteins
(B) Structural proteins
(C) Storage proteins
(D) Receptor proteins

45. In this organelle, sugar side chains on proteins and lipids are modified.

(A) Rough endoplasmic reticulum
(B) Golgi complex
(C) Nuclear lamella
(D) Smooth endoplasmic reticulum

46. During which stage of the cell cycle is DNA replicated?

(A) G_1 phase
(B) S phase
(C) G_2 phase
(D) M phase

47. The amount of energy needed to carry out basic body functions when you are at rest is known as

(A) intermediate metabolism.
(B) complex metabolism.
(C) catabolic metabolism.
(D) basal metabolism.

48. What is the function of the middle ear?

   (A) It contains hair cells that detect specific frequencies of sound.
   (B) It transmits sound vibrations to the tympanic membrane.
   (C) It amplifies sound transmitted to the cochlea.
   (D) It externally collects sound waves from the environment.

49. Blood is delivered to the heart from the lungs by the

   (A) renal veins.
   (B) pulmonary veins.
   (C) mitral arteries.
   (D) pulmonary arteries.

QUESTIONS 50 THROUGH 53 REFER TO THE FOLLOWING PASSAGE:

A man is at the doctor's office for his yearly physical. During his physical last year, he was given a good bill of health. After performing a physical exam and reviewing the man's urinalysis from this year, his physician becomes concerned. The man's urine analysis shows higher than normal levels of glucose as well as the presence of ketones and bilirubin. The specific gravity of the man's urine is also abnormally high.

   The man's blood analysis is also reviewed. Like his urine results, he has elevated levels of glucose and the presence of bilirubin. His high density lipoprotein cholesterol is abnormally low compared to last year, and his white blood cell count is slightly below normal for his sex and age. The physician is concerned for many reasons.

50. Which of the following would indicate that the man is not drinking enough water?

   (A) The presence of ketones in the urine
   (B) The presence of bilirubin in the urine and blood
   (C) The higher than normal levels of glucose in the urine and blood
   (D) The higher than normal specific gravity of the urine

51. The man has lost weight since the previous year and is now underweight for his age and height. Which of the following indicates that he is breaking down fat reserves?

   (A) The presence of ketones in the urine
   (B) The lower than normal levels of white blood cells
   (C) The higher than normal levels of glucose in the urine and blood
   (D) The higher than normal specific gravity of the urine

52. The physician fears the man may be hyperglycemic. What result likely led the physician to that conclusion?

   (A) The higher than normal levels of glucose in the urine and blood
   (B) The presence of bilirubin in the urine and blood
   (C) The lower than normal levels of white blood cells
   (D) The lower than normal levels of high density lipoprotein cholesterol

53. The physician tells the man that she is concerned about his liver. What symptom is the cause of her concern?

(A) The presence of ketones in the urine
(B) The presence of bilirubin in the urine
(C) The higher than normal levels of glucose in the urine
(D) The higher than normal specific gravity of the urine

_____

54. The long chain of carbons and hydrogens that form the "tails" of phospholipids is

(A) hydrophobic.
(B) hydrophilic.
(C) both hydrophobic and hydrophilic.
(D) neither hydrophobic nor hydrophilic.

55. Which of the following is found in gram-positive bacteria?

(A) Pseudomurein
(B) Sterol-rich membranes
(C) Peptidoglycan
(D) Amniotransports

56. What is the role of oxygen in cellular respiration?

(A) Oxygen provides electrons for the electron transport chain.
(B) Oxygen provides hydrogen ions for the production of ATP.
(C) Oxygen is an electron acceptor for the electron transport chain.
(D) Oxygen is an electron acceptor for the citric acid cycle.

57. The movement of an action potential along the axon of a neuron is caused by the opening and closing of what type of voltage-gated membrane channels?

(A) Sodium and potassium
(B) Potassium and calcium
(C) Calcium and sodium
(D) Sodium, potassium, and calcium

58. The process in which two bacteria exchange DNA via a pilus is called

(A) translation.
(B) transduction.
(C) conjugation.
(D) transformation.

59. Bacterial meningitis affects what part of the body?

    (A) The nervous system
    (B) The respiratory system
    (C) The urinary tract
    (D) The integumentary system

QUESTIONS 60 THROUGH 63 REFER TO THE FOLLOWING PASSAGE:

The digestive system is responsible for the breakdown and absorption of nutrients to fuel the cells of the human body. Complex macromolecules are ingested, then specific enzymes target and break those macromolecules down into smaller monomers for absorption. A majority of digestive enzymes are produced by epithelial cells of the small intestine.

    When digestive enzymes are absent or produced in small amounts, specific foods cannot be digested by the body. For example, low levels of the enzyme lactase lead to an intolerance of milk and dairy products that contain the sugar lactose. Fortunately, someone who is lactose intolerant can supplement their diet with lactase pills when consuming lactose rich foods.

60. What enzyme, found in saliva, begins the digestion of starch?

    (A) Pepsin
    (B) Lipase
    (C) Amylase
    (D) Maltase

61. What enzyme, secreted by the stomach, digests protein?

    (A) Maltase
    (B) Pepsin
    (C) Trypsin
    (D) Amylase

62. What enzyme, secreted into the small intestine, digests fats?

    (A) Lipase
    (B) Trypsin
    (C) Nuclease
    (D) Maltase

63. Fiber, a complex carbohydrate, is found in many of the plant foods we eat such as grains, fruits, and vegetables. Cells of the human digestive system are not able to break down fiber. However, our guts are home to a variety of anaerobic bacteria which secrete fiber-digesting enzymes. Which of the following enzymes would target fiber?

(A) Cellulase
(B) Nuclease
(C) Protease
(D) Chitinase

64. What component(s) do all viruses possess?

(A) Nucleic acids only
(B) Protein coat only
(C) Protein coat and nucleic acids
(D) Protein coat, nucleic acids, and plasma membrane

65. Prions are disease-causing agents that are composed of

(A) DNA only.
(B) protein only.
(C) proteins and DNA.
(D) proteins, DNA, and a plasma membrane.

66. The chemical component of a nucleotide that forms hydrogen bonds with another nucleotide on the complementary strand of DNA is the

(A) amino group.
(B) phosphate group.
(C) deoxyribose sugar.
(D) nitrogenous base.

67. Bacteria that are transmitted via insects fall into which of the following categories?

(A) Contact transmission
(B) Fluid transmission
(C) Vector transmission
(D) Airborne transmission

68. Most nutrients are absorbed in which organ of the digestive system?

(A) Esophagus
(B) Stomach
(C) Small intestine
(D) Large intestine

69. Animal viruses are classified into taxonomic groups based on

(A) their type of genetic material.
(B) the kind of cells they infect.
(C) their replication strategy.
(D) whether they are naked or enveloped.

QUESTIONS 70 THROUGH 73 REFER TO THE FOLLOWING PASSAGE:

The immune system is composed of a series of organs, tissues, and specialized cells that fight infection. To better understand the immune system, researchers created four strains of mice with specific mutations in their genome. Each set of mutations disrupts the function of one of four immune cells. Table 3 below indicates which strain of mouse contains functional (+) or non-functional (–) immune cells.

Table 3

	Dendritic cells	B lymphocytes	Neutrophils	Helper T lymphocytes
Strain 1	+	+	–	+
Strain 2	+	–	+	+
Strain 3	+	+	+	–
Strain 4	–	+	+	+

70. Which strain of mouse cannot produce antibodies in response to an infection as a part of acquired immunity?

(A) Strain 1
(B) Strain 2
(C) Strain 3
(D) Strain 4

71. Which strain of mouse will not produce an inflammatory response when infected?

(A) Strain 1
(B) Strain 2
(C) Strain 3
(D) Strain 4

72. Which strain of mouse will not be able to engulf and kill bacteria or viruses present at a site of injury during innate immunity?

(A) Strain 1
(B) Strain 2
(C) Strain 3
(D) Strain 4

73. Which strain of mouse lacks the cells that are stimulated by antigens as a part of acquired immunity?

(A) Strain 1
(B) Strain 2
(C) Strain 3
(D) Strain 4

---

74. A sample of blood of three males, Mark, Richard, and Steve, was taken at rest and a second sample was taken after each watched a scary movie clip. Based on the data in the table below, who hyperventilated when they saw the scary movie clip?

	Blood pH at rest	Blood pH after
Mark	7.4	7.2
Richard	7.4	7.4
Steve	7.4	7.6

(A) Mark
(B) Richard
(C) Steve
(D) No one hyperventilated

75. Prokaryotes that thrive in extremely high temperatures are considered to be

(A) bacteria.
(B) archaea.
(C) fungi.
(D) protists.

76. Malaria is a disease caused by a _____ and spread by [a] _____.

(A) bacterium; mosquito
(B) plasmodium; mosquito
(C) bacterium; contact
(D) plasmodium; contact

77. Rumen bacteria that live in the digestive tracts of animals such as cows are

(A) antagonists.
(B) pathogens.
(C) anaerobes.
(D) aerobes.

78. Which of the following drugs is considered to be a depressant?

   (A) Alcohol
   (B) Nicotine
   (C) Amphetamines
   (D) Cocaine

79. Koch's postulate defines the criterion used to demonstrate that

   (A) an organism is a heterotroph.
   (B) an organism causes a specific disease.
   (C) a disease-causing organism also has harmless variants.
   (D) organisms that lack cell walls undergo lyses in hypotonic solutions.

QUESTIONS 80 THROUGH 83 REFER TO THE FOLLOWING PASSAGE:

A healthy diet and lifestyle are essential for proper human development and continued maintenance over the course of a lifetime. For example, osteoporosis is a condition in which mature bones weaken and become brittle. People with osteoporosis are often slow to recover from bone breaks or fractures, and can even display height decline due to loss of bone in the spine. A diet that lacks calcium may result in osteoporosis.

   Vitamins are critical components of a healthy diet. Vitamins are typically small molecules that are found in a variety of plant and animal foods. Once ingested, vitamins pair up with enzymes involved in numerous metabolic pathways. Diets that are deficient in vitamins can lead to a myriad of medical conditions.

80. A diet that lacks enough vitamin C is associated with

   (A) anemia.
   (B) scurvy.
   (C) neural tube birth defect.
   (D) night blindness.

81. Consumption of too little vitamin A may result in

   (A) anemia.
   (B) reduced blood clotting.
   (C) neural tube birth defect.
   (D) night blindness.

82. The absence of vitamin D may result in

   (A) an increased risk of bone fracture.
   (B) reduced blood clotting.
   (C) scurvy.
   (D) night blindness.

83. A diet that lacks folic acid, or vitamin B, may result in

   (A) anemia.
   (B) scurvy.
   (C) neural tube birth defect.
   (D) an increased risk of bone fracture.

---

84. Which of the following nutrients has the highest caloric value per gram?

   (A) Protein
   (B) Glucose
   (C) Fat
   (D) Carbohydrates

85. If Y represents yellow (dominant color) and y represents green (recessive color), which of the following crosses would be expected to result in 75 percent yellow offspring?

   (A) $Yy \times yy$
   (B) $YY \times yy$
   (C) $Yy \times Yy$
   (D) $Yy \times YY$

86. Many animal viruses contain a membrane-like envelope structure that includes viral proteins protruding from a lipid bilayer. When does a newly formed virus acquire an envelope?

   (A) During the entry of the virus into the host cell
   (B) During the removal of the viral proteins inside the host cell
   (C) During replication of the virus inside the host cell
   (D) During the exiting of the virus from the host cell

87. Which of the following ecological terms best describes a virus in relation to the cell that it infects?

   (A) Mutualist
   (B) Parasite
   (C) Obligate parasite
   (D) Symbiotic partner

88. Which of the following diseases/disorders is caused by a fungal pathogen?

   (A) Phenomena
   (B) Common cold
   (C) Ringworm
   (D) Influenza

89. The peptide bond formed between amino acids in a protein involves the

(A) amino and the carboxyl groups.
(B) central carbon and the carboxyl groups.
(C) amino and the variable R-groups.
(D) hydrogen and the variable R-groups.

QUESTIONS 90 THROUGH 93 REFER TO THE FOLLOWING PASSAGE:

Genetic mutations occur when a DNA sequence is altered. Some mutations lead to a new allele, or variation, in the same gene. For example, mutations in which a single nucleotide is changed often will code for a different amino acid. This alteration of the amino acid sequence of the resulting protein may alter the protein's function, creating a new allele.

Other mutations can lead to loss of function of the resulting protein. For example, many cancers are linked to a deleterious mutation in the gene for the p53 protein. This protein is responsible for pausing the cell cycle so that damaged DNA can be fixed or, in the case of extensive damage, the cell can undergo apoptosis. Cancer resulting from a mutation in p53 does not stop progressing through the cell cycle, despite DNA damage.

90. If a point mutation causes a change in the sequence of DNA but does not change the protein sequence produced, it is called a

(A) missense mutation.
(B) frameshift mutation.
(C) nonsense mutation.
(D) silent mutation.

91. Which of the following mRNA sequences is an example of a nonsense mutation based on the original sequence UCCCGAGUCAUUACG? (Note that the three stop codons in RNA are UAG, UGA, and UAA.)

(A) UACCGAGUCAUUACG
(B) UCCCGAGUCAUACG
(C) UCCCGAGUCAUUACUC
(D) UCCUGAGUCAUUACG

92. Which of the following mRNA sequences is an example of a frameshift mutation based on the original sequence UCCCGAGUCAUUACG?

(A) UACCGAGUCAUUACG
(B) UCCGAGUCAUUACG
(C) UCCCGAGUCAUUACC
(D) UCCUGAGUCAUUACG

93. If a mutation causes a change in one nucleotide which results in a new amino acid in the protein sequence, it is called a

    (A) missense mutation.
    (B) frameshift mutation.
    (C) nonsense mutation.
    (D) silent mutation.

---

94. Blue (B) is the dominant color for the Figbird, whereas white (b) is the alternative recessive color. When a homozygous blue bird is crossed with a homozygous white bird, what percentage of the offspring is expected to be blue heterozygous?

    (A) 0
    (B) 25
    (C) 50
    (D) 100

95. A person who is heterozygous at the gene locus related to a disorder, but shows no signs of the disorder, is called a(n) _____ of the disorder.

    (A) infector
    (B) carrier
    (C) infection
    (D) holder

96. Sickle-cell anemia develops in individuals who inherit two copies of a recessive gene(s). If a man with sickle-cell anemia marries a woman who does not have the disease but is a carrier of it, what percentage of their offspring is expected to have the disease or to be a carrier of it?

    (A) 25
    (B) 50
    (C) 75
    (D) 100

QUESTIONS 97 THROUGH 100 REFER TO THE FOLLOWING PASSAGE:

The membrane of a cell serves as a barrier between the inside of the cell and the outside world. The membrane forms a bilipid layer that can be selective, allowing certain materials into or out of the cell. Fluidity is a unique characteristic of cell membranes. Fluidity allows for the formation and fusion of vesicles during endocytosis and exocytosis, the growth of a cell in preparation for cell division, and the diffusion of membrane components through the membrane.

In certain situations, fluidity of a cell plasma membrane is unfavorable. A cell may require that components in the membrane, such as proteins, no longer diffuse. A cell can anchor or attach proteins to the cell's cortex to prevent diffusion. A cell can also form a lipid raft, a temporary structure which will prevent one or more proteins from diffusing.

97. Which of the following is the most common component of cell membranes?

   (A) Sterols
   (B) Phospholipids
   (C) Protein channels
   (D) Protein transporters

98. Which of the following regulates the movement of ions across the membrane by forming an opening in the cell membrane?

   (A) Glycolipids
   (B) Glycoproteins
   (C) Protein channels
   (D) Protein transporters

99. Which of the following binds and moves ions and molecule materials through a cell membrane?

   (A) Glycolipids
   (B) Glycoproteins
   (C) Protein channels
   (D) Protein transporters

100. Which of the following reduces the fluidity of a cell membrane when present, such as in lipid rafts?

   (A) Sterols
   (B) Phospholipids
   (C) Protein channels
   (D) Protein transporters

ANSWER KEY
Biological Processes

1.	C	26.	B	51.	A	76.	B
2.	A	27.	D	52.	A	77.	C
3.	C	28.	B	53.	B	78.	A
4.	D	29.	C	54.	A	79.	B
5.	D	30.	A	55.	C	80.	B
6.	A	31.	C	56.	C	81.	D
7.	A	32.	D	57.	A	82.	A
8.	D	33.	B	58.	C	83.	C
9.	C	34.	B	59.	A	84.	C
10.	B	35.	A	60.	C	85.	C
11.	D	36.	D	61.	B	86.	D
12.	C	37.	C	62.	A	87.	C
13.	A	38.	A	63.	A	88.	C
14.	B	39.	A	64.	C	89.	A
15.	D	40.	B	65.	B	90.	D
16.	D	41.	C	66.	D	91.	D
17.	B	42.	A	67.	C	92.	B
18.	A	43.	A	68.	C	93.	A
19.	D	44.	A	69.	C	94.	D
20.	D	45.	B	70.	B	95.	B
21.	A	46.	B	71.	D	96.	D
22.	D	47.	D	72.	A	97.	B
23.	A	48.	C	73.	C	98.	C
24.	D	49.	B	74.	C	99.	D
25.	A	50.	D	75.	B	100.	A

ANSWERS EXPLAINED

1. **(C)** Nucleoplasm, meaning protoplasm of the nucleus, is the fluid medium of the nucleus.

2. **(A)** The active sites of ATP synthase function in the matrix of the mitochondria.

3. **(C)** If your drug is mimicking testosterone, then it would bind to testosterone's receptor inside the cell and move into the nucleus.

4. **(D)** Protein localization is determined by the sorting signal sequence within the protein sequence.

5. **(D)** Ionic bonding includes the unequal share of one or more electrons between atoms. Electrostatic interactions (choice A) occur when an atom with a negative charge is attracted to an atom with a positive charge. An example is two ionized R-groups on amino acids. Hydrophobic interactions (choice B) occur between two nonpolar, hydrophobic molecules. Van der Waals interactions (choice C) are due to the weak, short range attraction of two atoms.

6. **(A)** Hydrophobic interactions occur between two nonpolar, hydrophobic molecules, in this case two nonpolar R-groups. Cohesion (choice B) is the attraction between two different types of substances and is not found in protein folding. Adhesion (choice C) is the attraction between two like molecules and is not found in protein folding. Ionic bonding (choice D) includes the unequal share of one or more electrons between atoms.

7. **(A)** Electrostatic interactions occur when an atom with a negative charge is attracted to an atom with a positive charge. An example is two ionized R-groups on amino acids. Adhesion (choice B) is the attraction between two like molecules and is not found in protein folding. Hydrophobic interactions (choice C) occur between two nonpolar, hydrophobic molecules. Van der Waals interactions (choice D) are due to the weak, short range attraction of two atoms.

8. **(D)** While substrate concentration has an effect on the reaction rate of an enzyme, it has no bearing on protein folding. Changes in pH can affect the forces that maintain the folded shape of a protein; therefore, choice A is incorrect. High levels of sodium can affect the forces that maintain the folded shape of a protein; therefore, choice B is incorrect. High temperatures can break the bonds that maintain the folded shape of a protein; therefore, choice C is incorrect.

9. **(C)** Microbial ecology is the term used to describe the study of the relationship of microorganisms with one another and with their environment.

10. **(B)** All chemical reactions must overcome a certain amount of energy (the "activation energy") in order to begin. Enzymes reduce the activation energy needed, therefore encouraging the chemical reaction to occur.

11. **(D)** The pituitary gland produces FSH. Low levels will indirectly reduce sperm production. The thyroid (choice A) controls metabolism, not reproduction. While testes (choice B) are involved in reproduction, they do not produce FSH. The parathyroid (choice C) is involved with bone development.

12. **(C)** The luteinizing hormone signals the release of an egg from the ovary. Estrogen (choice A) is not directly involved in ovulation. Testosterone (choice B) is not involved in ovulation. Progesterone (choice D) helps prepare the endometrial lining in case of fertilization.

13. **(A)** Progesterone helps prepare the endometrial lining in case of fertilization. Estrogen (choice B) is not directly involved in building the endometrium. The gonadotropin-releasing hormone (choice C) is not involved in building the endometrium. The luteinizing hormone (choice D) signals the release of an egg from the ovary, but does not affect the endometrium.

14. **(B)** Estrogen, specifically estradiol, is involved in the development of the ovaries during puberty. Progesterone (choice A) helps prepare the endometrial lining in case of fertilization. The gonadotropin-releasing hormone (choice C) and testosterone (choice D) are not involved in the development of the sex organs during puberty.

15. **(D)** The nucleolus, a small area within the nucleus, is where ribonucleoproteins such as ribosomes are produced.

16. **(D)** Gases such as O_2 are small and neutral, allowing them to easily move through the phospholipid bilayer without issue. Glucose (choice A) and amino acids (choice B) are too large to pass through a membrane. They need a protein transporter to do so. While ions (choice C) are small, their charge (hydrophilic quality) does not allow them to pass through the hydrophobic layer of the phospholipid membrane.

17. **(B)** A person with blood type AB does not have antibodies for either type A or B antigens. A person with blood type O (choice A) has antibodies for both A and B antigens. A person with blood type A (choice C) has antibodies for type B antigens. A person with blood type B (choice D) has antibodies for type A antigens.

18. **(A)** Blood type O lacks antigens on the surface of red blood cells; therefore, no immune response will be triggered. Blood type AB (choice B) has AB antigens on the surface of red blood cells and will trigger an immune response in A, B, and O blood types. Blood type A (choice C) has A antigens on the surface of red blood cells and will trigger an immune response in AB, B, and O blood types. Blood type B (choice D) has B antigens on the surface of red blood cells and will trigger an immune response in A, AB, and O blood types.

19. **(D)** The presence of Rh proteins determines + (positive) blood type and its absence determines – (negative) blood type. Hemoglobin (choice A) is found in red blood cells but is not the surface antigen that determines + and – blood types. Spectrin (choice B) is a protein found inside of red blood cells but is not the surface antigen that determines + and – blood types. Aquaporins (choice C) are found in red blood cells but are not the surface antigens that determine + and – blood types.

20. **(D)** The offspring can inherit AO or BO, meaning blood type A or B are the possibilities.

21. **(A)** The theory of spontaneous generation states that certain living things arise from vital forces present in living or nonliving decomposers.

22. **(D)** mRNA binds to ribosomes during translation, or protein production. If siRNA binds to mRNA, it prevents translation from occurring. mRNA is not involved in DNA replication (choice A). Viral mRNA is present in the cell so RNA replication (choice B)

has not been blocked. Viral mRNA is present in the cell so transcription (choice C) has not been blocked.

23. **(A)** (–)ssRNA uses RNA polymerase to build an mRNA. The mRNA will then be used to build the capsid protein.

24. **(D)** (+)ssRNA is equivalent to mRNA so it can be used directly to build a protein.

25. **(A)** dsDNA viruses insert their DNA into the host's DNA in the nucleus (a step missing from choice B, making it incorrect). That viral dsDNA is used as a template to form mRNA and then the viral capsid protein. The dsDNA virus does not form a (–)ssRNA at any point, thus eliminating choices C and D.

26. **(B)** Eukaryotic DNA is bound by histones and condensed to form chromatin. The regions of the DNA that are transcribed into RNA are not condensed.

27. **(D)** Iron is the atom at the center of the heme groups found within hemoglobin proteins on red blood cells. Oxygen binds to the iron.

28. **(B)** UV radiation can damage DNA, leading to cancer.

29. **(C)** Organic molecules, at the very least, must be composed of carbon and hydrogen.

30. **(A)** Crossing over occurs during prophase I of meiosis, the stage where the homologous chromosomes first interact with one another.

31. **(C)** The cyclin concentrations vary in dividing cells. For example, M cyclin is produced in high levels to move a cell into the M (mitosis) phase of the cell cycle. Protein kinases and cyclins blend to form a mitosis-promoting complex that activates other proteins, leading to initiation of the M phase.

32. **(D)** Node 4 represents the most recent common ancestor of fungi and animals. Node 1 (choice A) represents the most recent common ancestor of insects and other animals. Node 2 (choice B) represents the most recent common ancestor of plants and other eukaryotes. Node 3 (choice C) represents the most recent common ancestor of bacteria and eukaryotes.

33. **(B)** Mammals share the closest common ancestor with birds. Fish (choice A) are closely related to birds, but mammals share a more recent ancestor. Dragonflies (choice C) and beetles (choice D) do not share the most recent common ancestor with birds.

34. **(B)** Divergent evolution is best described as the evolution of one group into two groups through the evolution of differing characteristics. Convergent evolution (choice A) is when two groups that are not related to each other independently evolve similar structures or abilities. Parallel evolution (choice C) is when two groups with a recent common ancestor evolve the same characteristics. Coevolution (choice D) is the evolution of two groups as a result of the symbiotic relation between the two groups.

35. **(A)** Convergent evolution is when two groups that are not related to each other independently evolve similar structures or abilities. Divergent evolution (choice B) is best described as the evolution of one group into two groups through the evolution of differing characteristics. Parallel evolution (choice C) is when two groups with a recent common ancestor evolve the same characteristics. Coevolution (choice D) is the evolution of two groups as a result of the symbiotic relation between the two groups.

36. **(D)** The lac operon is usually in the off position and is activated by an inducer molecule.

37. **(C)** The process of splitting glucose into two molecules of pyruvate while creating ATP is called glycolysis.

38. **(A)** The stages of cellular division include prophase, metaphase, anaphase, and telophase. During prophase (choice C), the chromosomes condense, the nuclear membrane deteriorates, and the spindle microtubules attach to the chromosomes. During metaphase (choice B), the chromosomes move to the center of the cell. During anaphase (choice A), each kinetochore divides, and the chromosomes separate. During telophase (choice D), the nuclear membrane reforms around each new daughter cell's nucleus.

39. **(A)** Apoptosis, or programmed cell death, occurs when a cell (1) has DNA damage beyond repair, (2) is infected, or (3) is old or unnecessary.

40. **(B)** Receptors are the proteins that bind and recognize signal molecules. Enzymes (choice A) may be involved in signal pathways, but they do not have binding sites for signal molecules. Transcription regulators (choice C) can bind signal molecules directly, but they are not found in the cell membrane. Transporters (choice D) may be involved in signal pathways, but they do not have binding sites for signal molecules.

41. **(C)** Transcription regulators affect gene expression. Enzymes (choice A), receptors (choice B), and transporters (choice D) do not affect gene expression.

42. **(A)** Many sterol hormones, such as cortisol, pass directly through the cell plasma membrane to bind to their receptor intracellularly. Proteins (choice B) require a cell surface receptor and are too large to pass through the cell plasma membrane. Nucleotides (choice C) require a cell surface receptor and are also too large to pass through the cell plasma membrane. Neurotransmitters (choice D) require a cell surface receptor and are often too large to pass through the cell plasma membrane.

43. **(A)** Nitric oxide is the only known gas molecule that is involved in smooth muscle relaxation. Acetylcholine (choice B) causes smooth muscles to contract. Testosterone (choice C) and insulin (choice D) are not involved in smooth muscle contraction.

44. **(A)** Myosin moves and is therefore considered to be a motor protein. It does not provide any structure to the cell like structural proteins (choice B) do nor does it store materials for the cell (choice C). It is not involved in cell signaling like receptor proteins (choice D).

45. **(B)** The Golgi complex modifies carbohydrate chains of glycosylated proteins and lipids. The original sugar chain is added in the endoplasmic reticulum first, and then it is modified in the Golgi.

46. **(B)** The G phases (choices A and C) are periods of growth. The M phase (choice D) is the stage where DNA condenses, the nuclear envelope dissolves, chromosomes are divided, and two new cells form.

47. **(D)** The amount of energy needed to carry out basic body functions when you are at rest is known as basal metabolism.

48. **(C)** The middle ear amplifies the sound energy transmitted to the cochlea.

49. **(B)** To answer this question correctly, it is important to remember two principles: (1) arteries carry blood away from the heart, while veins carry blood to the heart; and (2) pulmonary circulation consists of blood vessels that transport blood to the lungs and then to the heart. Therefore, the correct choice is pulmonary veins (choice B), not pulmonary arteries (choice D). Choices A and C are irrelevant.

50. **(D)** High specific gravity of urine indicates that the urine is concentrated and the person is likely not drinking enough fluids. Ketones (choice A) are produced and excreted in urine when fat cells are broken down for energy. Bilirubin (choice B) is made by the liver and stored in the gallbladder. The presence of bilirubin in the urine indicates an issue with the liver. High glucose levels (choice C) indicate a high carbohydrate diet or the possibility of hyperglycemia. This does not directly explain dehydration.

51. **(A)** Ketones are produced and excreted in urine when fat cells are broken down for energy. White blood cells (choice B) are involved in the immune response and do not play a role in the breakdown of fat. High glucose levels (choice C) indicate a high carbohydrate diet or the possibility of hyperglycemia. This does not explain his weight loss. High specific gravity of urine (choice D) indicates that urine is concentrated and the person is likely not drinking enough fluids.

52. **(A)** High glucose levels indicate a high carbohydrate diet or the possibility of hyperglycemia. The presence of bilirubin (choice B) indicates an issue with the liver. White blood cells (choice C) are involved in the immune system and are not directly related to hyperglycemia. High density lipoprotein cholesterol (choice D) is involved in cardiovascular health, not in hyperglycemia.

53. **(B)** Bilirubin is made by the liver and stored in the gallbladder. The presence of bilirubin in the urine indicates an issue with the liver. Ketones (choice A) are produced and excreted in urine when fat cells are broken down for energy. High glucose levels (choice C) indicate a high carbohydrate diet or the possibility of hyperglycemia. High specific gravity of urine (choice D) indicates that urine is concentrated and that the person may be dehydrated.

54. **(A)** The long chain of carbons and hydrogens that form the "tails" of phospholipids is hydrophobic.

55. **(C)** In gram-positive bacteria, peptidoglycan is found within the cell wall.

56. **(C)** In cellular respiration, oxygen is an electron acceptor for the electron transport chain.

57. **(A)** Sodium and potassium channels are opened and closed as voltage changes during an action potential in neurons.

58. **(C)** Transduction (choice B) occurs when bacteriophages inject new DNA into a bacterium. Transformation (choice D) is when a bacterium takes up free DNA from the environment. Translation (choice A) is not a means of DNA exchange between bacteria.

59. **(A)** Bacterial meningitis affects the nervous system.

60. **(C)** Amylase targets starch and breaks it down into glucose. Pepsin (choice A) is released by the stomach and breaks down polypeptides. Lipase (choice B) is released

by the small intestine and breaks down fats. Maltase (choice D) targets maltose sugar and breaks it down into glucose.

61. **(B)** Pepsin is released by the stomach and breaks down polypeptides. Maltase (choice A) targets maltose sugar and breaks it down into glucose. While trypsin (choice C) does digest proteins, it is secreted in the pancreas. Amylase (choice D) targets starch and breaks it down into glucose.

62. **(A)** Lipase is released into the small intestine where it breaks down fats. Trypsin (choice B) is released in the pancreas and breaks down polypeptides. Nuclease (choice C) targets nucleotides, not fats. Maltase (choice D) targets maltose sugar and breaks it down into glucose.

63. **(A)** Cellulase is a carbohydrate that is part of fibrous plants and is broken down by cellulose. Nuclease (choice B) breaks down nucleotides, not carbohydrates. Protease (choice C) breaks down proteins, not carbohydrates. Chitinase (choice D) is a carbohydrate, but it is not found in plants.

64. **(C)** All viruses possess a protein coat and nucleic acids.

65. **(B)** Prions are misfolded proteins that cause diseases like Mad Cow Disease.

66. **(D)** When paired, the nitrogenous bases of adenine and thymine form two hydrogen bonds, while the bases of cytosine and guanine form three hydrogen bonds.

67. **(C)** Insects carry, or vector, the pathogen and therefore spread disease. This process is called vector transmission. Contact transmission (choice A) requires direct contact with the pathogen (e.g., touching). Fluid transmission (choice B) requires that the pathogen contact the host via fluid (e.g., saliva), and airborne transmission (choice D) includes pathogen movement to the host on air current (e.g., cough).

68. **(C)** The small intestine absorbs most nutrients. The esophagus (choice A) is a passage for food from the mouth to the stomach and does not absorb any nutrients. The stomach (choice B) mostly absorbs sugars. The large intestine (choice D) absorbs mostly water.

69. **(C)** Animal viruses are classified on the basis of their replication strategy.

70. **(B)** Mouse strain 2 lacks the B lymphocytes which are responsible for making antibodies. Mouse strains 1 (choice A), 3 (choice C), and 4 (choice D) have B cells or lymphocytes which make antibodies.

71. **(D)** Mouse strain 4 lacks dendritic cells which produce inflammatory cytokines. Mouse strains 1 (choice A), 2 (choice B), and 3 (choice C) have dendritic cells which produce inflammatory cytokines.

72. **(A)** Mouse strain 1 lacks neutrophils which arrive at sites of infection to engulf and kill pathogens. Mouse strains 2 (choice B), 3 (choice C), and 4 (choice D) have neutrophils which arrive at sites of infection to engulf and kill pathogens.

73. **(C)** Mouse strain 3 lacks T cells which are stimulated by antigens as a part of acquired immunity. Mouse strains 1 (choice A), 2 (choice B), and 4 (choice D) make T cells.

74. **(C)** The answer is Steve because his pH increased. The pH of the blood will increase after hyperventilating due to a low level of carbon dioxide.

75. **(B)** Bacteria (choice A) are prokaryotes but do not live in extreme environments. Fungi and protists (choices C and D) are eukaryotes, not prokaryotes.

76. **(B)** Malaria is caused by plasmodium and spread by a mosquito.

77. **(C)** Because rumen bacteria live inside the digestive tracts where there is little oxygen, these bacteria are anaerobic (choice C), not aerobic (choice D). They are also symbiotic with the cow, not antagonistic (choice A) or pathogenic (choice B).

78. **(A)** All the other options (choices B through D) are stimulants.

79. **(B)** Koch's postulate defines the criterion used to demonstrate that an organism is responsible for causing a specific disease.

80. **(B)** A lack of vitamin C can lead to scurvy. A lack of iron is associated with anemia (choice A). A lack of folic acid is associated with neural tube birth defect (choice C). Eyesight maintenance is dependent on vitamin A (choice D).

81. **(D)** Eyesight maintenance is dependent on vitamin A. A lack of iron is associated with anemia (choice A). A lack of vitamin K, not vitamin A, can lead to reduced blood clotting (choice B). A lack of folic acid is associated with neural tube birth defect (choice C).

82. **(A)** Weak bones that fracture easily are associated with a vitamin D deficiency. A lack of vitamin K, not vitamin D, can lead to reduced blood clotting (choice B). A lack of vitamin C can lead to scurvy (choice C). Eyesight maintenance is dependent on vitamin A (choice D).

83. **(C)** A lack of folic acid is associated with neural tube birth defect. A lack of iron is associated with anemia (choice A). A lack of vitamin C can lead to scurvy (choice B). Weak bones that fracture easily are associated with a vitamin D deficiency (choice D).

84. **(C)** Fats have the highest caloric value with 9 calories/gram. Proteins (choice A) and sugars (choice B) have 4 calories per gram, while carbohydrates (choice D) are negligible.

85. **(C)** The best way to solve this problem is to find the cross that will most likely result in 75 percent yellow offspring given that yellow is dominant over green. After making your selection from the four possible choices, you should perform the cross by using a Punnett square. For example, let's cross choice C (Yy and Yy):

	Y	y
Y	YY	Yy
y	Yy	yy

YY = homozygous yellow;
Yy = heterozygous yellow;
yy = green

This cross will result in 75 percent yellow offspring. To check the other choices, set up each of them in a Punnett square. Choice A will result in 50 percent yellow and 50 percent green. Choice B will result in 100 percent yellow offspring. Choice D will result in 100 percent yellow.

86. **(D)** Viruses obtain their envelope via exocytosis at the host cell membranes at sites where viral proteins have been inserted in the membrane.

87. **(C)** Viruses require the help of a host cell in order to replicate. This definition makes it an obligate parasite.

88. **(C)** Phenomena (choice A) is caused by a bacterium, the common cold (choice B) is caused by a virus, and the flu (choice D) is caused by the influenza virus.

89. **(A)** Peptide bonds are formed between the amino and the carboxyl groups of amino acids. The central carbon (choice B) is full with four bonds. Choices C and D are incorrect because the R-groups are never involved in peptide bonding.

90. **(D)** A silent mutation does not change the resulting protein sequence. Missense mutations (choice A) lead to a change in the resulting protein sequence. A frameshift mutation (choice B) occurs when one or more nucleotides are inserted or deleted. This leads to a shift in frame of the sequence and, ultimately, a change in the protein sequence. A nonsense mutation (choice C) occurs when a change in DNA codes for a stop codon instead of an amino acid.

91. **(D)** A nonsense mutation occurs when a change in DNA codes for a stop codon instead of an amino acid. Choice D shows a change in the second codon from "CGA" to "UGA," a stop codon. The sequence in choice A had a change in the second nucleotide, but it did not result in a premature stop codon which is expected in nonsense mutations. The addition or deletion of nucleotides to a sequence is a frameshift mutation. The example in choice B is shorter so it had one base removed. The example in choice C is longer so it had one base added.

92. **(B)** The addition or deletion of nucleotides to a sequence is a frameshift mutation. Choice B is shorter because it had one base removed, which is an example of a frameshift mutation. Choice A shows a sequence with a change in the second nucleotide. Choice C shows a sequence with a change in one nucleotide. Choice D shows a change in the second codon from "CGA" to "UGA," which is the introduction of a stop codon.

93. **(A)** Missense mutations lead to a change in the resulting protein sequence. A frameshift mutation (choice B) occurs when one or more nucleotides are inserted or deleted. This leads to a shift in frame of the sequence and, ultimately, a change in the protein sequence. A nonsense mutation (choice C) occurs when a change in DNA codes for a stop codon instead of an amino acid. A silent mutation (choice D) does not change the resulting protein sequence.

94. **(D)** Follow the same procedure as in question 85:

	b	b
B	Bb	Bb
B	Bb	Bb

Bb = blue

A cross between a homozygous blue bird and a homozygous white bird will result in 100 percent blue heterozygous (Bb) birds, 0 percent white birds.

95. **(B)** A carrier is a person who is heterozygous at the gene locus related to a disorder, but shows no signs of the disorder.

96. **(D)** Set up the cross between the individual carrying the disease (Ss) and the individual with the disease (ss):

	S	s
s	Ss	ss
s	Ss	ss

Ss = carrier of disease;
ss = have the disease

Therefore, 100 percent are expected to either be a carrier or have the disease.

97. **(B)** Phospholipids form the bilipid layer of the membrane and are the most common component found in membranes.

98. **(C)** Channels typically move ions by creating an opening or pore. Glycolipids (choice A) and glycoproteins (choice B) do not move ions across a membrane; instead they are often used in cell-to-cell recognition. While protein transporters (choice D) may move ions, they do not create an opening. Instead, they have binding sites for what they move.

99. **(D)** While protein transporters may move ions, they do not create an opening. Instead, they have binding sites for what they move. Glycolipids (choice A) and glycoproteins (choice B) do not move ions across a membrane; instead they are often used in cell-to-cell recognition. Channels (choice C) typically move ions by creating an opening or pore; they do not bind what they move.

100. **(A)** Sterols, like cholesterol in animal membranes, stiffen the membrane and reduce fluidity as seen in the formation of lipid rafts. Phospholipids (choice B) create the fluidity of a membrane. Channels (choice C) and transporters (choice D) do not alter the fluidity of a membrane.

Chemical Processes Review and Practice

5

TIPS FOR THE CHEMICAL PROCESSES SECTION

The chemical processes section of the PCAT consists of 48 questions. Some questions will be based on brief passages. You should read through each passage and then answer its associated questions, referring back to the passage as needed. You will have 40 minutes to complete the chemical processes section. To prepare for the chemical processes section of the PCAT, review textbooks and notes used in chemistry courses. General chemistry, organic chemistry, and biochemistry questions are asked.

GENERAL CHEMISTRY REVIEW OUTLINE

I. **Matter and the Periodic Table**
   A. States of Matter
      1. Solid
      2. Liquid
      3. Gas
   B. Chemical and Physical Properties
   C. Elements, Compounds, and Mixtures
   D. Metals and Nonmetals
   E. Periodic Properties
      1. Atomic radius
      2. Ionization energy
      3. Electron affinity
      4. Electronegativity
   F. Phase Changes

II. **Simple Mathematics**
   A. Unit Conversions (Metric, English)
   B. Density
   C. Percent Composition
   D. Weighted Average Atomic Mass
   E. Moles, Avogadro's Number
   F. Limiting Reactant
   G. Percent Yield
   H. Formal Charge

III. **Atomic Structure**
  A. Subatomic Particles from Atomic Number and Atomic Mass
     1. Protons
     2. Neutrons
     3. Electrons
  B. Formula Weight
  C. Isotopes
  D. Allotropes

IV. **Oxidation and Reduction**
  A. Oxidation Number
  B. Oxidizing and Reducing Agents

V. **Balancing Equations**
  A. Double Displacement Reactions
  B. Acid-Base Reactions
  C. Oxidation-Reduction Reactions

VI. **Solutions**
  A. Electrolytes/Nonelectrolytes
  B. Expressions of Concentration
     1. Molarity
     2. Molality
     3. Percent composition
     4. Mole fraction
  C. Dilutions of Solutions
  D. Colligative Properties
     1. Freezing point depression
     2. Boiling point elevation
     3. Vapor pressure
     4. Osmotic pressure
  E. Solubility Rules

VII. **Gases**
  A. Kinetic Molecular Theory
  B. Gas Laws
     1. Boyle's law
     2. Charles's law
     3. Ideal gas law
     4. Dalton's law of partial pressures
  C. Effusion and Diffusion

VIII. **Bonding and Intermolecular Forces**
  A. Ionic
  B. Covalent
     1. Nonpolar
     2. Polar

C. Intermolecular Forces
   1. London forces (dispersion)
   2. Dipole-dipole
   3. Hydrogen bonds
   4. Ion-dipole forces

IX. **Stoichiometry and Equations**
   A. Molar Relationships
   B. Volume Relationships
   C. Limiting Reactant
   D. Percent Yield

X. **Nomenclature and Formulas of Compounds**

XI. **Molecular Geometry**
   A. Lewis Dot Structure
   B. Valence Shell Repulsion Theory
   C. Bond Angles
   D. Hybrid Orbitals
   E. Molecular Polarity

XII. **Resonance**

XIII. **Electromagnetic Spectrum**
   A. Quantum Theory and Quantum Numbers
   B. Electron Configuration and Orbital Diagram

XIV. **Calorimetry**
   A. Specific Heat
   B. Heat Capacity
   C. Hess's Law

XV. **Acids and Bases**
   A. Arrhenius, Brønsted-Lowry, Lewis Definitions
   B. Strong and Weak Acids and Bases
   C. pH
   D. Buffers
   E. Acidic and Basic Oxides

XVI. **Kinetics**
   A. First-order Reactions
   B. Second-order Reactions
   C. Half-life

XVII. **Equilibrium**
   A. Equilibrium Constant
      1. Acid
      2. Base
      3. Solubility product
      4. Complex ion formation
   B. Le Châtelier's Principle

XVIII. **Electrochemistry**
   A. Electrolytic and Galvanic Cells
   B. Oxidation and Reduction Half Reactions

XIX. **Radioactivity**
   A. Alpha, Beta, and Gamma
   B. Balancing Equations
   C. Fission and Fusion

ORGANIC CHEMISTRY REVIEW OUTLINE

I. **Functional Groups**
   A. Structures
   B. Nomenclature of Families
      1. Alkanes, alkyl halides, alkenes, alkynes
      2. Alcohols
      3. Arenes
      4. Aldehydes and ketones
      5. Carboxylic acids, esters, amides
   C. Hybridization of Carbon
      1. Types: sp^3, sp^2, sp
      2. Geometries

II. **Isomerism**
   A. Constitutional
   B. Stereoisomers
      1. Enantiomers (R/S)
      2. Diastereomers (E/Z and others)
      3. Meso forms

III. **Simple Reactions: Reagents and Mechanisms**
   A. Addition
      1. Electrophilic addition to alkenes/alkynes
      2. Nucleophilic addition to carbonyl compounds
   B. Substitution
      1. Electrophilic substitution of arenes
      2. Nucleophilic substitution of alkyl halides (S_N2 and S_N1) and carboxylic acid derivatives
      3. Alpha substitution of carbonyl compounds

C. Oxidation
   1. Oxidative cleavage of alkenes/alkynes
   2. Oxidation of alcohols and aldehydes
D. Reduction
   1. Catalytic hydrogenation of alkenes/alkynes
   2. Hydride reduction of carbonyl compounds
E. Elimination (E2 and E1)
F. Condensations of Carbonyl Compounds
   1. Aldol
   2. Claisen
   3. Michael

IV. **Resonance**
   A. Benzene
   B. Cations
   C. Anions
   D. Radicals

V. **Spectroscopy**
   A. Infrared (IR)
      1. Quadrants of spectrum and functional groups indicated
      2. Interpretation
   B. ^1H Nuclear Magnetic Resonance (NMR)
      1. Information regarding kinds of hydrogens, relative quantity of each kind, neighbors, environment
      2. Interpretation

BIOCHEMISTRY REVIEW OUTLINE

I. **Nucleic Acids (DNA, RNA)**
   A. Structures
      1. Ribonucleotides, deoxyribonucleotides
      2. Polymerization of nucleotides
      3. Parallel and antiparallel
      4. Hydrogen bonding between nitrogenous bases
   B. Processes
      1. Transcription
      2. Translation
      3. Replication

II. **Lipids**
   A. Structures
      1. Fatty acids and triglycerides
      2. Phosphoglycerides
      3. Prostaglandins
      4. Steroids

B. Processes
1. Storage of fatty acids
2. Energy production via beta-oxidation
3. Membrane formation

III. Proteins
A. Structure
1. Amino acid names and structures
2. Peptide bond
3. Levels of protein structure
B. Processes
1. Conformations and biological activity
2. Translation
3. Degradation and excretion

IV. Carbohydrates
A. Structure
1. Monosaccharides
   a. Fischer projections
   b. Haworth projections
2. Di- and polysaccharides
   a. Glycosidic bonds
   b. Reducing/nonreducing
B. Processes
1. Glycolysis
2. Citric acid cycle
3. Oxidative phosphorylation

ANSWER SHEET
Chemical Processes

1. Ⓐ Ⓑ Ⓒ Ⓓ	26. Ⓐ Ⓑ Ⓒ Ⓓ	51. Ⓐ Ⓑ Ⓒ Ⓓ	76. Ⓐ Ⓑ Ⓒ Ⓓ
2. Ⓐ Ⓑ Ⓒ Ⓓ	27. Ⓐ Ⓑ Ⓒ Ⓓ	52. Ⓐ Ⓑ Ⓒ Ⓓ	77. Ⓐ Ⓑ Ⓒ Ⓓ
3. Ⓐ Ⓑ Ⓒ Ⓓ	28. Ⓐ Ⓑ Ⓒ Ⓓ	53. Ⓐ Ⓑ Ⓒ Ⓓ	78. Ⓐ Ⓑ Ⓒ Ⓓ
4. Ⓐ Ⓑ Ⓒ Ⓓ	29. Ⓐ Ⓑ Ⓒ Ⓓ	54. Ⓐ Ⓑ Ⓒ Ⓓ	79. Ⓐ Ⓑ Ⓒ Ⓓ
5. Ⓐ Ⓑ Ⓒ Ⓓ	30. Ⓐ Ⓑ Ⓒ Ⓓ	55. Ⓐ Ⓑ Ⓒ Ⓓ	80. Ⓐ Ⓑ Ⓒ Ⓓ
6. Ⓐ Ⓑ Ⓒ Ⓓ	31. Ⓐ Ⓑ Ⓒ Ⓓ	56. Ⓐ Ⓑ Ⓒ Ⓓ	81. Ⓐ Ⓑ Ⓒ Ⓓ
7. Ⓐ Ⓑ Ⓒ Ⓓ	32. Ⓐ Ⓑ Ⓒ Ⓓ	57. Ⓐ Ⓑ Ⓒ Ⓓ	82. Ⓐ Ⓑ Ⓒ Ⓓ
8. Ⓐ Ⓑ Ⓒ Ⓓ	33. Ⓐ Ⓑ Ⓒ Ⓓ	58. Ⓐ Ⓑ Ⓒ Ⓓ	83. Ⓐ Ⓑ Ⓒ Ⓓ
9. Ⓐ Ⓑ Ⓒ Ⓓ	34. Ⓐ Ⓑ Ⓒ Ⓓ	59. Ⓐ Ⓑ Ⓒ Ⓓ	84. Ⓐ Ⓑ Ⓒ Ⓓ
10. Ⓐ Ⓑ Ⓒ Ⓓ	35. Ⓐ Ⓑ Ⓒ Ⓓ	60. Ⓐ Ⓑ Ⓒ Ⓓ	85. Ⓐ Ⓑ Ⓒ Ⓓ
11. Ⓐ Ⓑ Ⓒ Ⓓ	36. Ⓐ Ⓑ Ⓒ Ⓓ	61. Ⓐ Ⓑ Ⓒ Ⓓ	86. Ⓐ Ⓑ Ⓒ Ⓓ
12. Ⓐ Ⓑ Ⓒ Ⓓ	37. Ⓐ Ⓑ Ⓒ Ⓓ	62. Ⓐ Ⓑ Ⓒ Ⓓ	87. Ⓐ Ⓑ Ⓒ Ⓓ
13. Ⓐ Ⓑ Ⓒ Ⓓ	38. Ⓐ Ⓑ Ⓒ Ⓓ	63. Ⓐ Ⓑ Ⓒ Ⓓ	88. Ⓐ Ⓑ Ⓒ Ⓓ
14. Ⓐ Ⓑ Ⓒ Ⓓ	39. Ⓐ Ⓑ Ⓒ Ⓓ	64. Ⓐ Ⓑ Ⓒ Ⓓ	89. Ⓐ Ⓑ Ⓒ Ⓓ
15. Ⓐ Ⓑ Ⓒ Ⓓ	40. Ⓐ Ⓑ Ⓒ Ⓓ	65. Ⓐ Ⓑ Ⓒ Ⓓ	90. Ⓐ Ⓑ Ⓒ Ⓓ
16. Ⓐ Ⓑ Ⓒ Ⓓ	41. Ⓐ Ⓑ Ⓒ Ⓓ	66. Ⓐ Ⓑ Ⓒ Ⓓ	91. Ⓐ Ⓑ Ⓒ Ⓓ
17. Ⓐ Ⓑ Ⓒ Ⓓ	42. Ⓐ Ⓑ Ⓒ Ⓓ	67. Ⓐ Ⓑ Ⓒ Ⓓ	92. Ⓐ Ⓑ Ⓒ Ⓓ
18. Ⓐ Ⓑ Ⓒ Ⓓ	43. Ⓐ Ⓑ Ⓒ Ⓓ	68. Ⓐ Ⓑ Ⓒ Ⓓ	93. Ⓐ Ⓑ Ⓒ Ⓓ
19. Ⓐ Ⓑ Ⓒ Ⓓ	44. Ⓐ Ⓑ Ⓒ Ⓓ	69. Ⓐ Ⓑ Ⓒ Ⓓ	94. Ⓐ Ⓑ Ⓒ Ⓓ
20. Ⓐ Ⓑ Ⓒ Ⓓ	45. Ⓐ Ⓑ Ⓒ Ⓓ	70. Ⓐ Ⓑ Ⓒ Ⓓ	95. Ⓐ Ⓑ Ⓒ Ⓓ
21. Ⓐ Ⓑ Ⓒ Ⓓ	46. Ⓐ Ⓑ Ⓒ Ⓓ	71. Ⓐ Ⓑ Ⓒ Ⓓ	96. Ⓐ Ⓑ Ⓒ Ⓓ
22. Ⓐ Ⓑ Ⓒ Ⓓ	47. Ⓐ Ⓑ Ⓒ Ⓓ	72. Ⓐ Ⓑ Ⓒ Ⓓ	97. Ⓐ Ⓑ Ⓒ Ⓓ
23. Ⓐ Ⓑ Ⓒ Ⓓ	48. Ⓐ Ⓑ Ⓒ Ⓓ	73. Ⓐ Ⓑ Ⓒ Ⓓ	98. Ⓐ Ⓑ Ⓒ Ⓓ
24. Ⓐ Ⓑ Ⓒ Ⓓ	49. Ⓐ Ⓑ Ⓒ Ⓓ	74. Ⓐ Ⓑ Ⓒ Ⓓ	99. Ⓐ Ⓑ Ⓒ Ⓓ
25. Ⓐ Ⓑ Ⓒ Ⓓ	50. Ⓐ Ⓑ Ⓒ Ⓓ	75. Ⓐ Ⓑ Ⓒ Ⓓ	100. Ⓐ Ⓑ Ⓒ Ⓓ

PRACTICE QUESTIONS

100 Questions

The periodic table is provided below, if needed.

H																	He
Li	Be											B	C	N	O	F	Ne
Na	Mg											Al	Si	P	S	Cl	Ar
K	Ca	Sc	Ti	V	Cr	Mn	Fe	Co	Ni	Cu	Zn	Ga	Ge	As	Se	Br	Kr
Rb	Sr	Y	Zr	Nb	Mo	Tc	Ru	Rh	Pd	Ag	Cd	In	Sn	Sb	Te	I	Xe
Cs	Ba	La	Hf	Ta	W	Re	Os	Ir	Pt	Au	Hg	Tl	Pb	Bi	Po	At	Rn
Fr	Ra	Ac	Rf	Ha	Sg	Ns	Hs	Mt									
			Ce	Pr	Nd	Pm	Sm	Eu	Gd	Tb	Dy	Ho	Er	Tm	Yb	Lu	
			Th	Pa	U	Np	Pu	Am	Cm	Bk	Cf	Es	Fm	Md	No	Lr	

Directions: Select the best answer to each of the following questions.

QUESTIONS 1 THROUGH 4 REFER TO THE FOLLOWING PASSAGE:

Proteins are used to catalyze biological reactions. Their three-dimensional shape and function are determined by their amino acid sequence. The polarity of the amino acid side chain affects whether that portion of the protein favorably interacts with water (i.e., it is a hydrophilic side chain) or unfavorably interacts with water (i.e., it is hydrophobic). These interactions will direct the folding of the protein chain causing it to assume a three-dimensional shape that is unique to the sequence of amino acids.

The sequence of amino acids is coded in the nucleotide sequence of the cell's genes, the DNA. However, proteins are not synthesized directly from the DNA genetic sequence. The information in DNA is first used to synthesize RNA. The nucleotide sequence of the RNA is then used to dictate the amino acid sequence in the resultant proteins. Changes in the DNA sequence may result in changes in the amino acid sequence of the protein produced. These amino acid changes may adversely affect the protein's three-dimensional shape and function—particularly if the amino acid changes are in the protein's active site.

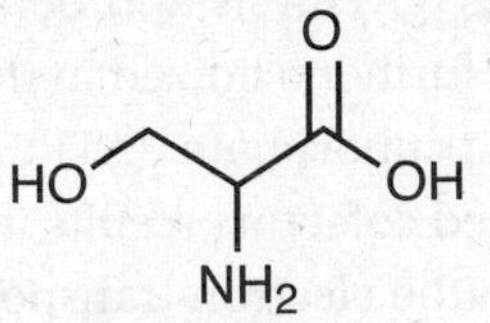

serine
(hydrophilic)

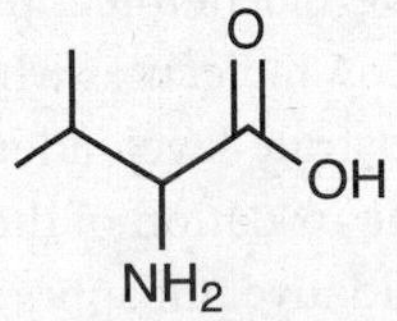

valine
(hydrophobic)

1. The process by which an RNA molecule is synthesized based on the nucleotide sequence in DNA is called

   (A) transcription.
   (B) translation.
   (C) replication.
   (D) respiration.

2. The intermolecular force that holds the two strands of DNA in a helical form is called

   (A) London forces.
   (B) covalent bonding.
   (C) hydrogen bonding.
   (D) dipole-dipole interactions.

3. Which of the following statements is true concerning DNA?

   (A) It contains ribonucleotides.
   (B) It contains adenine, guanine, cytosine, and uracil.
   (C) It exists as a double helix in the cell.
   (D) It is commonly found in the cytoplasm of animal cells.

4. RNA differs from DNA in that it

   (A) cannot base pair.
   (B) doesn't contain phosphate groups.
   (C) is used as the template for DNA synthesis.
   (D) contains uracil rather than thymine found in DNA.

QUESTIONS 5 THROUGH 8 REFER TO THE FOLLOWING PASSAGE:

Organic compounds (carbohydrates, lipids, and proteins) found in food are used as energy sources for cells. They may also be used, along with vitamins found in food, to synthesize cofactors like nicotinamide adenine dinucleotide (NAD^+) and flavin adenine dinucleotide (FAD). FAD is made from riboflavin (vitamin B2) and NAD^+ from niacin.

Different biochemical processes are used to oxidize organic compounds depending on the class of compound. Many of the enzymes in these processes require cofactors to facilitate catalysis. For example, NAD^+ is used as a cofactor in the sixth step of glycolysis in which glyceraldehyde-3-phosphate is oxidized to 1,3-bisphosphoglycerate with the simultaneous reduction of NAD^+ to NADH.

Two of the oxidative biochemical processes, glycolysis and beta oxidation, result in the production of acetyl CoA molecules which are further oxidized in the citric acid cycle (Krebs Cycle) producing substrate-level adenosine triphosphate (ATP) and reduced cofactors, NADH and $FADH_2$. The oxidation of the reduced cofactors results in the production of additional ATP through oxidative phosphorylation (the electron transport chain).

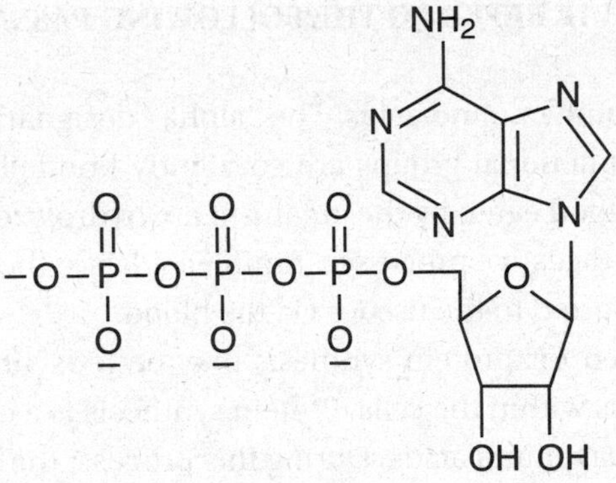

ATP

5. Beta oxidation is a metabolic pathway involving the oxidation of

    (A) polysaccharides.
    (B) nucleic acids.
    (C) fatty acids.
    (D) polypeptides.

6. Which of the following reactions is an oxidation?

    (A) $CH_2=CH_2 \rightarrow CH_3CH_2OH$
    (B) $CH_3CH_3 \rightarrow CH_2=CH_2$
    (C) $CH\equiv CH \rightarrow CH_2BrCH_2Br$
    (D) $CH_2Br-CH_2Br \rightarrow CH_2=CH_2$

7. All of the following are uses of lipids EXCEPT

    (A) hormones.
    (B) energy production.
    (C) cell membrane construction.
    (D) gene composition.

8. Adenosine triphosphate (ATP) is an important source of chemical energy in the cell and is produced

    (A) directly during translation.
    (B) from NADH and $FADH_2$ through oxidative phosphorylation (also known as the electron transport chain).
    (C) in the cell nucleus.
    (D) from DNA.

QUESTIONS 9 THROUGH 12 REFER TO THE FOLLOWING PASSAGE:

Proteins are polymers of alpha amino acids. The "alpha" designation indicates that the carboxylic acid and amine functional groups are covalently bonded to the same carbon, the alpha carbon. Proteins in food eaten by the organism are hydrolyzed to smaller peptides and free amino acids through digestive processes. Amino acids are then absorbed in the gastrointestinal tract and transported to the tissues via the blood.

The amino acids needed for protein synthesis may be biosynthesized or salvaged from the degradation of proteins within the cells. Protein synthesis is a complex process involving nucleic acids and individual amino acids. During this process, the alpha amino group of the one amino acid is condensed with the alpha carboxylic acid of a second amino acid. This condensation continues until the final protein has been synthesized. A shortage of the requisite amino acids can adversely impact protein synthesis and/or the amino acid sequence of resultant proteins.

9. Proteins are composed of twenty amino acids that

 (A) are joined by glycosidic bonds.
 (B) differ in the identity of a group at the alpha carbon.
 (C) are all essential.
 (D) are not water soluble.

10. What reagent is needed for the following conversion?

$$CH_3CH_2CH(CH_3)CH_2OH \rightarrow CH_3CH_2CH(CH_3)CO_2H$$

 (A) $NaBH_4$
 (B) $KMnO_4$
 (C) DMP (Dess-Martin periodinane)
 (D) $LiAlH_4$

11. The infrared spectrum of a substance has a strong absorption at 3300 cm^{-1} and at 1700 cm^{-1}. What functional group is present in the substance?

 (A) Ester
 (B) Alcohol
 (C) Acid
 (D) Aldehyde

12. What is the percentage of hydrogen in the amino acid glycine, $C_2H_5NO_2$?

 (A) <10%
 (B) 10–25%
 (C) 25–50%
 (D) >50%

QUESTIONS 13 THROUGH 16 REFER TO THE FOLLOWING PASSAGE:

Molecular polarity affects solubility. The adage "like dissolves like" describes solubility patterns. Polar molecules are soluble in polar solvents and nonpolar molecules are soluble in nonpolar solvents. For example, when using oil-based paint (nonpolar), turpentine (a nonpolar solvent) is required for cleanup while ethanol (polar) can be washed away with water (polar).

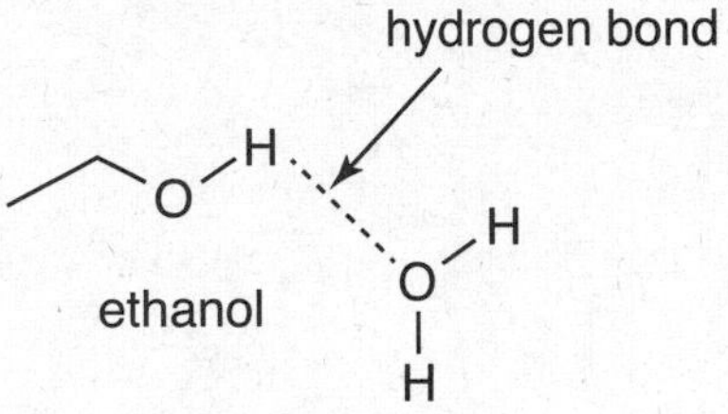

Water is a polar solvent ubiquitous in biological tissues. Polar biological molecules are soluble in water, while nonpolar biological molecules are not. To solubilize nonpolar molecules in an aqueous environment, surfactants are required. Surfactants are molecules with both nonpolar and polar areas, allowing them to solubilize nonpolar molecules as well as interact favorably with water. Biological surfactants include bile acids and lipoproteins. The water solubility of the major classes of biomolecules (proteins, lipids, carbohydrates, and nucleic acids) varies and is governed by the polarity of each.

13. Which of the following molecules is a lipid?

(A)

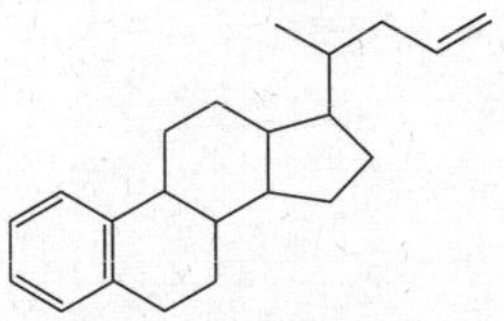

(B)

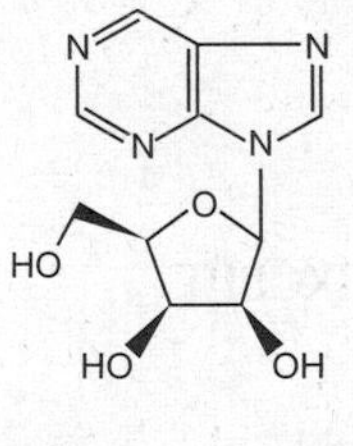

(C)

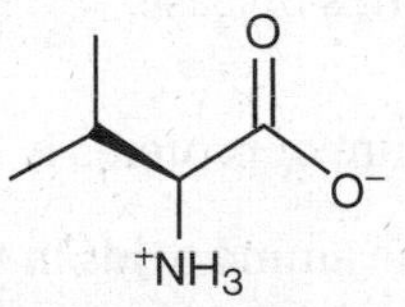

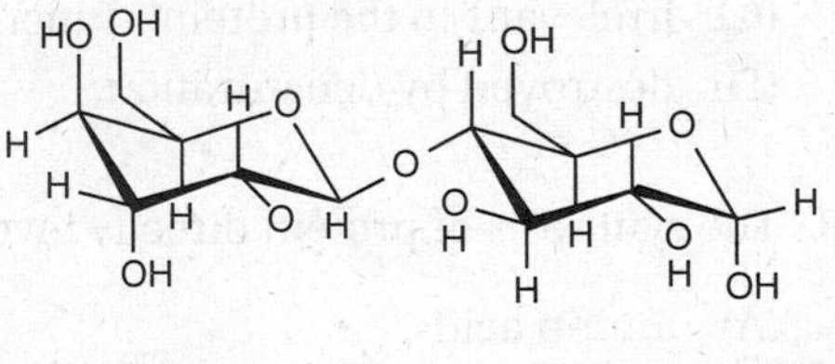

(D)

14. Which of the following is the most polar molecule?

(A) CO_2
(B) Li_2O
(C) CH_4
(D) NH_3

15. Which of the following molecules has a dipole moment of zero?

    (A) CO_2
    (B) H_2O
    (C) HF
    (D) NH_3

16. In which of the following solutions will aluminum hydroxide, $Al(OH)_3$, be the LEAST soluble?

    (A) H_2O
    (B) 0.5 M $Al(NO_3)_3$
    (C) 1.6 M NaOH
    (D) 0.3 M HCl

QUESTIONS 17 THROUGH 19 REFER TO THE FOLLOWING PASSAGE:

Proteins are important biological molecules involved in catalyzing reactions (enzymes) and in providing rigidity/support, among other things. Genetic mutations that result in changes in the primary structure of proteins can be harmful (or fatal) to the cell. For example, in the disorder phenylketonuria (PKU), a mutation in the gene coding for the enzyme phenylalanine hydroxylase results in irreversible mental retardation in newborns if undiagnosed. For this reason, a laboratory test (blood or urine analysis) is performed shortly after birth and dietary adjustments are made if PKU is diagnosed. Such adjustments are effective at preventing the damage associated with this disease.

17. The primary structure of proteins is

    (A) the order of the amino acids in the polymer.
    (B) the result of hydrogen bonding between amino acids.
    (C) irrelevant to the protein's function.
    (D) destroyed by denaturation.

18. The synthesis of protein directly involves all of the following EXCEPT

    (A) amino acids.
    (B) DNA.
    (C) ribosomes.
    (D) RNA.

19. What are the monomeric units of peptides and proteins?

    (A) Amino acids
    (B) Aminoalcohols
    (C) Aminals
    (D) β-hydroxyacids

A variety of laboratory methods are used to separate components of a mixture. Common among those is distillation. Industrially, distillation is used in petroleum refineries to separate the organic components found in crude petroleum. More than 100 operating refineries in the United States purify millions of barrels of crude petroleum each year. Gasoline, a mixture of organic compounds, is a commodity of increasing concern as a result of its cost and the environmental impact of its combustion products. Distillation separates the components of mixtures based on boiling point—the lowest boiling component evaporates at the lowest temperature and its vapor is removed and condensed, thus isolating that component from the mixture. This process continues to isolate the next lowest boiling component, and so on. Due to the low boiling point of gasoline, it will be removed from the crude oil earlier than diesel fuel, as shown in the figure below.

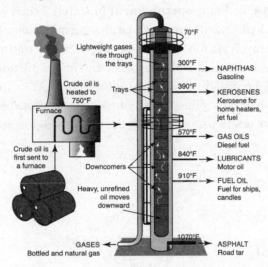

(Graphic courtesy of Bismarck State College
National Energy Center for Excellence)

20. Which of the following compounds would be expected to have the highest boiling point?

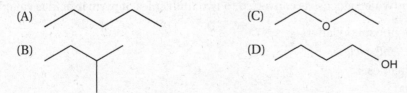

21. Boiling point and water solubility are affected by hydrogen bonding. Which of the following compounds is the most water soluble?

(A) Ethyl ether, $CH_3CH_2OCH_2CH_3$
(B) 1-chlorodecane, $CH_3(CH_2)_8CH_2Cl$
(C) Ethane, CH_3CH_3
(D) Benzene, C_6H_6

22. Which of the following statements is true concerning intermolecular forces?

    (A) Dipole-dipole forces are the strongest type of intermolecular force.
    (B) London forces or dispersion forces occur between all molecules.
    (C) Hydrogen bonding is a type of covalent bond.
    (D) Dipole-dipole forces occur between nonpolar molecules.

QUESTIONS 23 THROUGH 26 REFER TO THE FOLLOWING PASSAGE:

About 50% of the dry biomass on Earth is glucose. Glucose is a carbohydrate that is produced in plants from water and carbon dioxide. This process is called photosynthesis and requires sunlight as an energy source. The glucose molecules are polymerized to make long chains, two of which are amylose and amylopectin found in starch. When animals eat plants, the polymers of glucose are hydrolyzed to release free glucose molecules. After absorption in the digestive tract, glucose travels via the blood to the tissues and is transported into the cells.

Within cells, glucose is oxidized with the concomitant production of energy, stored in the phosphoanhydride bonds in adenosine triphosphate (ATP) molecules. Subsequent hydrolysis of these high-energy phosphoanhydride bonds provides the energy to drive nonspontaneous cellular reactions. In this way, the energy originating from the sun is used by the cell.

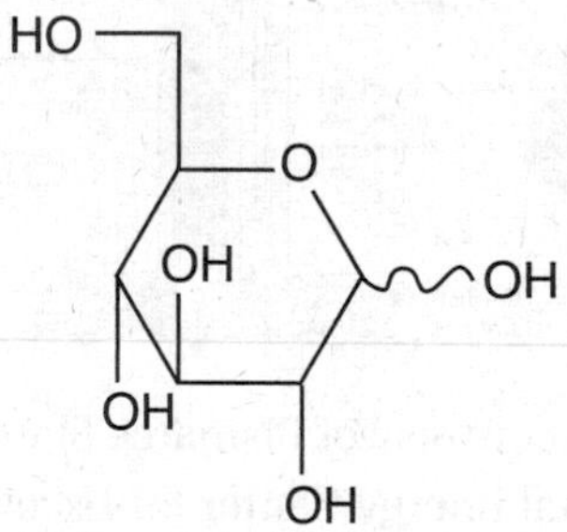

glucose

23. The process by which glucose is converted to two molecules of pyruvic acid is called

    (A) oxidative phosphorylation.
    (B) the citric acid cycle.
    (C) gluconeogenesis.
    (D) glycolysis.

24. The classification of macromolecules as carbohydrates is primarily based on the

    (A) cellular function of the molecule.
    (B) nonpolarity of the molecule.
    (C) presence of alcohol groups and an aldehyde or ketone.
    (D) presence of peptide bonds.

25. What is the molarity of a solution prepared by dissolving 1.8 g of glucose, $C_6H_{12}O_6$, in enough water to make 1000 mL of solution?

   (A) 0.01 M
   (B) 1.80 M
   (C) 0.0018 M
   (D) 0.10 M

26. What is the approximate value of the bond angle in carbon dioxide?

   (A) 105°
   (B) 120°
   (C) 180°
   (D) 90°

_____

QUESTIONS 27 THROUGH 30 REFER TO THE FOLLOWING PASSAGE:

Protein function is intimately linked to the three-dimensional conformation assumed by the protein in aqueous solution. A loss of that conformation ordinarily results in a loss of function. Extreme changes in temperature or pH can cause these changes because the intermolecular forces responsible for the protein's conformation are adversely affected. An important intermolecular force involved is hydrogen bonding. When hydrogen bonding is disrupted, the protein's secondary and tertiary structures are affected. A protein's secondary structure involves hydrogen bonding between the partial negative oxygen of a peptide bond and the hydrogen covalently bonded to the nitrogen of another peptide bond. The tertiary structure involves hydrogen bonding between polar side chains of amino acids and the water molecules within the cell.

27. An example of secondary structure in proteins includes a

   (A) tetramer.
   (B) peptide bond.
   (C) beta sheet.
   (D) double helix.

28. Which of the following theories would describe the covalent bond in water as the overlap of a half-filled 1s orbital with a half-filled sp³ orbital?

   (A) Molecular Orbital Theory
   (B) Valence Shell Electron Pair Repulsion Theory (VSEPR)
   (C) Valence Bond Theory
   (D) Kinetic Molecular Theory

29. Which of the following types of RNA carries amino acids to the ribosome for protein synthesis?

(A) mRNA
(B) rRNA
(C) tRNA
(D) aRNA

30. Amino acids used in translation may come from

(A) biosynthesis reactions.
(B) digestion of dietary fats.
(C) degradation of cellular nucleic acids.
(D) the citric acid cycle.

QUESTIONS 31 THROUGH 35 REFER TO THE FOLLOWING PASSAGE:

Vitamins are organic compounds that are needed in small amounts as part of a healthy diet. A vitamin important in fatty acid metabolism is biotin, also known as vitamin B7 or vitamin H.

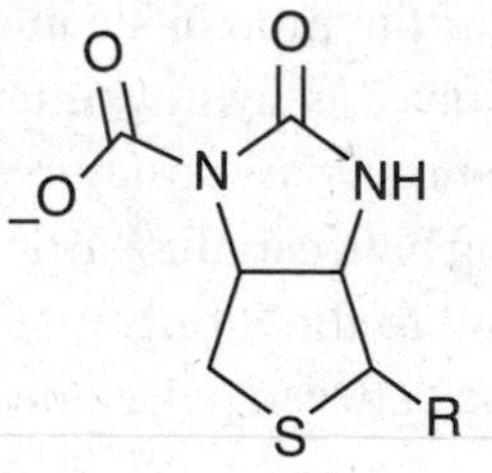

carboxylated biotin

Foods rich in biotin include eggs, avocado, and meats. Physical manifestations of biotin deficiency include dermatitis and alopecia—both of which are related to biotin's role in fatty acid synthesis. Hair follicles and skin cells require fatty acids to function normally.

Fatty acids are long chain carboxylic acids. They are found in foods and synthesized in the liver when amounts of acetyl CoA exceed the requirements for ATP production. ATP is produced with the concomitant oxidation of NADH and $FADH_2$, which results in part from acetyl CoA's entry into the citric acid cycle. Cellular quantities of acetyl CoA in excess of those needed for the citric acid cycle may be used to synthesize fatty acids, the long-term storage of two carbon units. The synthetic pathway begins with the conversion of acetyl CoA to malonyl CoA, a reaction requiring carboxylated biotin as the carboxylate source.

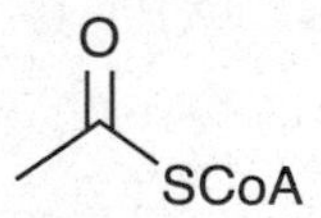

acetyl CoA 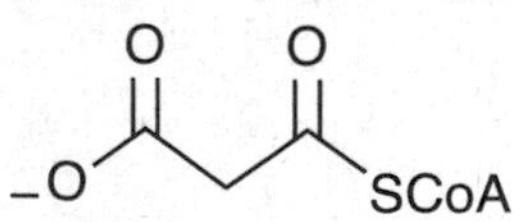   malonyl CoA

The mechanism of the reaction involves the enol form of acetyl CoA acting as a nucleophile on the carbonyl carbon of the carboxylated biotin. After malonyl CoA is formed, since it is a beta-carbonyl carboxylic acid, it is easily decarboxylated to yield a nucleophilic carbon alpha to the thioester, which adds two carbons to the growing fatty acid chain in fatty acid biosynthesis. Thus the biosynthesis of fatty acids yields chains that are an even number of carbons.

31. As stated above, malonyl CoA is able to undergo decarboxylation, activating the alpha carbon of acetyl CoA for the condensation of the two-carbon unit with the growing fatty acid chain. Which of the following statements is true concerning decarboxylation of carboxylic acids?

   (A) Beta-carbonyl carboxylic acids are able to undergo decarboxylation due to the fact that they are more acidic than other types of carboxylic acids.
   (B) Only enzyme catalyzed decarboxylations occur with beta-carbonyl carboxylic acids.
   (C) The beta-carbonyl group allows resonance stabilization of the anion formed following decarboxylation.
   (D) Resonance stabilization of the intermediate carbocation allows for decarboxylation.

32. Acetyl CoA, like all carbonyl compounds, exists in an equilibrium of two forms. This equilibrium is a keto-enol tautomerization. The % enol in a sample of a carbonyl compound can be determined using NMR spectroscopy. Consider the keto-enol tautomerization below.

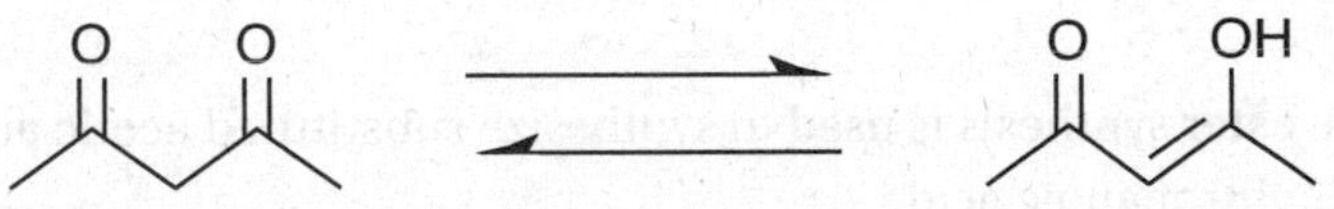

   Integration of the methylene signal and the methine signal allows the calculation of % enol. If the methylene signal integrates for 1 and the methine signal integrates for 4, what is the % enol?

   (A) 90%
   (B) 60%
   (C) 30%
   (D) 10%

33. Thioesters like acetyl CoA have a higher enol content than esters like methyl acetate.

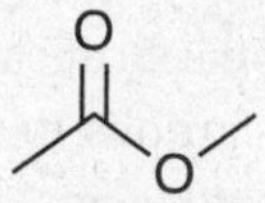

methyl acetate

Which of the following statements is true concerning enol content of these functional groups?

(A) The enol content of a carboxylic acid derivative is dependent on the steric bulk of the alcohol side of the ester or the thioester.

(B) The enol content of a carboxylic acid derivative is dependent on the partial positive charge on the carbonyl carbon with a smaller partial positive charge correlating to increased enol content.

(C) Thioesters have higher enol content because sulfur is more electronegative than oxygen.

(D) Thioesters have higher enol content because the electron donation of sulfur through resonance is less than that of oxygen.

34. Fatty acids are synthesized to store excess acetyl units. Which of the following lipids are the primary storage form of fatty acids?

(A) Steroids
(B) Triacylglycerols
(C) Waxes
(D) Prostaglandins

35. The malonic ester synthesis is used to synthesize substituted acetic acid derivatives such as methylpropanoic acid.

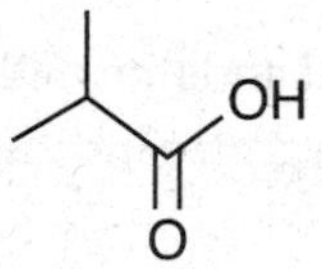

methylpropanoic acid

Which of the following synthetic procedures would yield methylpropanoic acid from diethyl malonate?

(A) Ethoxide followed by 2-bromopropane followed by acid catalyzed hydrolysis with heat.

(B) Ethoxide followed by methyl iodide followed by ester hydrolysis.

(C) Ethyl bromide followed by ethoxide followed by acid catalyzed hydrolysis with heat.

(D) Ethoxide followed by methyl iodide followed by ethoxide followed by methyl iodide followed by acid catalyzed hydrolysis with heat.

QUESTIONS 36 THROUGH 38 REFER TO THE FOLLOWING PASSAGE:

The element sulfur is commonly found in the proteins of living things. In fact, it is the formation of disulfide bonds in proinsulin that results in the active form of the hormone insulin (see the figure below). Because of its position in the periodic table, it is not a surprise that many of sulfur's properties are similar to those of oxygen. Unlike oxygen, sulfur's valence shell (the third shell) has available d orbitals so it can exceed the "octet rule" in Lewis structures. The ease with which sulfur is oxidized (as in the formation of the disulfide bonds in insulin) is related to sulfur's increased size, relative to oxygen. Common polyatomic ions containing sulfur are sulfate (SO_4^{2-}) and sulfite (SO_3^{2-}).

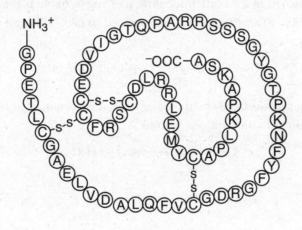

36. What is the reducing agent in the following equation?

$$Zn + CuSO_4 \longrightarrow ZnSO_4 + Cu$$

   (A) Zn
   (B) $CuSO_4$
   (C) $ZnSO_4$
   (D) Cu

37. How many liters of oxygen gas, O_2, will react completely with 3.5 liters of carbon disulfide gas, CS_2, in the following reaction?

$$CS_2 + 3O_2 \longrightarrow CO_2 + 2SO_2$$

   (A) 14.0
   (B) 3.5
   (C) 10.5
   (D) 1.8

38. The electron configuration for the sulfide ion, S^{2-}, is

   (A) $1s^2 2s^2 2p^6 3s^2 3p^6$.
   (B) $1s^2 2s^2 2p^6 3s^2 3p^4$.
   (C) $1s^2 2s^2 2p^6 3s^2 3p^2$.
   (D) $1s^2 2s^2 2p^6 3s^2 3p^6 4s^2$.

QUESTIONS 39 THROUGH 42 REFER TO THE FOLLOWING PASSAGE:

Nitrogen oxides (NOx) are compounds containing the elements nitrogen and oxygen. They are produced in a number of industrial processes. The Environmental Protection Agency regulates the emission of these compounds because they can precipitate respiratory symptoms in humans and are implicated in the production of acid rain. Acid rain occurs when these compounds (or other compounds containing sulfur and oxygen) combine with water in the atmosphere.

An industrial process involving the production of NOx is the Ostwald process. This process is used to produce nitric acid through a series of reactions beginning with the gases, ammonia and oxygen. As shown in the equation below, a nitrogen oxide is the product of the first step in the process. The NO formed is further oxidized to NO_2 followed by its reaction with water to form HNO_3.

$$4NH_3(g) + 5O_2(g) \dashrightarrow 4NO(g) + 6H_2O(g)$$

39. In the following reaction, how many moles of O_2 are necessary to react with 5 moles of NH_3? (O = 16 amu, N = 14 amu, H = 1 amu)

$$4NH_3 + 5O_2 \longrightarrow 4NO + 6H_2O$$

(A) 4.0
(B) 5.0
(C) 5.5
(D) 6.3

40. In the following reaction, how many grams of H_2O are produced from 17.0 g of NH_3? (O = 16 amu, N = 14 amu, H = 1 amu)

$$4NH_3 + 5O_2 \longrightarrow 4NO + 6H_2O$$

(A) 1.5
(B) 18
(C) 27
(D) 2.4

41. In the following reaction, how many liters of NO are produced from 1.70 g of NH_3 at standard temperature and pressure conditions? (O = 16 amu, N = 14 amu, H = 1 amu)

$$4NH_3 + 5O_2 \longrightarrow 4NO + 6H_2O$$

(A) 2.24
(B) 1.70
(C) 8.96
(D) 0.026

42. In the following reaction, how many molecules of NO are produced from 0.17 g of NH_3? ($O = 16$ amu, $N = 14$ amu, $H = 1$ amu)

$$4NH_3 + 5O_2 \longrightarrow 4NO + 6H_2O$$

(A) 6.0×10^{21}
(B) 1.4×10^{22}
(C) 4.0×10^{23}
(D) 2.9×10^{23}

QUESTIONS 43 THROUGH 46 REFER TO THE FOLLOWING PASSAGE:

Early in the 20th century, Brønsted and Lowry described acid-base reactions as those involving the exchange of a proton. An acid was defined as a proton donor, and a base was defined as a proton acceptor. The magnitude of the equilibrium constant for proton donation (Ka) is used as a measure of acid strength. Tabulation of these equilibrium constants is facilitated by converting them to pKas by the following equation:

$$pKa = -\log Ka$$

Similarly, Kb and pKb tables are used to compare bases. Acids and bases affect the pH of solutions by raising or lowering the proton concentration.

43. If the value of Ka for an acid, HY, is 3.7×10^{-4}, what is the value of Kb for the conjugate base, Y^-?

(A) 2.7×10^{-11}
(B) 2.5×10^{-10}
(C) 4.0×10^{-8}
(D) 6.3×10^{-6}

44. Which of the following acids is the strongest?

(A) Para-toluic acid, $Ka = 5.0 \times 10^{-5}$
(B) Acetic acid, $Ka = 1.8 \times 10^{-4}$
(C) Para-nitrobenzoic acid, $Ka = 4.0 \times 10^{-4}$
(D) Formic acid, $Ka = 1.7 \times 10^{-4}$

45. What is the pH of a solution with a hydroxide ion concentration of 0.001 M?

(A) 3
(B) 1
(C) 11
(D) 13

46. What is the hydroxide ion concentration in a solution that is 3.0 M $Mg(OH)_2$?

    (A) 3.0 M

    (B) 1.5 M

    (C) 6.0 M

    (D) 4.5 M

---

47. Calculate the formula weight, in atomic mass units (amu), of ammonium nitrate.

    (A) 80

    (B) 45

    (C) 66

    (D) 98

48. The mass of 1 mole of magnesium atoms equals 24.3 grams. What is the weight, in grams, of one atom of Mg?

(Avogadro's number $= 6 \times 10^{23}$)

    (A) 4×10^{-23}

    (B) 2.5×10^{22}

    (C) 1.5×10^{-21}

    (D) 4×10^{-22}

49. How many neutrons are contained in the following atom of the element germanium, ^{74}Ge?

    (A) 40

    (B) 32

    (C) 74

    (D) 42

50. Which of the following is NOT a nuclear reaction?

    (A) A sodium atom becomes a sodium ion.

    (B) A uranium atom becomes a barium atom and a krypton atom.

    (C) A thorium atom releases a gamma particle.

    (D) An iodine atom becomes a different isotope of iodine.

51. If the volume of a sample of gas at 1 atm and 25°C is reduced and the temperature remains constant, then

    (A) the pressure will decrease.

    (B) the gas particles will slow down.

    (C) Boyle's law will be demonstrated.

    (D) Charles's law will be demonstrated.

52. Which of the following statements describes a physical property?

   (A) Liquid water is converted to water vapor by the application of heat.
   (B) Gasoline combusts in the presence of O_2.
   (C) Ozone is formed from O_2 during lightning strikes.
   (D) Milk sours more readily at room temperature than in the refrigerator.

53. When the following equation is balanced with the smallest set of whole numbers, what is the coefficient of CO_2?

   $$\_\_Na_2CO_3 + \_\_H_2SO_4 \longrightarrow \_\_NaHSO_4 + \_\_H_2O + \_\_CO_2$$

   (A) 1
   (B) 2
   (C) 3
   (D) 5

54. A 100-milliliter sample of oxygen, O_2, is collected over water at 25°C and 750 mm Hg pressure. The pressure of water vapor at 25°C is 23.76 mm Hg. Which of the following equations is correct to calculate the number of grams of oxygen collected? (R = 0.082 L-atm/K-mole)

   (A) $750 \text{ mm}(100 \text{ mL}) = \dfrac{x}{16 \text{ g/mole}}\left(\dfrac{0.082 \text{ L-atm}}{\text{K-mole}}\right)(25°C)$

   (B) $\dfrac{726.24 \text{ mm}(0.100 \text{ liter})}{760 \text{ mm/atm}} = \dfrac{16 \text{ g/mole}}{x}\left(\dfrac{0.082 \text{ L-atm}}{\text{K-mole}}\right)(25°C)$

   (C) $\dfrac{750 \text{ mm}(100 \text{ mL})}{760 \text{ mm/atm}} = \dfrac{x}{32 \text{ g/mole}}\left(\dfrac{0.082 \text{ L-atm}}{\text{K-mole}}\right)(298K)$

   (D) $\dfrac{726.24 \text{ mm}(0.100 \text{ liter})}{760 \text{ mm/atm}} = \dfrac{x}{32 \text{ g/mole}}\left(\dfrac{0.082 \text{ L-atm}}{\text{K-mole}}\right)(298K)$

55. How many grams of nitrogen gas, N_2, are present in a bulb of volume 1.0 liter, at 27°C and 1 atmosphere? (R = 0.082 liter-atm/K-mole, N = 14 amu)

   (A) 7.9×10^{-2}
   (B) 1.0×10^5
   (C) 1.1
   (D) 8.4×10^{-3}

56. How many milliliters of 5.0 M, sodium hydroxide, NaOH, solution must be used to prepare 500 milliliters of 2.5 M solution?

   (A) 1,000
   (B) 750
   (C) 250
   (D) 150

57. How many milliliters of 2.5 M lithium hydroxide, LiOH, solution are necessary to neutralize 10 milliliters of 2.0 M sulfuric acid, H_2SO_4, according to the following equation?

$$2LiOH + H_2SO_4 \longrightarrow Li_2SO_4 + 2H_2O$$

(A) 60
(B) 30
(C) 15
(D) 16

58. A bubble of gas (1.4 mL) is at the bottom of a lake where the temperature and pressure are 7°C and 2.0 atmospheres, respectively. The temperature and pressure at the surface of the lake are 27°C and 1.0 atmosphere. What is the volume, in milliliters, of a gas bubble at the surface of the lake?

(A) 2.6
(B) 3.0
(C) 0.75
(D) 0.65

59. Specify the absolute configuration of each chiral center in:

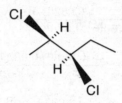

(A) 2R
(B) 2S
(C) 2R, 3R
(D) 2S, 3S

60. The specific heat of copper, Cu, is 0.385 joule per gram °C. What is the heat capacity, in joules per °C, of 10.0 grams of copper?

(A) 0.03
(B) 15.4
(C) 3.85
(D) 38.9

61. Radium undergoes beta decay producing what element?

$$^{228}_{88}Ra \longrightarrow ^{0}_{-1}e + ?$$

(A) Fr
(B) Rn
(C) Ac
(D) Ra

62. Which species below has the valence shell electron configuration $2s^2 2p^6$?

  (A) Be^{2+}
  (B) F^-
  (C) C
  (D) Ar

63. How many unshared electrons are on the sulfur atom in the Lewis dot structure for SF_6?

  (A) 5
  (B) 2
  (C) 0
  (D) 8

64. What is the formal charge on the nitrogen atom in the nitrate ion, NO_3^-?

  (A) 0
  (B) +1
  (C) −1
  (D) −3

65. What is the molecular geometry of the nitrogen trifluoride, NF_3, molecule?

  (A) Linear
  (B) Bent
  (C) Triangular planar
  (D) Trigonal pyramidal

66. What is the hybridization state of the boron atom in BF_3?

  (A) sp
  (B) sp^2
  (C) sp^3
  (D) $sp^3 d^2$

67. What is the product of the following reaction?

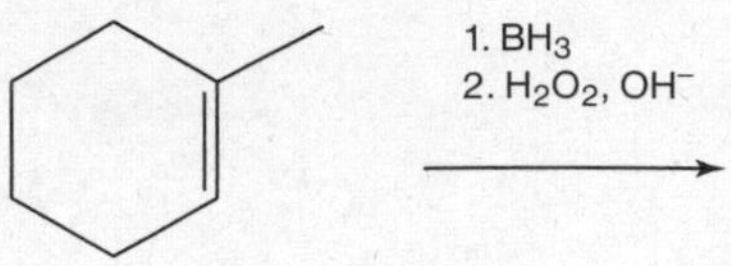

(A)

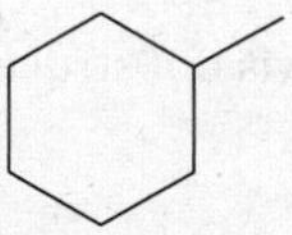

(C)

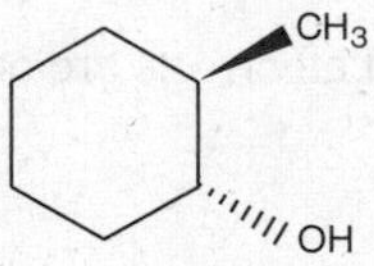

(B)

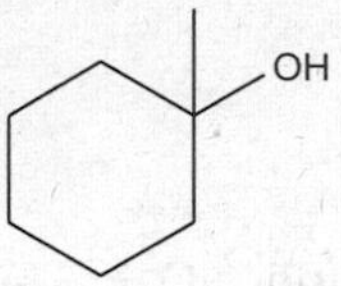

(D)

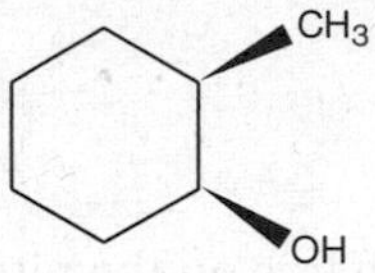

68. In the process of replication,

(A) the DNA duplex does not melt (unwind).
(B) the two resulting DNA molecules are identical.
(C) both new DNA molecules are synthesized discontinuously.
(D) the raw material nucleotides are carried by tRNA.

69. Which of the following sets of quantum numbers is possible?

(A) $n = 2, \ell = 0, m_\ell = 0, m_s = +\dfrac{1}{2}$

(B) $n = 1, \ell = 1, m_\ell = 0, m_s = -\dfrac{1}{2}$

(C) $n = 3, \ell = -2, m_\ell = -1, m_s = +\dfrac{1}{2}$

(D) $n = 2, \ell = 1, m_\ell = 1, m_s = -1$

70. What reagent would accomplish the following conversion?

$$CH_3CH_2CHO \rightarrow CH_3CH_2CH_2OH$$

(A) PCC (pyridinium chlorochromate)
(B) $NaBH_4$
(C) H_2
(D) $KMnO_4$

71. What is a product of the following reaction?

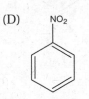

Br₂, FeBr₃

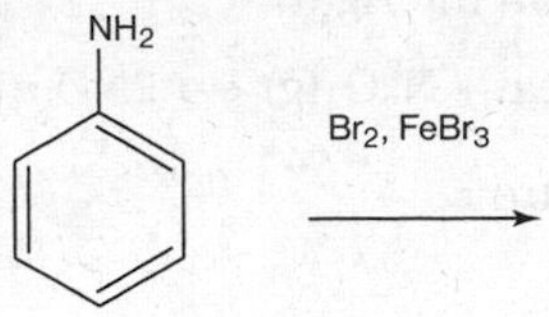

(A)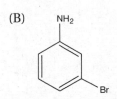

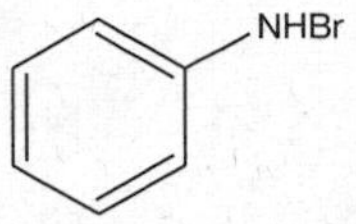

(C)

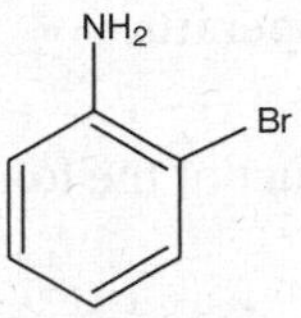

(B)

(D)

72. The major kind of lipid found in food is

(A) triglycerides.
(B) phospholipids.
(C) waxes.
(D) starch.

73. What is the half-life, in seconds, for a first-order reaction having a rate constant of 6.93×10^2 per second?

(A) $1.0 \times 10^{+1}$
(B) 1.0×10^{-3}
(C) 1.0×10^{-1}
(D) $1.0 \times 10^{+5}$

74. What functional group is formed by the following reaction?

$$CH_3OH + (CH_3)_2CHCOBr \longrightarrow$$

(A) Ester
(B) Acid
(C) Acid anhydride
(D) Ketone

75. What is the equilibrium constant for the following reaction when $[H_2] = 0.25$ M, $[I_2] = 0.25$ M, and $[HI] = 0.50$ M?

$$H_2 + I_2 \longleftrightarrow 2HI$$

(A) 4.0
(B) 0.25
(C) 8.0
(D) 0.13

76. Which of the following changes will NOT cause the reaction equilibrium shown below to shift toward the products on the right?

$$Heat + N_2O_4(g) \leftrightarrow 2NO_2(g)$$

(A) A decrease in temperature
(B) Addition of more N_2O_4
(C) Removal of some NO_2
(D) An increase in temperature

77. What is the major product of the following elimination?

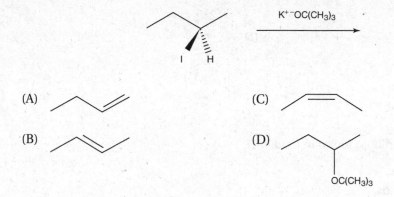

(A)

(C)

(B)

(D)

78. What kind of condensation reaction is demonstrated by the following reaction under basic conditions?

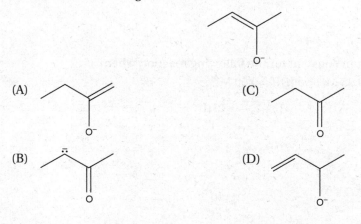

(A) Claisen
(B) Williamson
(C) Michael
(D) Aldol

79. Which of the following is a resonance structure of

(A)

(C)

(B)

(D)

80. Which statement describes triglycerides?

 (A) They are stored in smooth muscle.
 (B) Acid catalyzed hydrolysis yields soap.
 (C) They are triesters of glycerol.
 (D) Their long carbon chains are used to generate ATP via gluconeogenesis.

81. Which of the following statements is true concerning the acid-base reaction below?

$$NH_3 + H_2O \rightarrow NH_4^+ + OH^-$$

 (A) The equilibrium lies far to the left.
 (B) Water is acting as a base.
 (C) Ammonium is the conjugate base of ammonia.
 (D) Hydroxide is the conjugate acid of water.

82. Which structure for a compound with the formula $C_9H_{10}O$ is consistent with the following ^1H NMR data?

 δ 1.4 ppm, triplet, 3H
 δ 4.1 ppm, quartet, 2H
 δ 7.0 ppm, doublet, 2H
 δ 7.8 ppm, doublet, 2H
 δ 9.8 ppm, singlet, 1H

 (A) CHO

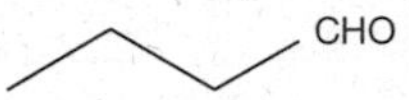

 (C) CHO

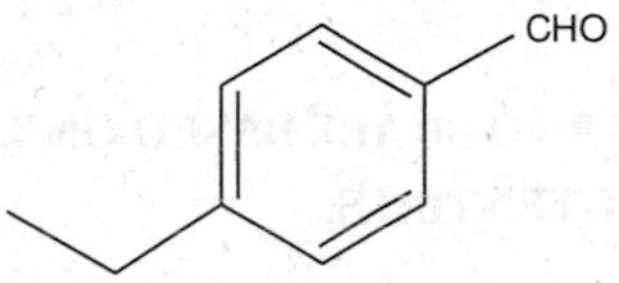

 (B) CH2OH

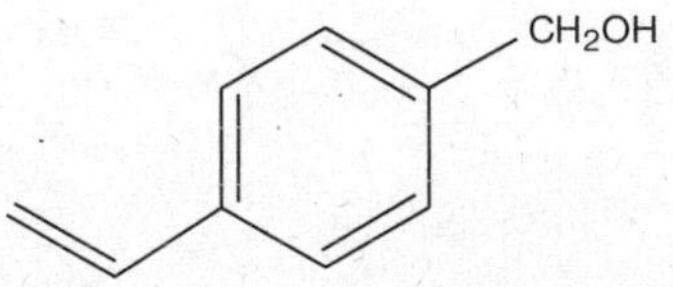

 (D) CHO

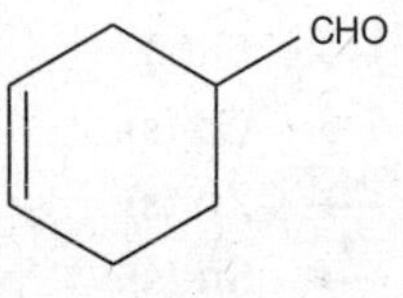

83. Which is a product of the following reaction?

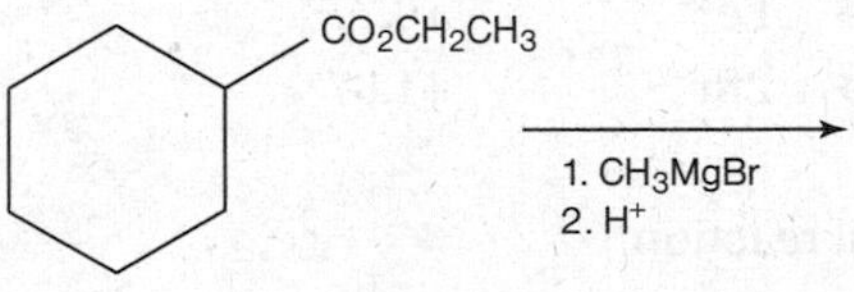

CO2CH2CH3

1. CH3MgBr
2. H⁺

 (A) OH

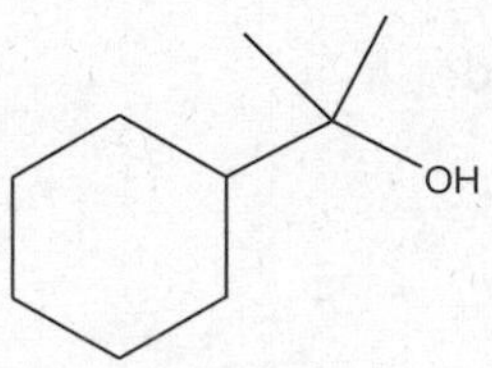

 (C) OH

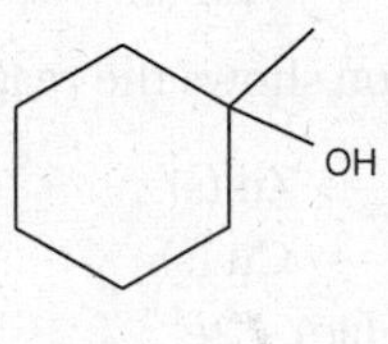

 (B) OH

 (D) OH

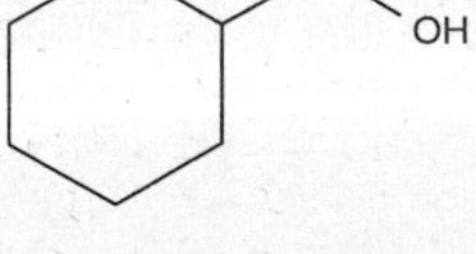

84. Which of the following compounds is insoluble in water?

(A) NaOH

(B) NH_4Cl

(C) $LiNO_3$

(D) $CaCO_3$

85. Which of the following slightly soluble salts is the most soluble?
(The solubility product constants are given.)

		K_{sp}
(A)	Copper (II) sulfide	6.0×10^{-37}
(B)	Nickel (II) sulfide	1.4×10^{-24}
(C)	Silver chloride	1.6×10^{-10}
(D)	Lead (II) chromate	2.0×10^{-14}

86. Which of the following complex ions is the most stable? (The formation constants, K_f, are given.)

		K_f
(A)	$Ag(NH_3)_2^{+1}$	1.5×10^7
(B)	$Zn(NH_3)_4^{2+}$	2.0×10^9
(C)	HgI_4^{2-}	2.0×10^{30}
(D)	$Cd(CN)_4^{2-}$	7.1×10^{16}

QUESTIONS 87 AND 88 ARE BASED ON THE FOLLOWING TABLE OF STANDARD REDUCTION POTENTIALS:

						emf°
Li^+	(aq)	+	e^-	$\longrightarrow$	Li (s)	-3.05
Ca^{2+}	(aq)	+	$2e^-$	$\longrightarrow$	Ca (s)	-2.87
Zn^{2+}	(aq)	+	$2e^-$	$\longrightarrow$	Zn (s)	-0.76
Sn^{+2}	(aq)	+	$2e^-$	$\longrightarrow$	Sn (s)	-0.14
$2H^+$	(aq)	+	$2e^-$	$\longrightarrow$	H_2 (g)	0.00
Cu^{2+}	(aq)	+	$2e^-$	$\longrightarrow$	Cu (s)	$+0.34$
Fe^{3+}	(aq)	+	e^-	$\longrightarrow$	Fe^{2+}	$+0.77$
Br_2	(ℓ)	+	$2e^-$	$\longrightarrow$	$2Br^{-1}$	$+1.07$

87. In the following overall reaction:

$$Zn\ (s) + Cu^{2+} \longrightarrow Zn^{2+} + Cu\ (s)$$

which partial reaction shows the reagent that is oxidized?

(A) $Zn^{2+}\ (aq) + 2e^- \longrightarrow Zn\ (s)$

(B) $Cu^{2+}\ (aq) + 2e^- \longrightarrow Cu\ (s)$

(C) $Zn\ (s) \longrightarrow Zn^{2+}\ (aq) + 2e^-$

(D) $Cu\ (s) \longrightarrow Cu^{2+}\ (aq) + 2e^-$

88. Which of the following species is the strongest reducing agent?

(A) Li^+

(B) Br_2

(C) Br^{-1}

(D) Li

---

89. Which of the following statements describes the reaction which occurs at the cathode in an electrochemical cell?

(A) The cathode is the electrode at which electrons are lost and oxidation occurs.

(B) The cathode is the electrode at which electrons are lost and reduction occurs.

(C) The cathode is the electrode at which electrons are gained and oxidation occurs.

(D) The cathode is the electrode at which electrons are gained and reduction occurs.

90. Which of the following groups is expected to have the greatest 1,3-diaxial energy in a monosubstituted cyclohexane?

(A) Methyl

(B) Hydrogen

(C) Isopropyl

(D) Fluorine

91. How many different structural isomers can be formed by the compound having the molecular formula C_4H_9Cl?

(A) 1

(B) 2

(C) 3

(D) 4

92. How many different compounds (ignoring stereoisomers) can be formed by the monochlorination of propane?

(A) 1

(B) 2

(C) 3

(D) 4

93. What is the name of the following compound?

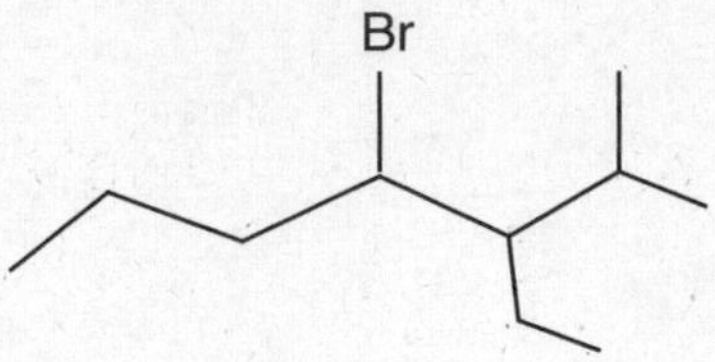

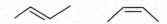

(A) 4-bromo-3-ethyl-2-methylheptane
(B) 4-bromo-3-isopropylheptane
(C) 4-bromo-5-isopropylheptane
(D) 4-bromodecane

94. A stereocenter is one that

(A) is attached to four different groups.
(B) is a meso compound.
(C) has a plane of symmetry.
(D) gives rise to conformational isomers.

95. The two formulas shown below represent

(A) constitutional isomers.
(B) a racemic mixture.
(C) enantiomers.
(D) diastereomers.

96. The carbon atoms in benzene C_6H_6 have the hybridization

(A) sp.
(B) sp^2.
(C) sp^3.
(D) sp^3d^2.

97. Oxidation of the secondary alcohol 2-propanol

$$CH_3-CH-CH_3$$
$$|$$
$$OH$$

yields:

(A) ethanol.
(B) propanone.
(C) propanal.
(D) dimethyl ether.

98. After workup, the reaction of the Grignard reagent, methyl magnesium bromide, CH_3MgBr, with the aldehyde, butanal, $CH_3CH_2CH_2CHO$, produces as a product

(A) an ether.
(B) an alcohol.
(C) a carboxylic acid.
(D) a ketone.

99. Which of the following is true concerning the dehydration of an alcohol?

(A) It may occur through an SN2 mechanism.
(B) It may occur through an E1 mechanism with a primary alcohol.
(C) It may occur through an SN1 mechanism with a secondary alcohol.
(D) It may occur through an E1 mechanism with a tertiary alcohol.

100. A mixture of unequal amounts of a pair of enantiomers is

(A) a meso mixture.
(B) a disastereomic mixture.
(C) optically active.
(D) a racemic mixture.

1.	A	26.	C	51.	C	76.	A
2.	C	27.	C	52.	A	77.	B
3.	C	28.	C	53.	A	78.	D
4.	D	29.	C	54.	D	79.	B
5.	C	30.	A	55.	C	80.	C
6.	B	31.	C	56.	C	81.	A
7.	D	32.	A	57.	D	82.	C
8.	B	33.	D	58.	B	83.	A
9.	B	34.	B	59.	C	84.	D
10.	B	35.	D	60.	C	85.	C
11.	C	36.	A	61.	C	86.	C
12.	A	37.	C	62.	B	87.	C
13.	A	38.	A	63.	C	88.	D
14.	B	39.	D	64.	B	89.	D
15.	A	40.	C	65.	D	90.	C
16.	C	41.	A	66.	B	91.	D
17.	A	42.	A	67.	C	92.	B
18.	B	43.	A	68.	B	93.	A
19.	A	44.	C	69.	A	94.	A
20.	D	45.	C	70.	B	95.	D
21.	A	46.	C	71.	C	96.	B
22.	B	47.	A	72.	A	97.	B
23.	D	48.	A	73.	B	98.	B
24.	C	49.	D	74.	A	99.	D
25.	A	50.	A	75.	A	100.	C

ANSWERS EXPLAINED

1. **(A)** Transcription is the synthesis of RNA. Translation (choice B) is the synthesis of protein. Replication (choice C) is the synthesis of DNA. Respiration (choice D) is the oxidation of molecules for energy production.

2. **(C)** The DNA helix is composed of two molecules of DNA (strands) that are intertwined and held together by hydrogen bonding between the purine and pyrimidine bases of each strand. This type of hydrogen bonding is called base-pairing.

3. **(C)** DNA (deoxyribonucleic acid) is composed of two nucleic acid polymers hydrogen bonded together, forming a double helix. DNA contains deoxyribose, a carbohydrate without an alcohol group at C2; RNA (ribonucleic acid) contains ribose (choice A). DNA contains the nitrogenous bases adenine, guanine, cytosine, and thymine while RNA contains adenine, guanine, cytosine, and uracil (choice B). DNA is found in the nucleus of animal cells, not in the cytoplasm (choice D).

4. **(D)** See the answer for question 3. Although RNA does not exist as a pair of nucleic acid polymers like DNA, it can fold back on itself and assume a hydrogen bonded structure in which the nitrogenous bases are base paired. This eliminates choice A. All nucleic acids contain phosphate groups in the polymer chain, so choice B is incorrect. DNA is the template for RNA and DNA synthesis, so choice C is incorrect as well.

5. **(C)** Beta oxidation refers to the series of reactions that results in the oxidation of the carbons of fatty acids resulting in ATP synthesis (through oxidative phosphorylation). Polysaccharides (after conversion to monosaccharides) are oxidized through glycolysis followed by the citric acid cycle resulting in ATP synthesis.

6. **(B)** Oxidation is the loss of electron density. We can assign oxidation numbers to the carbons in a molecule to tell if oxidation has occurred. If the oxidation number gets smaller, a reduction has occurred. If the oxidation number gets larger, an oxidation has occurred. To assign oxidation numbers, look at what is bonded to each carbon and give a +1 for each bond to an electronegative atom and a –1 for each bond to hydrogen. In choice A, each of the two carbons in the reactant molecule have oxidation numbers of –2, so the reactant molecule has a total oxidation number of –4. In the product in choice A, one carbon has an oxidation number of –3 and one carbon has an oxidation number of –1, so the molecule's oxidation number is still –4. No net oxidation or reduction has occurred (although one of the carbons has been oxidized, the other one has been reduced so there has not been a net change). In choice B, the reactant molecule has a total oxidation number of –6 while the product has a total oxidation number of –4. Since the oxidation number has gotten larger (–4 is a larger number than –6), oxidation has occurred.

7. **(D)** Genes are composed of DNA.

8. **(B)** Adenosine triphosphate (ATP) is produced from NADH and $FADH_2$ through oxidative phosphorylation (also known as the electron transport chain). To explain further, oxidative phosphorylation is the oxidation of reduced cofactors (NADH, $FADH_2$) from glycolysis and the citric acid cycle coupled to the phosphorylation of ADP to ATP.

9. **(B)** Proteins are polymers of amino acids joined by peptide bonds, a kind of amide bond. The different amino acids differ in a group attached to the alpha carbon (the

carbon to which the amine and acid groups are attached)—this group is often called the side chain. (The term "essential," when used in reference to amino acids, specifically means amino acids that cannot be biosynthesized and are therefore essential in the diet.)

10. **(B)** Oxidation of a primary alcohol can be accomplished with $KMnO_4$ or with DMP (an alternative to DMP is PCC, pyridinium chlorochromate). DMP (and PCC) have the distinction that since they are not used in aqueous solution, they can oxidize primary alcohols to aldehydes without further oxidation to carboxylic acids. Potassium permanganate (and chromic acid) are used in aqueous solutions and thus when used to oxidize primary alcohols to aldehydes, further oxidation to carboxylic acids cannot be avoided. Note that choices A and D are hydride donors. Hydride donors are used to reduce carbonyls to alcohols.

11. **(C)** The most important infrared (IR) absorptions are around 3000 cm^{-1} for O–H or N–H, around 2100 cm^{-1} for triple bonds, and around 1600–1700 cm^{-1} for double bonds. The only functional group that would have bands at both 3300 and 1700 is the acid.

12. **(A)** Determine the formula weight; then divide the mass of hydrogen by the formula weight and multiply by 100. For glycine, the formula weight is 75 (calculated as $24 + 5 + 14 + 32 = 75$). To determine the percentage of hydrogen, divide 5 by 75 and then multiply by 100: $5/75 = 0.067 \times 100 = 6.7\% = {<}10\%$.

13. **(A)** Lipids are nonpolar molecules meaning they have lots of carbon–hydrogen bonds (which are nonpolar) and very few, if any, polar bonds (like carbon–oxygen, nitrogen–hydrogen, or oxygen–hydrogen bonds).

14. **(B)** The farther two elements are from each other in the periodic table, the more ionic the bond between them. The metals are on the left side of the table and the nonmetals are on the right side. Hydrogen is an exception in that it can act as a metal or a nonmetal. Carbon, oxygen, and nitrogen are all nonmetals. Lithium is definitely a metal so when it forms a compound with a nonmetal like oxygen, their electronegativities (and ionization energies and electron affinities) are different enough that one or more electrons will be exchanged, leaving the metal and going to the nonmetal, forming ions and thus an ionic compound. Ionic compounds are more polar than covalent compounds.

15. **(A)** The dipole moment is a measure of the polarity of a molecule; that is, one part of the molecule is partially positive and one part is partially negative. The greater the dipole moment, the more polar a molecule is. Carbon dioxide, CO_2, has a dipole moment of zero because the molecule is linear with carbon in the middle and one oxygen atom on either side of the carbon. Although each individual C–O bond is polar, the two bonds balance each other to produce a nonpolar molecule.

H_2O (choice B), HF (choice C), and NH_3 (choice D) are all polar molecules. The water molecule is bent with the electrons being drawn toward the oxygen. The hydrogen fluoride molecule is linear, but the H–F bond is polar with the electrons drawn toward the fluorine. The ammonia molecule is trigonal pyramidal with the electrons drawn toward the nitrogen.

16. **(C)** Aluminum hydroxide, $Al(OH)_3$, dissolves in water to produce aluminum ions, Al^{+3}, and hydroxide ions, OH^{-1}.

$$Al(OH)_3 \text{ (s)} \leftrightarrow Al^{+3} \text{ (aq)} + 3OH^{-1} \text{ (aq)}$$

An equilibrium exists in solution between undissolved aluminum hydroxide, $Al(OH)_3$ (s), and dissolved aluminum hydroxide, Al^{+3} (aq) $+ 3OH^{-1}$ (aq).

Dissolving aluminum hydroxide in either choice B, 0.5 M $Al(NO_3)_3$, or choice C, 1.6 M NaOH, will decrease its solubility relative to its solubility in water. Since aluminum nitrate, $Al(NO_3)$, is a soluble salt, the concentration of the aluminum ion, Al^{+3}, will be 0.5 M (0.5 mole/liter) in a solution of 0.5 M $Al(NO_3)_3$.

$$Al(NO_3)_3 \text{ (s)} \quad \longrightarrow \quad Al^{+3} \text{ (aq)} \quad + \quad 3NO_3^{-1} \text{ (aq)}$$

$\dfrac{0.5 \text{ mole}}{\text{liter}}$	$\dfrac{0.5 \text{ mole}}{\text{liter}}$	$\dfrac{3(0.5 \text{ mole})}{\text{liter}}$

In the same way, the concentration of the hydroxide ion, OH^{-1}, in a solution of 1.6 M sodium hydroxide, NaOH (s), a soluble base, will be 1.6 M.

$$NaOH \text{ (s)} \quad \longrightarrow \quad Na^{+1} \text{ (aq)} \quad + \quad OH^{-1} \text{ (aq)}$$

$\dfrac{1.6 \text{ moles}}{\text{liter}}$	$\dfrac{1.6 \text{ moles}}{\text{liter}}$	$\dfrac{1.6 \text{ moles}}{\text{liter}}$

Both the aluminum and hydroxide ions result in solution from dissolving solid aluminum hydroxide in water. According to Le Châtelier's Principle, increasing the concentration of either ion on the right side of the equation will shift the equilibrium to the left and decrease the solubility of $Al(OH)_3$ (s). Therefore, the presence of aluminum ions in the aluminum nitrate solution and the presence of hydroxide ions in the sodium hydroxide solution decrease the solubility of aluminum hydroxide in either of these solutions. The concentration of hydroxide in the sodium hydroxide solution is 1.6 M, which is larger than the concentration of the aluminum ion, 0.5 M, in the aluminum nitrate solution. The 1.6 M sodium hydroxide solution will decrease the solubility of aluminum hydroxide more than the 0.5 M aluminum nitrate solution will.

Adding solid aluminum hydroxide to the 0.3 M hydrochloric acid, HCl (choice D), will increase the solubility of the aluminum hydroxide relative to its solubility in water, since the hydroxide ion concentration would be reduced by reacting with the hydrogen ion, H^{+1}, of the hydrochloric acid, HCl, and the equilibrium would shift to the right. More aluminum hydroxide would dissolve.

17. **(A)** With respect to proteins, the primary structure is the sequence of amino acids in the protein, the secondary structure is localized patterns that arise due to hydrogen bonding between peptide bonds in the protein, the tertiary structure is the overall folding pattern of the protein, and the quaternary structure is the association of multiple proteins (not all proteins exhibit quaternary structure). All of the levels of structure are important in the protein's function. Denaturation disrupts the noncovalent interactions in the protein (secondary through quaternary structure), but the primary structure (which involves covalent bonds) is not affected.

18. **(B)** Protein synthesis (translation) involves the covalent connection of amino acids associated with the cellular structure called the ribosome. Several types of RNA are involved in the process: mRNA (messenger RNA) provides the "instructions" for the

amino acid sequence, rRNA (ribosomal RNA) is part of the ribosome structure, and tRNA (transfer RNA) brings the appropriate amino acids to the ribosome for incorporation into the growing protein. DNA is not directly involved in protein synthesis.

19. **(A)** Proteins and peptides are polymers of amino acids joined by amide bonds (called peptide bonds).

20. **(D)** Boiling point is based on molecular weight (how heavy the molecule is) and the strength of the intermolecular forces of attraction that occur between molecules. The heavier the molecule, the more energy will be required to get it into the gaseous state and the boiling point will increase. The stronger the intermolecular forces of attraction between molecules, the more energy it will take to break these forces and liberate the molecules in the gas form, so the higher the boiling point. All of the selections have about the same molecular weight, so the determining factor will be the strength of the intermolecular forces possible in a sample of each. Since the molecule in choice D has an alcohol functional group that can hydrogen bond (the strongest of all the available intermolecular forces) with other alcohol functional groups on nearby molecules, it will have the highest boiling point. Remember that in order for a molecule to be capable of hydrogen bonding, it must have a hydrogen atom covalently attached to a small electronegative element (N, O, halogen)—so the molecule in choice D is the only one capable of hydrogen bonding.

21. **(A)** Water solubility and boiling point are affected by the ability of molecules to hydrogen bond with water (as in water solubility) or with other molecules of themselves (as in raising the boiling point). Although both choices A and B have atoms with unshared electrons that might be able to participate in hydrogen bonding with water, choice B has a longer nonpolar hydrocarbon chain that would impede its water solubility.

22. **(B)** There are three main types of intermolecular forces: hydrogen bonding, dipole-dipole interactions, and London (or dispersion) forces. London forces are the weakest type and consist of induced dipoles secondary to reduced intermolecular distances. They are transient and weak and occur between all molecules. Dipole-dipole interactions are the attraction between the partial positive part of one molecule and the partial negative part of a second molecule. Only polar molecules have permanent areas of partial positive and partial negative charges, thus only polar molecules can participate in dipole-dipole interactions. Hydrogen bonds are an extreme type of dipole-dipole interaction (they are about 5 times stronger than ordinary dipole-dipole interactions [choice A]). Hydrogen bonds occur between an electronegative atom with unshared electrons and a highly partial positive hydrogen of a second molecule (the only types of hydrogen that are sufficiently partial positive to qualify for a hydrogen bond are hydrogen atoms covalently bonded to an N, O, or halogen atom).

23. **(D)** In glycolysis, one glucose molecule (6 carbons) is converted to two pyruvic acid molecules (3 carbons each). The pyruvic acid molecules are then converted to acetyl coenzyme A molecules that enter the citric acid cycle (choice B) for oxidation. Gluconeogenesis (choice C) is the synthesis of glucose from noncarbohydrate precursors. Oxidative phosphorylation (choice A) is the oxidation of reduced cofactors (NADH, $FADH_2$) from glycolysis and the citric acid cycle coupled to the phosphorylation of ADP to ATP.

24. **(C)** Carbohydrates are polyhydroxy aldehydes or ketones. Monosaccharides can be drawn in a Fischer projection in which the aldehyde or ketone functional group is explicit, or in a cyclic Haworth projection in which the carbonyl group is involved in a hemiacetal functional group and therefore not explicitly seen. When monosaccharides are connected to form chains (polysaccharides), the hemiacetal functional group is converted to an acetal. Thus, sometimes it is difficult to spot the aldehyde or ketone because it has been converted to a hemiacetal or an acetal, but multiple alcohol groups are always evident. Upon hydrolysis of the acetal, a hemiacetal would be regenerated and the reaction between an aldehyde or ketone and an alcohol to form a hemiacetal is easily reversible. You should view a hemiacetal or acetal as a "hidden" aldehyde or ketone and use the presence of multiple alcohol groups to confirm that the structure is a carbohydrate.

25. **(A)** Molarity is moles of solute divided by liters of solution. Glucose has a formula weight of 180 so 1.8 g is 0.010 moles. Since the question asks about making 1000 mL of solution (1 L), then the molarity is 0.01 M.

26. **(C)** To determine bond angles, draw the Lewis structure. For carbon dioxide (CO_2), the Lewis structure has carbon as the central atom with an oxygen atom on each side of it. To complete the octets of all three atoms, there must be a double bond (two pairs of shared electrons) between carbon and each of the two oxygen atoms. Thus, in the Lewis structure, there are two sets of electrons (each double bond counts as a set) around the carbon atom. The Valence Shell Electron Pair Repulsion Theory (VSEPR) states that the two sets will spread out as far as possible, which means they will be 180° apart, and the molecule will be linear.

27. **(C)** See question 17. The two most common examples of secondary structure are alpha helices and beta (pleated) sheets. A tetramer (choice A) would be an example of quaternary structure, and peptide bonds (choice B) are what connect amino acids so they are involved in the primary structure. A double helix (choice D) refers to the arrangement of DNA molecules (which aren't proteins).

28. **(C)** The Valence Bond Theory is a theory concerning how atoms share electrons in covalent bonds. It views covalent bonds as being the overlap of an atomic orbital from each of the involved atoms. The Molecular Orbital Theory (choice A) is also a theory of covalent bonding but it views the covalent bonding in molecules as being the addition of the individual atoms' atomic orbitals, creating new orbitals that encompass the molecule (called molecular orbitals) that replace the atomic orbitals. The Valence Shell Electron Pair Repulsion Theory (choice B) is used to predict the geometry of molecules and says that the electron pairs around a central atom in a molecule will spread out as far as possible. The Kinetic Molecular Theory (choice D) is the theory that brings together the observed properties of gases.

29. **(C)** See question 18.

30. **(A)** One source of amino acids for protein synthesis is cellular biosynthesis (the other source is dietary protein).

31. **(C)** Decarboxylation of beta carbonyl carboxylic acids occurs fairly easily even without enzyme catalysts. The mechanism involves the movement of the electrons on the negatively charged oxygen toward the carbonyl carbon, which pushes the electrons

of the bond between the carboxyl carbonyl carbon, toward the carbon alpha to the thioester. The resulting anion is resonance stabilized by the thioester carbonyl group. A similar type of decarboxylation occurs in the last step of the malonic ester synthesis and the acetoacetic ester synthesis, a topic typically part of the second semester of the organic chemistry sequence.

32. **(A)** The methylene (CH_2) signal represents the quantity of the keto form (the left structure in the equilibrium). Since the methylene group has two hydrogens, the integration of 1 must be divided by 2 to give 0.5. The methine (CH) signal represents the quantity of the enol form (the right structure in the equilibrium). The methine group has just one hydrogen, and it integrates for 4. That means in the mixture of the two forms, the quantity of the enol form is 4/4.5 (the amount of that form divided by the total of both forms) or approximately 90%.

33. **(D)** The percent enol present with any carboxylic acid derivative (including esters and thioesters) is dependent on the amount of partial positive charge on the carbonyl carbon. You can think of it this way: the more partial positive charge on the carbonyl carbon, the more the electrons of the neighboring C–H bond are pulled toward the carbonyl carbon moving toward the enol form. When esters and thioesters are compared, the carbonyl carbon of thioesters is more partial positive than that of esters. This is due to the fact that sulfur, being in the third row of the periodic table, is bigger than carbon, a second row element. That means that when sulfur donates electron density to the carbonyl carbon, the donation through resonance is minimal due to a mismatch of the sizes of the p orbitals of the two atoms (C and S). When oxygen donates electron density to the carbonyl carbon, since oxygen and carbon are both second row elements, their p orbitals are the same size, allowing good overlap and effective electron donation through resonance.

34. **(B)** Triacylglycerols are triesters of fatty acids and glycerol. Lipolysis results in ester hydrolysis to give fatty acids that yield acetyl units upon beta oxidation. Steroids (choice A) are also lipids but they do not contain fatty acids. Waxes (choice C) contain fatty acids but they are not the primary storage form of fatty acids. Prostaglandins (choice D) are formed from the 20 carbon fatty acid, arachidonic acid, and are involved in the inflammatory process.

35. **(D)** The malonic ester synthesis begins with malonic ester.

diethyl malonate

The addition of ethoxide (or any alkoxide) deprotonates the carbon alpha to both esters, creating a nucleophilic carbon. Addition of methyl iodide would place a methyl on that carbon. A second deprotonation with ethoxide followed by methyl iodide would place two methyl groups on that carbon. Acid catalyzed hydrolysis with heat will result in hydrolysis of both esters to carboxylic acids and then, since a beta carbonyl acid is present, decarboxylation of one of them. Subsequent tautomerization of the enol form yields the disubstituted acetic acid derivative, methylpropanoic acid.

36. **(A)** Oxidation is the loss of electrons; the substance oxidized is the reducing agent. Reduction is the gain of electrons; the substance reduced is the oxidizing agent. In the given equation, Zn loses electrons while Cu^{2+} gains electrons. Thus, Zn^0 (which is oxidized to Zn^{2+}) is the reducing agent; Cu^{2+} (which is reduced to Cu^0) is the oxidizing agent.

$$Zn + CuSO_4 \longrightarrow ZnSO_4 + Cu$$
$$Zn^0 \longrightarrow Zn^{2+} + 2e^-$$
$$Cu^{2+} + 2e^- \longrightarrow Cu$$

37. **(C)** Refer to the explanation for question 39.

38. **(A)** The correct electron configuration for the sulfide ion, S^{2-}, is $1s^2 2s^2 2p^6 3s^2 3p^6$. The letters s, p, d, and f indicate the type of orbital. The number in front of the symbols, as in 1s, indicates the number of the orbital, in this case 1. The superscript, as in $1s^2$, indicates the number of electrons present in the orbital, in this case 2. The electron configuration for the sulfur atom, S, which is $1s^2 2s^2 2p^6 3s^2 3p^4$, shows the 16 electrons present in the atom. The sulfur ion, S^{2-}, has two more electrons in the p orbital: $1s^2 2s^2 2p^6 3s^2 3p^6$.

39. **(D)** The coefficients of the reactants and products in a balanced equation represent *volume* for gases, as well as *molecules* and *moles*. These are the only direct relationships involving coefficients that exist in a balanced equation. Use the factor-label method to calculate the number of moles of oxygen formed when the reaction begins with 4 moles of ammonia.

$$4NH_3 \text{ (g)} + 5O_2 \text{ (g)} \longrightarrow 4NO \text{ (g)} + 6H_2O \text{ (g)}$$

Two fractions are possible from the relationship that 4 moles of NH_3 require 5 moles of O_2:

$$\frac{4 \text{ moles } NH_3}{5 \text{ moles } O_2} \qquad \frac{5 \text{ moles } O_2}{4 \text{ moles } NH_3}$$

Having 5 moles of NH_3, multiply by the appropriate fraction so that only moles of O_2 remain.

$$5 \text{ moles } NH_3 \times \frac{5 \text{ moles } O_2}{4 \text{ moles } NH_3} = 6.3 \text{ moles } O_2$$

40. **(C)** Convert 17.0 g of NH_3 to moles of NH_3:

$$17.0 \text{ g} \times \frac{1 \text{ mol } NH_3}{17.0 \text{ g } NH_3} = 1 \text{ mol } NH_3$$

Use the coefficients in the equation to find moles of H_2O:

$$1 \text{ mol } NH_3 \times \frac{6 \text{ mol } H_2O}{4 \text{ mol } NH_3} = 1.5 \text{ mol } H_2O$$

Convert mol H_2O to grams H_2O:

$$1.5 \text{ mol } H_2O \times \frac{18 \text{ g } H_2O}{1 \text{ mol } H_2O} = 27 \text{ g } H_2O$$

41. **(A)** Follow the same method as shown in the explanation to question 40, except convert from moles of NO to liters of NO. Remember, 1 mole of any gas at standard temperature and pressure, STP, 0°C and 1 atm, occupies 22.4 liters.

$$g\ NH_3 \rightarrow \text{moles } NH_3 \rightarrow \text{moles } NO \rightarrow \text{liters } NO$$

g NH_3

1.7 g NH_3

moles NH_3

$$\frac{1.70\ g}{17\ g/mole} = 0.10 \text{ mole } NH_3$$

moles NO

$$0.10 \text{ mole } NH_3 \times \frac{4 \text{ moles } NO}{4 \text{ moles } NH_3} = 0.10 \text{ mole } NO$$

liters NO

$$0.10 \text{ mole } NO \times \frac{22.4 \text{ liters } NO}{1 \text{ mole } NO} = 2.24 \text{ liters } NO$$

42. **(A)** Follow the same method as shown in the explanations to questions 40 and 41, except convert from moles of NO to molecules of NO. Remember, 1 mole of any substance contains 6×10^{23} particles.

$$g\ NH_3 \rightarrow \text{moles } NH_3 \rightarrow \text{moles } NO \rightarrow \text{molecules } NO$$

g NH_3

0.17 g NH_3

moles NH_3

$$\frac{0.17\ g\ NH_3}{17\ g/mole} = 0.01 \text{ mole } NH_3$$

moles NO

$$0.01 \text{ mole } NH_3 \times \frac{4 \text{ moles } NO}{4 \text{ moles } NH_3} = 0.01 \text{ mole } NO$$

molecules NO

$$0.01 \text{ mole } NO \times \frac{6 \times 10^{23} \text{ molecules } NO}{1 \text{ mole } NO} = 6 \times 10^{21} \text{ molecules } NO$$

43. **(A)** Recall that Ka times Kb equals Kw (1×10^{-14}). To determine Kb for the conjugate base, Y^-, divide 1×10^{-14} by 3.7×10^{-4}. If you don't have a calculator, you can roughly determine which option to select by dividing 1 by 3.7 (about a third) and then 10^{-14} by 10^{-4} (10^{-10}). At this point, you have about 0.3×10^{-10}. To get the number in correct scientific notation, convert 0.3 to 3 by moving the decimal one place, which means you must change 10^{-10} to 10^{-11}. The actual value is 2.7×10^{-11}.

44. **(C)** The stronger the acid, the larger the Ka. Remember that the more negative the exponent, the smaller the number.

45. **(C)** Recall that pH + pOH equals 14. Since the question gives the hydroxide ion concentration, calculating pOH is straightforward.

$$pOH = -\log [OH^-]$$

The log of 0.001 is –3, so the pOH is 3 and thus the pH is 11.

46. **(C)** Magnesium hydroxide will dissociate completely in aqueous solution. There are two hydroxide ions per magnesium hydroxide unit; so, if the solution is 3.0 M in magnesium hydroxide, it will be 6.0 M OH^-.

47. **(A)** To calculate the formula weight, add up the atomic masses of the atoms in the formula (NH_4NO_3). In this case, the formula weight is $(1 \times 14) + (4 \times 1) + (1 \times 14) + (3 \times 16)$.

48. **(A)** To solve this problem, use the factor label method.

$$1 \text{ atom } (1 \text{ mole}/6 \times 10^{23} \text{ atoms}) (24.3g/1 \text{ mole}) = 24.3g/6 \times 10^{23} \text{ atoms}$$

At this point you have about 24 in the numerator divided by 6 in the denominator, which equals about 4, so you can narrow down the answer to choices A or D. Since 10^{23} is in the denominator, it becomes 10^{-23}, making choice A the correct answer.

49. **(D)** Germanium has an atomic number of 32 (it is the 32nd element in the Periodic Table), meaning it contains 32 protons. The mass number for the germanium in the question is 74, meaning that there are 32 protons plus 42 neutrons in the nucleus.

50. **(A)** Nuclear reactions are reactions involving the nucleus. When a sodium atom becomes a sodium ion, an electron is lost from the valence shell of sodium (not from the nucleus). All of the other reactions are nuclear reactions. Choice B is an example of fission (two nuclei are produced from one). Emission of gamma particles and conversion of one isotope of an element into another are both nuclear processes.

51. **(C)** If the volume of a gas is reduced (and the temperature remains constant), then the pressure must increase. This is stated formally in Boyle's law ($P_1V_1 = P_2V_2$). The movement of the gas particles is dependent on the temperature so choice B is not correct. Charles's law has to do with changes in volume and temperature ($V_1/T_1 = V_2/T_2$).

52. **(A)** Physical properties and physical changes do not describe or result in a new substance. Chemical properties and chemical changes describe or result in the formation of a new substance. When water evaporates (boils), the water molecules move from the liquid to the vapor or gas. If you trap the vapor (as on the underside of the lid on a pot of boiling water), the liquid water is reformed. No change into a new substance has occurred.

53. **(A)** To balance the equation, go from left to right, changing the coefficient (the big number in front of the formula) as needed. When balancing equations, you cannot change the subscripts in the formulas because that changes the substance. In this question, there are two sodiums on the left, so the coefficient for $NaHSO_4$ on the right becomes 2. Now there are 2 sulfurs on the right, so the coefficient of the H_2SO_4 on the left becomes 2. Now there are 4 hydrogens on the left side and 4 on the right. There are also 11 oxygens on the left and 11 on the right. Finally, there is one carbon on the left and one on the right. The equation is balanced and the coefficient for CO_2 is 1.

54. **(D)** The equation used to solve this problem is

$$PV = nRT$$

The symbol P is pressure in atmospheres, V is volume in liters, n is number of moles, which equals grams/molar mass, R is the gas constant, and T is temperature in Kelvin. Because the oxygen is collected over water, both water and oxygen contribute to the pressure of the gas. The contribution of water, 23.76 mm, must be subtracted from the total pressure, 750 mm, to determine the pressure contributed by the oxygen, 726.24 mm. Pressure must be converted to atmospheres, volume converted to liters, and temperature converted to Kelvin. In addition, oxygen is a diatomic gas and, consequently, its molar mass is 32 amu.

55. **(C)** The ideal gas law, $PV = nRT$, or

$$PV = \frac{\#g}{mol.\ wt.}(RT)$$

is used to solve this problem. Pressure is used in atmospheres, volume in liters, and temperature in Kelvin. Moles of gas is represented by n, which equals grams divided by molecular weight. The molar mass of nitrogen is 28 grams/mole since nitrogen is a diatomic molecule, N_2. Substituting the given data into the above formula gives:

$$1\ atm\ (1.0\ liter) = \frac{x}{28\ grams/mole}\left(0.082\frac{L\text{-}atm}{K\text{-}mole}\right)(273 + 27)\ K$$

$$x = 1.1\ g$$

56. **(C)** This question is one of diluting a 5.0 M solution to 2.5 M so the equation, $M_1V_1 = M_2V_2$, can be used.

$$5.0x = (2.5)(500),\ so\ x = 250$$

Rather than doing the math, if you notice that this is a one to two dilution (the new solution is half the concentration of the one given), then you will take half the desired volume of the more concentrated solution (5.0 M here) and then dilute it with the same amount of water.

57. **(D)** Solve this problem using the factor label method, the coefficients in the balanced equation, and the definition of molarity (moles solute/1000 mL solution). The advantage of using this method is that, if your units cancel out to give the units you are looking for, you know you have set it up correctly.

$$10\ mL\left(\frac{2.0\ moles\ H_2SO_4}{1000\ mL}\right)\left(\frac{2\ moles\ LiOH}{1\ mole\ H_2SO_4}\right)\left(\frac{1000\ mL}{2.5\ moles\ LiOH}\right) = 16\ mL$$

58. **(B)** The bubble at the bottom of the lake has a volume of 1.4 mL at (7 + 273) K and 2.0 atm pressure. To determine the volume of the bubble at the surface of the lake at (27 + 273) K and 1.0 atm pressure, use the equation shown below.

$$\frac{P_1V_1}{T_1} = \frac{P_2V_2}{T_2} = \frac{2.0\ atm\ (1.4\ mL)}{280\ K} = \frac{1\ atm\ V_2}{300\ K}\ \ V_2 = 3.0\ mL$$

Since pressure and volume are present on both sides of the equation, any pressure or volume term (atm, psi, mL, liters, etc.) can be used as long as the term is the same on both sides of the equation. The pressure units cancel, and the volume term is part of the answer.

Also, one can predict that the volume of the gas bubble will increase since, as temperature rises, volume increases, and as pressure decreases, volume increases.

59. **(C)** There are two chiral centers (a chiral center is a carbon with 4 different groups attached to it). One chiral center is at carbon 2 (it has a methyl, chlorine, hydrogen, and the rest of the molecule attached), and the other is at carbon 3 (it has a chlorine, a hydrogen, an ethyl, and the rest of the molecule attached). At this point, you can rule out choices A and B since they each have only one chiral center designation. To determine the absolute configuration of a chiral center, assign priorities based on atomic number to each of the four groups attached, orient the chiral center such that the #4 priority group is away from you, and then look at the order of the other 3 groups. If they are arranged clockwise, the chiral center is R; if counterclockwise, it is S. For the chiral center at C2, the chlorine is priority #1, the methyl is priority #3, the hydrogen is priority #4, and the rest of the molecule is priority #2. (When you are assigning priority, the four atoms attached to that carbon are Cl, H, C, and C. To break the tie between the two carbons, look at what each of them is attached to. One of the carbons is attached to three hydrogens while the other is attached to a chlorine, a hydrogen, and another carbon. The presence of the chlorine makes the carbon attached higher priority than the carbon with three hydrogens.) Therefore, the chiral center at C2 is R. Repeat this process for the chiral center at C3.

60. **(C)** The heat capacity, C, of a substance equals the specific heat, s, times the mass of the material, m.

$$C = ms$$

$$C = 10.0 \text{ g} \left(0.385 \frac{J}{g°C} \right) = 3.85 \text{ J/°C}$$

61. **(C)** To balance nuclear equations, the mass numbers on each side of the equation must be equal and the atomic numbers on each side of the equation must be equal. For the given equation, the atomic number of the element produced would have to be 89, meaning the element's symbol would be the one to the right of Ra in the periodic table.

62. **(B)** When reading the electron configuration from the periodic table, remember that for the representative elements (those in the two leftmost columns or the six rightmost columns), the valence shell is the row number of the element. Also, remember that the two leftmost columns represent filling s orbitals, and the six rightmost columns represent filling p orbitals. Finally, an atom loses electrons from its valence shell to form a cation and gains electrons to form an anion. Thus, when asked which option has a valence shell electron configuration of $2s^2 2p^6$, it would be anything with the same electron configuration of neon (and that would include F^-, Na^+, or Mg^{2+}).

63. **(C)** To draw the Lewis structure of SF_6, add up the valence electrons (6 for sulfur and 7 for each of the fluorines). The total is 48 electrons. Arrange the 7 atoms in a symmetrical arrangement with the first atom (S) in the middle. Complete the electron octets for

each of the peripheral atoms (the fluorines). That uses up all of the 48 valence electrons so there are no leftover valence electrons to put on the sulfur.

64. **(B)** To determine the formal charge on nitrogen, draw the Lewis structure for the nitrate ion. There are 24 valence electrons (5 for the nitrogen, 6 for each of the oxygens, and an extra one due to the negative charge). Arrange the oxygens around the nitrogen and complete the octets of the oxygens. That uses up all of the 24 valence electrons, but nitrogen doesn't have an octet around it so use one of the unshared pairs on an oxygen to make a double bond between nitrogen and one of the oxygen atoms. Now calculate the formal charge on the nitrogen. You can calculate formal charge by using the following equation:

> Formal charge =
> (number of valence electrons for the atom)
> − [(number of unshared electrons on the atom)
> + (number of bonds to the atom)]

Here, the formal charge on the nitrogen would equal $(5) − [(0) + (4)] = 1$.

65. **(D)** To determine the molecular geometry, first draw the Lewis structure. There are 26 valence electrons in NF_3. Place the fluorines around the nitrogen and complete the octets for the nitrogens. That uses up 24 of the 26 valence electrons. The remaining 2 electrons go on the nitrogen (now all four atoms in the molecule have an octet of electrons). After drawing the Lewis structure, the number of sets of electrons around the central atom will determine the 3D arrangement of the electron sets (the name of the molecular geometry, however, is given for the 3D arrangement of the atoms). There are four sets of electrons around the nitrogen, so the electron sets will be tetrahedral. The nitrogen will be in the middle of the tetrahedron, and the three fluorines plus the unshared pair of electrons will be directed toward the corners of the tetrahedron. The geometry of the molecule will be the 3D arrangement of the atoms. The atoms are at the corners of a pyramid with a triangular base; hence the molecule has a trigonal pyramidal molecular geometry.

66. **(B)** The hybridization of an atom can be determined from the geometry of the electron sets around it. In BF_3, there are 24 valence electrons. With the boron in the middle and the three fluorines around it, complete the octets for the fluorines which assign all 24 of the valence electrons. *Remember that boron violates the octet rule and forms a stable compound with only 6 electrons around it.* There are three electron sets around the boron, according to the VSEPR Theory; the three sets will spread out as far as possible, giving a triangular planar geometry. Triangular planar geometry of electron sets implies sp^2 hybridization. (Linear geometry of electron sets implies sp hybridization, and a tetrahedral geometry of electron sets implies sp^3 geometry.)

67. **(C)** These reagents represent hydroboration-oxidation, which is a method of hydrating an alkene (adding the components of water across the double bond). It occurs with anti-Markovnikov regiochemistry (meaning the H goes on the more highly substituted carbon of the alkene and the OH goes on the less highly substituted carbon of the alkene) and with syn stereochemistry (meaning the new H and OH add to the ring from the same side and will therefore be cis to each other). The other method of hydration

of alkenes, oxymercuration-demercuration, occurs with Markovnikov regiochemistry and antistereochemistry.

68. **(B)** Replication is the process whereby DNA is duplicated. The DNA duplex unwinds to expose its nucleotide sequence and new DNA molecules are synthesized complementary to each of the exposed DNA molecules, resulting in two molecules of DNA having identical nucleotide sequences. Since the involved synthetic enzymes (DNA polymerases) can synthesize new DNA in only one direction, and since the two DNA molecules composing the original duplex are antiparallel to each other, only one of the new DNA molecules can be synthesized continuously (without interruption). The other new DNA molecule is synthesized in pieces (called Okazaki fragments) or discontinuously.

69. **(A)** The allowed values for the quantum numbers of electrons are: n may be any whole number; ℓ may be from 0 up to n − 1; m_ℓ may be from negative ℓ to positive ℓ; and m_s may be either +1/2 or −1/2. Choice B is incorrect because the second quantum number cannot be equal to the first quantum number. Choice C is incorrect because the second quantum number cannot be negative. Choice D is incorrect because the fourth quantum number must be either +1/2 or −1/2.

70. **(B)** The conversion of an aldehyde to an alcohol is a reduction. Hydride donors like $NaBH_4$ and $LiAlH_4$ are used to perform this reduction. H_2 (choice C) is used to reduce alkenes and alkynes. PCC (choice A) and $KMnO_4$ (choice D) are both oxidizing agents.

71. **(C)** Bromine with $FeBr_3$ is used to accomplish electrophilic aromatic substitution on arene rings. A bromine atom will substitute for a hydrogen on the ring. The ring already has an amino group on it and an amino group is an ortho,para director (and also an activator by electron donation through resonance) so choice C is correct.

72. **(A)** Lipids include triglycerides, phospholipids, waxes, steroids, and prostaglandins among other nonpolar (water insoluble) biomolecules. The fat listed on food labels refers to triglycerides.

73. **(B)** In a first-order reaction, the half-life, that is, the length of time for one-half of the concentration to be reacted, is dependent only on the rate constant, not on the original concentration. If the rate constant, k, is 6.93×10^2/sec, the length of time needed for one-half of the starting material to be reacted is

$$t_{1/2} = \frac{0.693}{k}$$

$$t_{1/2} = \frac{0.693}{6.93 \times 10^2 / \text{sec}} = 1.0 \times 10^{-3} \text{ sec}$$

74. **(A)** When an alcohol reacts with an acid halide, an ester results through nucleophilic acyl substitution. All acid derivatives (acid halides, anhydrides, esters, and amides) undergo this type of reaction. In questions like this using condensed formulas, it is always a good idea to draw the line-bond structure before selecting an answer so that you can see clearly what types of functional groups are present (they are sometimes hard to see in a condensed structure).

75. **(A)** An equilibrium constant may be written for the following reaction. An equilibrium constant is equal to the product of the products divided by the product of the reactants, each raised to the power as indicated in the balanced equation.

$$H_2 + I_2 \leftrightarrow 2HI \qquad K = \frac{[HI]^2}{[I_2][H_2]} \qquad K = \frac{(0.5)^2}{(0.25)(0.25)} = 4$$

76. **(A)** According to Le Châtelier's Principle, any stress applied to a system in equilibrium will cause the equilibrium to shift so as to relieve the stress. For example, in the given system:

$$Heat + N_2O_4 (g) \leftrightarrow 2NO_2 (g)$$

think of heat as one of the reactants. An increase in any reactant concentration on the left will cause the equilibrium to shift to the right, to the products. An increase in the product concentration on the right will cause the equilibrium to shift to the left, to the reactants. A decrease in any reactant concentration will cause the equilibrium to shift to the left. A decrease in any product concentration will cause the equilibrium to shift to the right. Therefore, a decrease in temperature or heat will cause the reaction to shift to the left, NOT to the right.

An increase in the concentration of N_2O_4, a decrease in the concentration of NO_2, and an increase in temperature will all cause the equilibrium to shift to the right.

77. **(B)** Potassium t-butoxide is a strong base and is used to perform an E2 elimination by causing the removal of HI on this alkyl halide, creating an alkene. The most stable alkene will predominate. Remember, trans alkenes are more stable than cis alkenes, and more highly substituted alkenes are more stable than less highly substituted ones.

78. **(D)** When aldehydes and ketones condense in the presence of a base and either a beta-hydroxy carbonyl compound or an alpha beta-unsaturated carbonyl compound (as in this case) results, an aldol condensation has occurred. A Claisen (choice A) condensation involves an ester. A Williamson (choice B) is used to make an ether. A Michael (choice C) is the reaction between an enolate and an alpha beta-unsaturated carbonyl compound.

79. **(B)** Resonance structures have the same atom connections but different placements of pi and unshared electrons. Only choice B has all of the atoms in the same place.

80. **(C)** Triglycerides are a type of lipid biomolecule. They are stored in adipose tissue and yield soap upon basic hydrolysis (also called saponification). They are esters of fatty acids (long chain carboxylic acids) and glycerol. Their long carbon chains are oxidized to generate ATP through beta oxidation.

81. **(A)** Since ammonia is a weak base, the equilibrium would lie to the left for the deprotonation of water. In this reaction, water is acting as an acid. Ammonium is the conjugate acid of ammonia and hydroxide is the conjugate base of water.

82. **(C)** ^1H NMR gives information about the hydrogens in a molecule. Since there are five signals, there are five kinds of hydrogen in the molecule. Choice A can be excluded since the molecule has only four kinds of hydrogen and choice D can be excluded since the molecule has seven kinds of hydrogen. After comparing the number of signals in the spectrum to the number of different kinds of hydrogen in the molecule, look at

the splitting pattern and integration information. Simple splitting patterns follow the n + 1 rule, meaning that the splitting pattern for a group of hydrogens will be equal to the number of neighboring hydrogens (those on an adjacent carbon) plus one. For example, a triplet indicates that the hydrogens represented by that signal have two neighboring hydrogens, and a quartet indicates that the hydrogens represented by that signal have three neighboring hydrogens. Since the data include a triplet that integrates for 3H and a quartet that integrates for 2H, there must be an ethyl group, meaning choice C is correct.

83. **(A)** When a Grignard reagent reacts with an ester, a tertiary alcohol results. The Grignard reagent first attacks the ester, converting it into a ketone by nucleophilic acyl substitution, but a second Grignard reagent attacks the ketone carbonyl, resulting in an alcohol after protonation.

84. **(D)** Calcium carbonate, $CaCO_3$ (marble), is insoluble in water. The other compounds— NaOH, NH_4Cl, and $LiNO_3$—are all water soluble. The solubility rules include the following:

    All salts formed with the alkali metals, for example, any member of the lithium family, are soluble.

    All ammonium salts (NH_4^+) and all nitrate salts (NO_3^-) are soluble.

    Many chlorides (Cl^-), bromides (Br^-), and iodides (I^-) are soluble.

    Many sulfates (SO_4^{2-}) are soluble.

85. **(C)** The larger the value of K_{sp}, the more silver and chloride ions are present in the solution and hence the more soluble the salt. Of the salts listed, silver chloride is the most soluble.

86. **(C)** The formation constant for the formation of a complex ion, K_f, may be defined for the silver ammonia complex, $Ag(NH_3)_2^{+1}$, as shown below.

$$Ag^{+1} + 2NH_3 \longleftrightarrow Ag(NH_3)_2^{+1} \qquad K_f = \frac{\left[Ag(NH_3)_2^{+1}\right]}{\left[Ag^{+1}\right]\left[NH_3\right]^2}$$

The concentration of each of the species in the equation is raised to the power shown in the balanced equation. As can be seen from the equation above, K_f will have a large value when the concentration of the complex ion, $[Ag(NH_3)_2^{+1}]$, is high. When a lot of complex ion is formed, the ion must be stable. Hence the largest value for the formation complex, 2.0×10^{30} for HgI_4^{-2}, gives the most stable ion.

87. **(C)** Oxidation is the loss of electrons; reduction is the gain of electrons. The oxidizing agent is the material reduced, and the reducing agent is the material oxidized.

    In the given reaction between zinc and the ion Cu^{2+}:

$$Zn + Cu^{2+} \longrightarrow Zn^{2+} + Cu$$

    Zn is oxidized because it has lost electrons to form Zn^{2+} as in choice C, and consequently is the reducing agent. The ion Cu^{2+} has gained electrons to form copper, Cu, and is the oxidizing agent.

88. **(D)** Refer to the answer given to question 87. The reducing agent is the species that loses electrons, Li or Br^{-1}. The equation with the more negative value for emf^0

indicates the species with the greater tendency to lose electrons, Li. The equation with the more positive value indicates the species with the greater tendency to gain the electrons, Br_2.

89. **(D)** An electrochemical cell is made up of two electrodes connected in solution and by wires. One of the chemical species in solution loses electrons, the process of oxidation, to an electrode, the anode. Oxidation occurs at the anode. The electrons travel from the anode, through the wire, to the cathode where another species in solution gains the electrons, the process of reduction, supplied by the cathode. Reduction occurs at the cathode.

90. **(C)** The magnitude of 1,3-diaxial interactions is dependent on group size. The isopropyl group is larger than the other choices so it would be expected to have the greatest 1,3-diaxial energy.

91. **(D)** Four different structural isomers can be formed by C_4H_9Cl.

$CH_3 - CH_2 - CH_2 - CH_2 - Cl$	1-chlorobutane
$CH_3 - CH_2 - CHCl - CH_3$	2-chlorobutane
$(CH_3)_2 - CH - CH_2Cl$	1-chloro-2-methylpropane
$(CH_3)_3 - C - Cl$	2-chloro-2-methylpropane

92. **(B)** To determine the number of monochlorinated products of an alkane (ignoring stereoisomers), determine how many different kinds of hydrogen there are in the molecule. For propane, there are two different kinds of hydrogens (the 6 methyl hydrogens are equivalent and are one kind, and the 2 hydrogens on the carbon in the middle are equivalent and are the second kind). Thus, there are two monochlorinated products: 1-chloropropane and 2-chloropropane.

93. **(A)** To name an alkane or an alkyl halide, count the longest chain of carbons (that is, the parent chain). Number the parent such that the first branch has the lower number. Name the branches and arrange alphabetically. For this compound, there are two chains of 7 carbons. Choose the one with more branches as the parent. Number from the end closest to the first branch, which is a methyl branch in this case.

94. **(A)** A stereocenter, also called a chiral center, is a carbon with four different groups attached. A meso compound (choice B), in the simplest case, is a compound with two chiral centers composed of the same four groups, with one being R and the other being S. Chiral compounds do not have a plane of symmetry. Meso compounds contain a plane of symmetry (choice C) so even though they contain chiral centers, they are not chiral molecules. Conformational isomers (choice D) are different spatial arrangements of ONE compound that come about by rotation about a carbon–carbon single bond. The most common conformational isomers are the two chair forms of cyclohexanes.

95. **(D)** Constitutional isomers (choice A) are molecules that have the same molecular formula but different atom connections. A racemic mixture (choice B) is a 50:50 mixture to two enantiomers (choice C, which is defined as nonsuperimposable mirror images that arise due to the presence of one or more chiral centers). Diastereomers (choice D) are stereoisomers (molecules that have the same atom connections but different spatial arrangements) that are not enantiomers. In this question, both molecules have 4 carbons in the sequence $CH_3CH=CHCH_3$. They have the same atom connections so

they are not constitutional isomers. Neither has chiral centers so choices B and C can be eliminated. That leaves choice D as the correct answer.

96. **(B)** When C_6H_6 is drawn (such that each carbon has 4 bonds and each hydrogen has 1 bond), there will be a double bond to each carbon. When carbon is involved in a double bond, it reserves a p orbital from its valence shell to form the side-to-side overlap of a pi bond. That means the other orbitals of carbon's valence shell hybridize, giving sp^2 hybridization. An alternative way to arrive at the correct answer is to look at each carbon in the structure and see that each carbon has three sets of electrons around it (it is bonded to three groups). The VSEPR Theory predicts that these three groups of electron sets will be as far apart as possible, giving a triangular planar geometry. Triangular planar geometry implies sp^2 hybridization.

97. **(B)** Oxidation may be defined as the loss of hydrogen. Oxidation of the secondary alcohol results in the loss of the two underlined hydrogen atoms, one bonded to the carbon atom and one bonded to the oxygen atom. A double bond forms between the two atoms that lost the hydrogen atoms. The product is a ketone.

$$CH_3 - \underline{CH} - CH_3 \qquad \qquad CH_3 - \overset{\displaystyle \|}{C} - CH_3$$
$$\quad\quad\quad\; | \qquad\qquad\qquad \rightarrow$$
$$\quad\quad\;\; O\underline{H} \qquad\qquad\qquad\qquad\quad O$$

2-propanol   Propanone or acetone

98. **(B)** When an aldehyde reacts with a Grignard reagent, the nucleophilic carbon of the Grignard reagent attacks the carbonyl of the aldehyde, causing the pi electrons of the carbonyl to roll up on the oxygen. After protonation, an alcohol results.

99. **(D)** Dehydration of alcohols yields alkenes. Elimination reactions are used to form alkenes. There are two major elimination mechanisms: E2 and E1. E2 occurs in the presence of a strong base. E1 occurs in the absence of a strong base. Since the E1 mechanism involves a carbocation intermediate, only molecules that can form relatively stable carbocations can undergo an E1 reaction. Recall that the most stable carbocations are tertiary, followed by secondary, followed by primary. Thus, a primary alcohol would not undergo E1 but a tertiary alcohol would.

100. **(C)** A mixture of equal amounts of a pair of enantiomers is called a racemic mixture. Single enantiomers are optically active, meaning when placed in a polarimeter, the plane of polarized light will be rotated. Since a racemic mixture has equal amounts of enantiomers, one enantiomer rotates the plane of polarized light a certain number of degrees in one direction and the other enantiomer rotates the plane of polarized light the same number of degrees in the opposite direction; thus, there is no net rotation of the plane of polarized light, and it is said to be optically inactive. The question describes an *unequal* mixture of enantiomers so the mixture would be optically active.

Quantitative Reasoning Review and Practice

6

TIPS FOR THE QUANTITATIVE REASONING SECTION

The quantitative reasoning section of the PCAT consists of 48 math problems. You will have 45 minutes to complete the quantitative reasoning section. This section is the one that most students say they are unable to finish. Therefore, it is important that you pace yourself and answer all questions. There are 100 questions in this section to give you sufficient practice.

Calculators are permitted for use on the PCAT as of July 2016. However, it is also important to brush up on your math skills!

QUANTITATIVE REASONING REVIEW OUTLINE

   I. **Basic Mathematic Calculations**

  II. **Whole Numbers and Their Operations**
     A. Addition of Negative and Positive Integers
     B. Subtraction of Negative and Positive Integers
     C. Multiplication of Negative and Positive Integers
     D. Division of Negative and Positive Integers
     E. Absolute Value
     F. Factorial
     G. Order of Operations

 III. **Fractions**
     A. Adding Fractions
     B. Subtracting Fractions
     C. Multiplying Fractions
     D. Dividing Fractions
     E. Comparing Fractions: Which Is Larger or Smaller?

 IV. **Decimals**
     A. Adding Decimals
     B. Subtracting Decimals
     C. Multiplying Decimals
     D. Dividing Decimals

V. **Percentages**
  A. Calculating Percents
  B. Adding Percentages
  C. Subtracting Percentages
  D. Multiplying Percentages
  E. Dividing Percentages
  F. Percent Increase and Decrease (Percent Change)
  G. Simple and Compound Interest

VI. **Converting Percents, Fractions, and Decimals**
  A. Converting Fractions to Percents
  B. Converting Percents to Fractions
  C. Converting Fractions to Decimals
  D. Converting Decimals to Fractions
  E. Converting Percents to Decimals
  F. Converting Decimals to Percents

VII. **Ratios and Proportions**

VIII. **Powers and Exponents**

IX. **Logarithms**
  A. Base 10 and Natural Logarithms
  B. Solving Equations with Logarithms or Exponents
  C. Laws of Logarithms
    1. Addition
    2. Subtraction
    3. Multiplication
    4. Division

X. **Roots and Radicals**
  A. Square Root
  B. Cube Root
  C. Addition of Radicals
  D. Subtraction of Radicals
  E. Multiplying Radicals

XI. **Statistics**
  A. Mean
  B. Median
  C. Mode
  D. Probability

XII. **Basic Algebra**
    A. Simplifying Variable Expressions
    B. Factoring
    C. Slope of a Line
    D. Linear Equations
    E. Quadratic Equations and the Discriminant
    F. Rational Equations
    G. Logarithmic Equations

XIII. **Precalculus**
    A. Functions and Graphs
    B. Domain, Range, Symmetry
    C. Inverse Functions
    D. Linear Functions
    E. Quadratic Functions
    F. Rational Functions and Asymptotes
    G. Function Composition
    H. Distance Formula, Midpoint Formula
    I. Circle Equations, Completing the Square
    J. Average Rate of Change
    K. Graphing via Transformations (shifting, stretching, compressing, reflecting)
    L. Piecewise Functions

XIV. **Calculus**
    A. Derivatives of Functions
    B. Product Rule, Quotient Rule
    C. Limits
    D. Slope of a Tangent Line to a Curve
    E. Instantaneous Rate of Change
    F. Integrals of Functions
    G. Area Under a Curve
    H. Inflection Points and Concavity

XV. **Operations Concerning the Conversion of Basic Units of Measure**
(see Appendix)

XVI. **Word-Problem Solving—Analytical Reasoning**

XVII. **Interpretation of Graphs and Figures**

XVIII. **Probabilities**
    A. Venn Diagrams and Set Operations
    B. Counting Combinations
    C. Counting Permutations
    D. Calculating Probabilities of Independent Events

ANSWER SHEET
Quantitative Reasoning

1. Ⓐ Ⓑ Ⓒ Ⓓ
2. Ⓐ Ⓑ Ⓒ Ⓓ
3. Ⓐ Ⓑ Ⓒ Ⓓ
4. Ⓐ Ⓑ Ⓒ Ⓓ
5. Ⓐ Ⓑ Ⓒ Ⓓ
6. Ⓐ Ⓑ Ⓒ Ⓓ
7. Ⓐ Ⓑ Ⓒ Ⓓ
8. Ⓐ Ⓑ Ⓒ Ⓓ
9. Ⓐ Ⓑ Ⓒ Ⓓ
10. Ⓐ Ⓑ Ⓒ Ⓓ
11. Ⓐ Ⓑ Ⓒ Ⓓ
12. Ⓐ Ⓑ Ⓒ Ⓓ
13. Ⓐ Ⓑ Ⓒ Ⓓ
14. Ⓐ Ⓑ Ⓒ Ⓓ
15. Ⓐ Ⓑ Ⓒ Ⓓ
16. Ⓐ Ⓑ Ⓒ Ⓓ
17. Ⓐ Ⓑ Ⓒ Ⓓ
18. Ⓐ Ⓑ Ⓒ Ⓓ
19. Ⓐ Ⓑ Ⓒ Ⓓ
20. Ⓐ Ⓑ Ⓒ Ⓓ
21. Ⓐ Ⓑ Ⓒ Ⓓ
22. Ⓐ Ⓑ Ⓒ Ⓓ
23. Ⓐ Ⓑ Ⓒ Ⓓ
24. Ⓐ Ⓑ Ⓒ Ⓓ
25. Ⓐ Ⓑ Ⓒ Ⓓ

26. Ⓐ Ⓑ Ⓒ Ⓓ
27. Ⓐ Ⓑ Ⓒ Ⓓ
28. Ⓐ Ⓑ Ⓒ Ⓓ
29. Ⓐ Ⓑ Ⓒ Ⓓ
30. Ⓐ Ⓑ Ⓒ Ⓓ
31. Ⓐ Ⓑ Ⓒ Ⓓ
32. Ⓐ Ⓑ Ⓒ Ⓓ
33. Ⓐ Ⓑ Ⓒ Ⓓ
34. Ⓐ Ⓑ Ⓒ Ⓓ
35. Ⓐ Ⓑ Ⓒ Ⓓ
36. Ⓐ Ⓑ Ⓒ Ⓓ
37. Ⓐ Ⓑ Ⓒ Ⓓ
38. Ⓐ Ⓑ Ⓒ Ⓓ
39. Ⓐ Ⓑ Ⓒ Ⓓ
40. Ⓐ Ⓑ Ⓒ Ⓓ
41. Ⓐ Ⓑ Ⓒ Ⓓ
42. Ⓐ Ⓑ Ⓒ Ⓓ
43. Ⓐ Ⓑ Ⓒ Ⓓ
44. Ⓐ Ⓑ Ⓒ Ⓓ
45. Ⓐ Ⓑ Ⓒ Ⓓ
46. Ⓐ Ⓑ Ⓒ Ⓓ
47. Ⓐ Ⓑ Ⓒ Ⓓ
48. Ⓐ Ⓑ Ⓒ Ⓓ
49. Ⓐ Ⓑ Ⓒ Ⓓ
50. Ⓐ Ⓑ Ⓒ Ⓓ

51. Ⓐ Ⓑ Ⓒ Ⓓ
52. Ⓐ Ⓑ Ⓒ Ⓓ
53. Ⓐ Ⓑ Ⓒ Ⓓ
54. Ⓐ Ⓑ Ⓒ Ⓓ
55. Ⓐ Ⓑ Ⓒ Ⓓ
56. Ⓐ Ⓑ Ⓒ Ⓓ
57. Ⓐ Ⓑ Ⓒ Ⓓ
58. Ⓐ Ⓑ Ⓒ Ⓓ
59. Ⓐ Ⓑ Ⓒ Ⓓ
60. Ⓐ Ⓑ Ⓒ Ⓓ
61. Ⓐ Ⓑ Ⓒ Ⓓ
62. Ⓐ Ⓑ Ⓒ Ⓓ
63. Ⓐ Ⓑ Ⓒ Ⓓ
64. Ⓐ Ⓑ Ⓒ Ⓓ
65. Ⓐ Ⓑ Ⓒ Ⓓ
66. Ⓐ Ⓑ Ⓒ Ⓓ
67. Ⓐ Ⓑ Ⓒ Ⓓ
68. Ⓐ Ⓑ Ⓒ Ⓓ
69. Ⓐ Ⓑ Ⓒ Ⓓ
70. Ⓐ Ⓑ Ⓒ Ⓓ
71. Ⓐ Ⓑ Ⓒ Ⓓ
72. Ⓐ Ⓑ Ⓒ Ⓓ
73. Ⓐ Ⓑ Ⓒ Ⓓ
74. Ⓐ Ⓑ Ⓒ Ⓓ
75. Ⓐ Ⓑ Ⓒ Ⓓ

76. Ⓐ Ⓑ Ⓒ Ⓓ
77. Ⓐ Ⓑ Ⓒ Ⓓ
78. Ⓐ Ⓑ Ⓒ Ⓓ
79. Ⓐ Ⓑ Ⓒ Ⓓ
80. Ⓐ Ⓑ Ⓒ Ⓓ
81. Ⓐ Ⓑ Ⓒ Ⓓ
82. Ⓐ Ⓑ Ⓒ Ⓓ
83. Ⓐ Ⓑ Ⓒ Ⓓ
84. Ⓐ Ⓑ Ⓒ Ⓓ
85. Ⓐ Ⓑ Ⓒ Ⓓ
86. Ⓐ Ⓑ Ⓒ Ⓓ
87. Ⓐ Ⓑ Ⓒ Ⓓ
88. Ⓐ Ⓑ Ⓒ Ⓓ
89. Ⓐ Ⓑ Ⓒ Ⓓ
90. Ⓐ Ⓑ Ⓒ Ⓓ
91. Ⓐ Ⓑ Ⓒ Ⓓ
92. Ⓐ Ⓑ Ⓒ Ⓓ
93. Ⓐ Ⓑ Ⓒ Ⓓ
94. Ⓐ Ⓑ Ⓒ Ⓓ
95. Ⓐ Ⓑ Ⓒ Ⓓ
96. Ⓐ Ⓑ Ⓒ Ⓓ
97. Ⓐ Ⓑ Ⓒ Ⓓ
98. Ⓐ Ⓑ Ⓒ Ⓓ
99. Ⓐ Ⓑ Ⓒ Ⓓ
100. Ⓐ Ⓑ Ⓒ Ⓓ

100 Questions

> **Directions:** Select the best answer to each of the following questions.

1. Given the function $h(x) = \dfrac{3e^x + 1}{x^2 - 2}$, compute $\dfrac{dy}{dx}$.

   (A) $\dfrac{(x^2 - 2)(3e^x) + (2x)(3e^x + 1)}{(x^2 - 2)^2}$

   (B) $\dfrac{(x^2 - 2)(3e^x) - (2x)(3e^x + 1)}{(x^2 - 2)^2}$

   (C) $\dfrac{(2x)(3e^x + 1) - (x^2 - 2)(3e^x)}{(x^2 - 2)^2}$

   (D) $\dfrac{3e^x}{2x}$

QUESTIONS 2 AND 3 ARE BASED ON THE FOLLOWING TABLE:

Cause of Death	# of Deaths
Accidents and adverse effects	400
Homicide and legal intervention	185
Suicide	88
Malignant neoplasms	34
Diseases of the heart	290
Human immunodeficiency virus infection	12
Congenital anomalies	99
Chronic obstructive pulmonary diseases	94
Pneumonia and influenza	125
Cerebrovascular diseases	20
All other causes	300

2. What percentage of deaths was due to suicide or diseases of the heart?

   (A) 24%
   (B) 22.95%
   (C) 18.95%
   (D) 21%

3. What percentage of deaths was not due to malignant neoplasms?

(A) 2.1%

(B) 84.6%

(C) 97.9%

(D) 15.4%

---

4. John has $2.40 in quarters and nickels. He has three times as many nickels as quarters. How many nickels does he have?

(A) 6

(B) 20

(C) 8

(D) 18

5. Simplify the expression $\dfrac{x^2 + 18x + 80}{x + 8}$.

(A) $x - 10$

(B) $x - 12$

(C) $x + 10$

(D) $x + 12$

QUESTIONS 6 THROUGH 8 ARE BASED ON THE GRAPH BELOW OF THE FUNCTION $y = f(x)$:

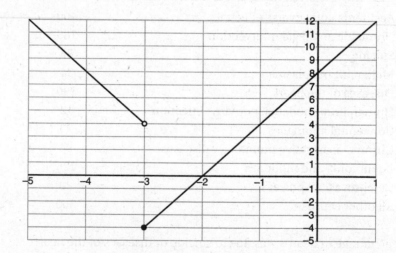

6. $\lim\limits_{x \to -3^+} f(x) =$

(A) 1 and –3

(B) does not exist

(C) 1 or –3

(D) –4

7. $\lim\limits_{x \to -3^-} f(x) =$

   (A) 4
   (B) does not exist
   (C) 1 or –3
   (D) 1 and –3

8. $\lim\limits_{x \to -3} f(x) =$

   (A) –4
   (B) does not exist
   (C) 4 or –4
   (D) 4 and –4

———————————————————

9. During a 6-hour flight, a plane flew 325 mph for the first 2 hours, 450 mph for the next 3 hours, and 300 mph for the last hour. What was the plane's approximate average speed for the entire flight?

   (A) 204 mph
   (B) 366 mph
   (C) 383 mph
   (D) 251 mph

10. $\log(8) + \log(6) =$

    (A) $\log(48)$
    (B) $\log(14)$
    (C) $\log(8) \cdot \log(6)$
    (D) $\log(8^6)$

11. $\sqrt{48} + \sqrt{300} =$

    (A) $14\sqrt{3}$
    (B) $\sqrt{348}$
    (C) $40\sqrt{3}$
    (D) $14\sqrt{6}$

12. Mike can wash a car in 45 minutes. His brother takes twice as long to do the same job. Working together, how many cars can they wash in 6 hours?

    (A) 12
    (B) 10
    (C) 8
    (D) 14

13. A fair coin is tossed 12 times. What is the probability that the fifth toss comes up heads?

(A) $\frac{1}{2}$

(B) $\frac{5}{12}$

(C) $\frac{1}{5}$

(D) $\frac{1}{12}$

14. A number is chosen at random from the set {1, 5, 9, 13, 15, 18, 20, 21, 30}. What is the probability that the chosen number is divisible by 5 or divisible by 9?

(A) 0.67%

(B) 33%

(C) 0.33%

(D) 67%

15. $\left(\frac{1}{x}\right)^6 + \left(\frac{2}{x^2}\right)^3 =$

(A) $3x^4$

(B) $\frac{9}{x^6}$

(C) $6x$

(D) $\frac{1}{2x^4}$

16. $\log_5(125) =$

(A) 3

(B) $\frac{1}{3}$

(C) 5

(D) $\frac{1}{5}$

17. $8 - 3^2(2 - 6 + [8 - 2]) + 1 =$

(A) 27

(B) 9

(C) −27

(D) −9

18. 300 cm is approximately

    (A) 3.28 yards
    (B) 2.86 yards
    (C) 3.68 yards
    (D) 2.28 yards

QUESTIONS 19 AND 20 ARE BASED ON THE GRAPH DATA SHOWN BELOW:

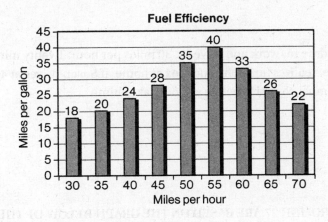

19. What is the mean value for miles per gallon?

    (A) 27.33
    (B) 26
    (C) 29
    (D) 25.24

20. What is the median value for miles per gallon?

    (A) 29
    (B) 24.89
    (C) 26
    (D) 25.24

21. $\int\limits_{1/e}^{e^3} \left(\dfrac{8}{x}\right) dx =$

    (A) 32

    (B) $\dfrac{8}{e^3} - \dfrac{8}{e^{-1}}$

    (C) 7

    (D) $\dfrac{8}{e^3} + \dfrac{8}{e^{-1}}$

22. Event A has a probability of $\frac{3}{8}$. What is the probability that event A does not occur?

   (A) $\frac{5}{8}$

   (B) $\frac{8}{3}$

   (C) $\frac{10}{3}$

   (D) $\frac{3}{10}$

23. Parks leaves home for work and drives at 30 miles per hour. Twenty minutes later, Susan, his wife, realizes he left his tool box at home. If Susan drives at 40 miles per hour, how far must she drive before she overtakes him?

   (A) 20 miles
   (B) 30 miles
   (C) 40 miles
   (D) 60 miles

QUESTIONS 24 THROUGH 27 ARE BASED ON THE GRAPH BELOW OF THE FUNCTION $y = f(x)$:

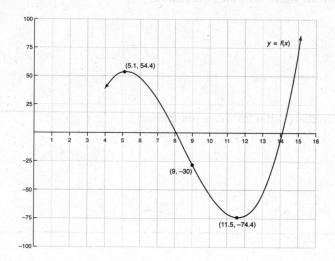

24. Identify the interval(s) for which $f' > 0$.

   (A) $(5.1, 11.5)$
   (B) $[5.1, 11.5]$
   (C) $(-\infty, 5.1) \cup (11.5, \infty)$
   (D) $[-\infty, 5.1] \cup [11.5, \infty]$

25. Identify the x value(s) at which the graph has a relative minimum.

   (A) $x = 5.1$
   (B) $x = 9$
   (C) $x = 11.5$
   (D) $x = 14$

26. Identify the interval(s) on which $f''(x) < 0$.

    (A) $[-\infty, 9]$
    (B) $(5.1, 11.5)$
    (C) $[5.1, 11.5]$
    (D) $(-\infty, 9)$

27. $\lim\limits_{x \to 9}\left(\dfrac{f(x) - f(9)}{x - 9} \right) \approx$

    (A) 0
    (B) -21
    (C) 21
    (D) Not enough information

---

28. A pair of fair six-sided dice is thrown. What is the probability that the sum of the numbers shown is equal to 7?

    (A) $\dfrac{1}{6}$

    (B) $\dfrac{1}{12}$

    (C) $\dfrac{1}{3}$

    (D) $\dfrac{2}{3}$

29. A computer password consists of 5 different characters chosen from the set $\{A, B, C, D, E, F, 1, 2, 3, 4, 5, 6\}$. How many different passwords are possible?

    (A) $\dfrac{12!}{5!}$

    (B) $\dfrac{12!}{7!}$

    (C) $\dfrac{12!}{7!5!}$

    (D) $\dfrac{5!}{12!7!}$

30. A box contains apples and oranges in a ratio of 8:5. If the box contains 45 oranges, how many apples does the box contain?

    (A) 72
    (B) 48
    (C) 36
    (D) 63

31. In a student survey, 300 students indicated that they would attend Summer Session I, and 220 students indicated that they would attend Summer Session II. If 90 students plan to attend both summer sessions and 115 students indicated that they would attend neither session, how many students participated in the survey?

    (A) 545
    (B) 635
    (C) 430
    (D) Not enough information

32. Find the extreme value of the given function and state whether that value represents a maximum or a minimum value for the function.

$$P(x) = 80x^2 - 320x + 500$$

    (A) 180, maximum
    (B) 2, minimum
    (C) 2, maximum
    (D) 180, minimum

33. A patient weighs 78 kilograms. What is the patient's approximate weight in pounds?

    (A) 171.60
    (B) 168.40
    (C) 176.20
    (D) 166.80

34. Find the vertex value for the given function.

$$f(x) = -14x^2 + 560x - 1$$

    (A) (-20, 5599)
    (B) (20, 0)
    (C) (-20, 5099)
    (D) (20, 5599)

35. A truck is 60 miles from its destination at 4:00 P.M. At what speed must the truck travel to arrive by 4:45 P.M.?

    (A) 80 mph
    (B) 75 mph
    (C) 70 mph
    (D) 85 mph

36. Given the following equation:

$$°C = \frac{5}{9} (°F - 32)$$

Convert 50°F to °C.

(A) 10
(B) 14
(C) 12
(D) 16

37. Find all the real solutions for the quadratic equation $3x^2 + 2x + 5 = 0$.

(A) $x = \dfrac{-2 \pm \sqrt{56}}{6}$

(B) No real solutions

(C) $x = \dfrac{-2 \pm \sqrt{-56}}{6}$

(D) $x = \dfrac{-2 \pm \sqrt{60}}{6}$

38. $6^2 \cdot 6^3 =$

(A) 46,656
(B) 7,776
(C) 1,296
(D) 248,832

39. $\dfrac{8}{9} - \dfrac{1}{2} =$

(A) $\dfrac{6}{18}$

(B) $\dfrac{7}{18}$

(C) $\dfrac{5}{18}$

(D) $\dfrac{3}{18}$

40. A dose of 400 milligrams of Drug A is equivalent to a dose of 900 milligrams of Drug B. A patient takes 650 milligrams of Drug B. What is the approximate equivalent dose of Drug A?

(A) 306 mg
(B) 312 mg
(C) 269 mg
(D) 289 mg

41. $4^3 + 4^{-1} =$

    (A) 16

    (B) 66

    (C) 8

    (D) $\dfrac{257}{4}$

42. A number is chosen at random from the set {1, 2, 3, 4, 5, 6, 7, 8, 9, 10, 11, 12}. What is the probability that the chosen number is NOT divisible by 2 and NOT divisible by 3?

    (A) $\dfrac{1}{3}$

    (B) $\dfrac{3}{5}$

    (C) $\dfrac{3}{4}$

    (D) $\dfrac{2}{5}$

43. 250 milligrams of aminophylline injection is equivalent to 200 milligrams of theophylline. The strength of aminophylline injection is 25 milligrams per milliliter. How many milliliters of aminophylline injection are needed to provide a dose of 320 milligrams of theophylline?

    (A) 10.67

    (B) 12.8

    (C) 16

    (D) 20

44. A patient's creatine clearance rate (CrCl) can be calculated by using the following formula:

$$\text{CrCl} = \frac{140 - \text{age in years}}{72 \cdot \text{SCr}} \cdot (\text{ideal body weight in kilograms})$$

What is the approximate CrCl for a 74-year-old patient who has a SCr of 3.2 and an ideal body weight of 84 kg?

    (A) 34

    (B) 24

    (C) 28

    (D) 38

45. The graph of function $y = f(x)$ contains the point $(3, -1)$. Determine which point must be on the graph of $y = 5 \cdot f(x + 2) - 3$.

    (A) $(1, -8)$

    (B) $(5, -8)$

    (C) $(1, -20)$

    (D) $(5, -20)$

46. Consider a circle centered at the origin with a radius equal to 5. Find the slope of the tangent line to the circle at the point (3, 4).

(A) $\dfrac{3}{4}$

(B) $-\dfrac{3}{4}$

(C) $\dfrac{4}{3}$

(D) $-\dfrac{4}{3}$

QUESTIONS 47 AND 48 ARE BASED ON THE GRAPH BELOW:

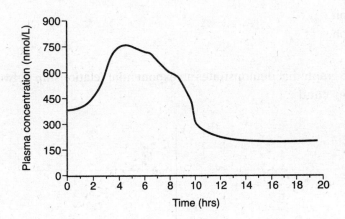

47. What is the maximum plasma concentration?

(A) 200 nmol/L
(B) 600 nmol/L
(C) 400 nmol/L
(D) 750 nmol/L

48. When does the maximum plasma concentration occur?

(A) after 4 hours
(B) after 2 hours
(C) after 10 hours
(D) after 12 hours

49. Determine the length of the line segment with endpoints (3, 6) and (–2, 5).

    (A) $\sqrt{24}$

    (B) $\sqrt{23}$

    (C) $\sqrt{26}$

    (D) $\sqrt{27}$

50. Larry's house is 12 miles from the park. Larry rode his bicycle from his house to the park at 12 miles per hour. He then walked the bicycle home from the park at 3 miles per hour. If he took the same route on both trips, what was his average speed?

    (A) 4.8 mph

    (B) 7.5 mph

    (C) 1.6 mph

    (D) 4.0 mph

51. Identify the graph that demonstrates an exponential relationship between the variables x and y.

(A) 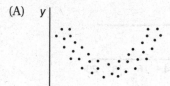   (B)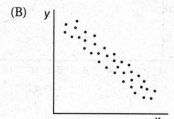

(C) 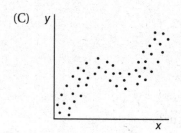   (D)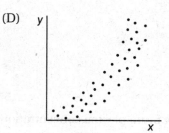

52. Determine the radius of a circle with the equation $x^2 + 6x + y^2 - 10y - 3 = 0$.

    (A) 37

    (B) $\sqrt{37}$

    (C) 34

    (D) $\sqrt{34}$

53. What is the mean of the given data set {10, 11, 9, 7, 5, 6}?

    (A) 9.5

    (B) 8

    (C) 8.5

    (D) 9

QUESTIONS 54 AND 55 ARE BASED ON THE FOLLOWING INFORMATION AND GRAPH:

Let $y = f(x)$ be a function whose first derivative yields the graph shown below.

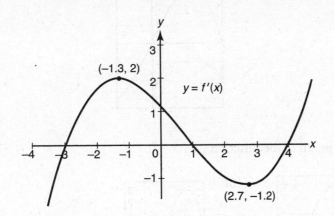

54. Determine the interval(s) on which the function $y = f(x)$ is increasing.

    (A) $(-\infty, -1.3) \cup (2.7, \infty)$

    (B) $(-3, 1) \cup (4, \infty)$

    (C) $[-\infty, -1.3] \cup [2.7, \infty]$

    (D) $[-3, 1] \cup [4, \infty]$

55. Determine the interval(s) on which the function $y = f(x)$ is concave down.

    (A) $(-\infty, 0)$

    (B) $[-1.3, 2.7]$

    (C) $[-\infty, 0]$

    (D) $(-1.3, 2.7)$

---

56. A particle moves along a horizontal line so that its position at time t is given by the function $p(t) = t^3 - 6t^2$. Determine the values of t for which the particle is moving to the left.

    (A) $0 < t < 4$

    (B) $0 \le t \le 4$

    (C) $t > 4$

    (D) $t \ge 4$

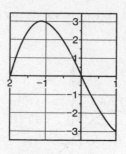

57. Identify the graph of the function $y = f(x - 2)$.

(A)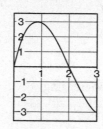

(B)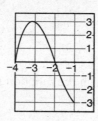

(C)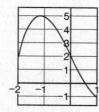

(D)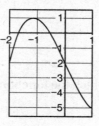

58. Identify the graph of the function $y = f(x) - 2$.

(A)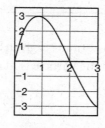

(B)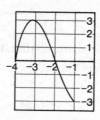

(C)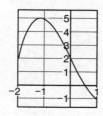

(D)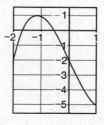

59. Lisa's gas tank is $\frac{2}{3}$ full. She completely fills the tank by putting in an additional

8 gallons. What is the capacity of the gas tank?

(A) 18 gallons
(B) 24 gallons
(C) 26 gallons
(D) 20 gallons

60. A walk-in clinic sees approximately 45% of its daily patients before noon. If the clinic sees a total of 40 patients on a given day, how many patients were seen **after** noon?

(A) 18
(B) 20
(C) 24
(D) 22

61. The height h of a projectile is given by $h(x) = -0.002x^2 + x$, where x is the horizontal distance the projectile travels. The projectile hits the ground after it has traveled a horizontal distance of

(A) 600 feet.
(B) 400 feet.
(C) 200 feet.
(D) 500 feet.

62. Express the distance from point P to point Q as a function of the x-coordinate of point P.

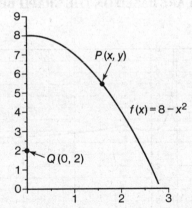

(A) $\sqrt{x^2 - \left(6 - x^2\right)^2}$

(B) $x^2 + \left(6 - x^2\right)^2$

(C) $\sqrt{x^2 + \left(6 - x^2\right)^2}$

(D) $x^2 - \left(6 - x^2\right)^2$

63. A bag contains four red balls and eight black balls. A ball is selected from the bag at random. What is the probability that the ball is red?

(A) $\dfrac{1}{3}$

(B) $\dfrac{1}{4}$

(C) $\dfrac{3}{4}$

(D) $\dfrac{2}{3}$

64. $\ln(100) - \ln(10) =$

(A) $\ln(90)$

(B) $\ln(10)$

(C) $\dfrac{\ln(100)}{\ln(10)}$

(D) $\ln(110)$

65. A jar contains 5 pennies, 4 nickels, and 6 dimes. What is the probability that a randomly chosen coin is NOT a dime?

(A) 60%

(B) 40%

(C) 0.40%

(D) 0.60%

QUESTIONS 66 THROUGH 71 ARE BASED ON THE GRAPH BELOW OF THE FUNCTION $y = f(x)$:

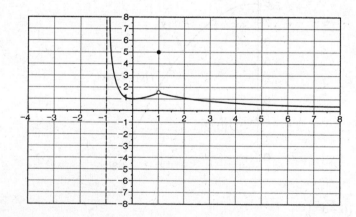

66. $\displaystyle\lim_{x \to 1^{+}} f(x) =$

(A) 1.5

(B) 5

(C) Does not exist

(D) 1.5 and 5

67. $\displaystyle\lim_{x \to -1^+} f(x) =$

   (A) ∞
   (B) $-\infty$
   (C) $\pm\infty$
   (D) -1

68. $\displaystyle\lim_{x \to \infty} f(x) =$

   (A) ∞
   (B) Undefined
   (C) $-\infty$
   (D) 0

69. The equation of the vertical asymptote is

   (A) $x = -1$.
   (B) $x = \infty$.
   (C) $x = -\infty$.
   (D) $x = 0$.

70. The equation of the horizontal asymptote is

   (A) $y = -1$.
   (B) $y = 0$.
   (C) $y = \infty$.
   (D) $y = -\infty$.

71. Determine the parabola with the equation $y = ax^2 + bx$ whose tangent line at the point $(1, 1)$ is given by $y = 3x - 2$.

   (A) $y = 2x^2 + x$
   (B) $y = 2x^2 - x$
   (C) $y = -2x^2 - x$
   (D) $y = -2x^2 + x$

_____

72. Determine the average rate of change of the function $f(x) = x^2$ on the interval $1 \le x \le 3$.

   (A) 4
   (B) 8
   (C) 3
   (D) 6

73. If 500 milligrams of drug A equal 400 milligrams of drug B, what is the equivalent dose of drug B for a patient taking 250 mg of drug A?

(A) 200 mg
(B) 240 mg
(C) 250 mg
(D) 300 mg

74. Determine the domain for the function $f(x) = \dfrac{x^2}{x^2 - 6}$.

(A) $\left\{ x : x = -\sqrt{6}, \, x = \sqrt{6} \right\}$
(B) $\left\{ x : x = -\sqrt{6}, \, x = 0 \right\}$
(C) $\left\{ x : x \neq -\sqrt{6}, \, x = 0, \, x \neq \sqrt{6} \right\}$
(D) $\left\{ x : x \neq -\sqrt{6}, \, x \neq \sqrt{6} \right\}$

75. $\dfrac{\sqrt{36} \cdot \sqrt{16}}{\sqrt{9}}$

(A) $\dfrac{6 \cdot 4}{3} = 12$

(B) $\dfrac{6 \cdot 4}{3} = 8$

(C) $\dfrac{4 \cdot 4}{4} = 4$

(D) $\dfrac{4 \cdot 3}{2} = 6$

76. The quadratic equation $bx^2 + cx + a = 0$ has solutions given by which of the following?

(A) $x = \dfrac{-c \pm \sqrt{c^2 - 4ba}}{2b}$

(B) $x = -c \pm \dfrac{\sqrt{c^2 - 4ba}}{2b}$

(C) $x = \dfrac{-b \pm \sqrt{b^2 - 4ac}}{2a}$

(D) $x = -b \pm \dfrac{\sqrt{b^2 - 4ac}}{2a}$

77. Given the function $f(x) = \begin{cases} 3x^2 & \text{for } x < 2 \\ 1 - 5x & \text{for } x > 2 \end{cases}$, evaluate the limit.

$\lim_{x \to 2} f(x) =$

(A) Undefined
(B) 12
(C) −9
(D) −9 and 12

78. The equation $5(x + 2)(x - 1) = 5x^2 + 6x$ has the solution

(A) $x = 10$.
(B) $x = -10$.
(C) $x = -\dfrac{2}{5}$.
(D) $x = \dfrac{2}{5}$.

QUESTIONS 79 AND 80 ARE BASED ON THE SURVEY DATA SHOWN IN THE TABLE BELOW:

Seat Belt Worn	Probability
Never	0.0416
Rarely	0.0532
Sometimes	0.1004
Most of the time	0.2238
Always	0.5810

79. What is the probability that someone sometimes wears a seat belt or most of the time wears a seat belt?

(A) 0.3422%
(B) 34.22%
(C) 0.3242%
(D) 32.42%

80. If 6,400 people participated in the survey, approximately how many people never wear a seat belt?

(A) 2,662
(B) 266
(C) 116
(D) 2,162

81. A pair of six-sided dice is thrown. What is the probability that the sum of the numbers shown is NOT equal to 7?

(A) $\dfrac{2}{3}$

(B) $\dfrac{1}{6}$

(C) $\dfrac{1}{3}$

(D) $\dfrac{5}{6}$

82. Find the exact value of the shaded area in the graph below.

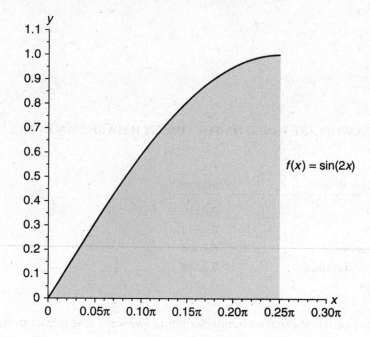

$f(x) = \sin(2x)$

(A) 4

(B) 1

(C) 2

(D) $\dfrac{1}{2}$

83. Consider the function $F(x) = g(h(x))$ where g and h are differentiable functions with the given properties.

$$
\begin{aligned}
h(4) &= 7 & h'(4) &= 11 \\
h(2) &= 4 & h'(2) &= 8 \\
g(2) &= 5 & g'(4) &= 9 \\
g(8) &= 6 & g'(8) &= 10
\end{aligned}
$$

Determine the exact value of $\dfrac{dF}{dx}$ when $x = 2$.

(A) 48
(B) 10
(C) 72
(D) 6

84. If $x < 10$, then $\dfrac{x^2 - 11x + 10}{|x - 10|} =$

(A) $-x + 1$
(B) $-x - 1$
(C) $x - 1$
(D) $x + 1$

85. Event A has a probability of 0.26. Event B has a probability of 0.42. The probability that events A and B both occur is 0.12. What is the probability that either event A or event B occurs?

(A) 0.68
(B) 0.44
(C) 0.56
(D) 0.32

86. Set A contains 20 elements. Set B contains 11 elements. Set $A \cap B$ contains 5 elements. Determine the number of elements in the set $A \cup B$.

(A) 26
(B) 31
(C) 36
(D) Not enough information

87. Determine the slope of the line passing through the points (2, 9) and (−5, 8).

(A) $\dfrac{1}{7}$

(B) $-\dfrac{1}{7}$

(C) $\dfrac{17}{3}$

(D) $-\dfrac{17}{3}$

88. If $\ln(w + 5x) = 3$, then

   (A) $x = \dfrac{e^3 - w}{5}$

   (B) $x = \dfrac{e^3 + w}{5}$

   (C) $x = \dfrac{3e - w}{5}$

   (D) $x = \dfrac{3e + w}{5}$

89. $\log(9) - \log(5)$ is the same as

   (A) $\log(4)$

   (B) $\log\left(\dfrac{9}{5}\right)$

   (C) $\dfrac{\log(9)}{\log(5)}$

   (D) $\log(45)$

90. Find the equation of the horizontal asymptote for the given function.

$$f(x) = \frac{3x + 1}{5 - 4x}$$

   (A) $y = -\dfrac{4}{5}$

   (B) $y = \dfrac{3}{4}$

   (C) $y = \dfrac{4}{5}$

   (D) $y = -\dfrac{3}{4}$

91. Write the equation of the line passing through the point $(5, -7)$ that is perpendicular to the line with the equation $y = 4$.

   (A) $x = -\dfrac{1}{4}$

   (B) $x = -4$

   (C) $x = 5$

   (D) $x = -7$

92. How many different ways can a 5-person committee be chosen from a group of 12 people?

   (A) $\dfrac{12!}{7!}$

   (B) $\dfrac{12!}{5!}$

   (C) $\dfrac{12!}{5!7!}$

   (D) $\dfrac{12!}{5!+7!}$

93. Convert 86°F to Kelvin.

   (A) 30
   (B) 243
   (C) 54
   (D) 303

94. Determine the domain of the function $f(x) = \ln(4x - 2)$.

   (A) $(-\infty, \infty)$
   (B) $[-\infty, \infty]$
   (C) $[0.5, \infty)$
   (D) $(0.5, \infty)$

95. A rental car company charges $25 per day, plus 12 cents per mile. Express the total rental cost of a 6-day rental as a function of the number of miles driven, x.

   (A) $C(x) = 25 + 12x$
   (B) $C(x) = 25 + 0.12x$
   (C) $C(x) = 150 + 12x$
   (D) $C(x) = 150 + 0.12x$

QUESTIONS 96 THROUGH 98 ARE BASED ON THE GRAPH BELOW OF THE FUNCTION $y = f(x)$:

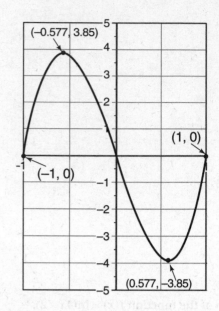

96. Choose the statement that best describes the function $y = f(x)$ with the given graph.

    (A) $y = f(x)$ is an even function.
    (B) $y = f(x)$ is a quadratic function.
    (C) $y = f(x)$ is an odd function.
    (D) $y = f(x)$ is a linear function.

97. Determine the domain of the function $y = f(x)$ with the given graph.

    (A) (–1, 1)
    (B) [–1, 1]
    (C) (–3.85, 3.85)
    (D) [–3.85, 3.85]

98. Determine the range of the function $y = f(x)$ with the given graph.

    (A) (–1, 1)
    (B) [–1, 1]
    (C) (–3.85, 3.85)
    (D) [–3.85, 3.85]

99. Kate had a box of red and blue crayons in a ratio of 5:9. If she had 20 red crayons, how many more blue crayons did she have than red?

   (A) 9
   (B) 16
   (C) 4
   (D) 11

100. $\frac{4}{11} - \frac{3}{8} =$

   (A) $\frac{1}{3}$

   (B) $\frac{1}{88}$

   (C) $-\frac{1}{3}$

   (D) $-\frac{1}{88}$

1.	B	26.	D	51.	D	76.	A
2.	B	27.	B	52.	B	77.	A
3.	C	28.	A	53.	B	78.	B
4.	D	29.	B	54.	D	79.	D
5.	C	30.	A	55.	D	80.	B
6.	D	31.	A	56.	A	81.	D
7.	A	32.	D	57.	A	82.	D
8.	B	33.	A	58.	D	83.	C
9.	C	34.	D	59.	B	84.	A
10.	A	35.	A	60.	D	85.	C
11.	A	36.	A	61.	D	86.	A
12.	A	37.	B	62.	C	87.	A
13.	A	38.	B	63.	A	88.	A
14.	D	39.	B	64.	B	89.	B
15.	B	40.	D	65.	A	90.	D
16.	A	41.	D	66.	A	91.	C
17.	D	42.	A	67.	A	92.	C
18.	A	43.	C	68.	D	93.	D
19.	A	44.	B	69.	A	94.	D
20.	C	45.	A	70.	B	95.	D
21.	A	46.	B	71.	B	96.	C
22.	A	47.	D	72.	A	97.	B
23.	C	48.	A	73.	A	98.	D
24.	C	49.	C	74.	D	99.	B
25.	C	50.	A	75.	B	100.	D

ANSWERS EXPLAINED

1. **(B)** We use the Quotient Rule for derivatives.

$$\frac{d}{dx}\left(\frac{f(x)}{g(x)}\right)=\frac{g(x)\cdot f'(x)-g'(x)\cdot f(x)}{\left(g(x)\right)^2}=\frac{\left(x^2-2\right)\left(3e^x\right)-(2x)\left(3e^x+1\right)}{\left(x^2-2\right)^2}$$

2. **(B)** There were $88 + 290 = 378$ deaths due to suicide or diseases of the heart. There were 1,647 total deaths. Thus, the desired probability is given by

$$\frac{378}{1647}\approx 0.2295 = 22.95\%.$$

3. **(C)** The percentage of deaths due to malignant neoplasms was $\frac{34}{1647}=0.021=2.1\%.$ Thus, the percentage of deaths not due to malignant neoplasms was $1-0.021=0.979=97.9\%.$

4. **(D)** Let $x =$ the number of quarters, and $3x =$ the number of nickels. This yields the equation $25\cdot x+5\cdot 3x =$ total money in cents. So we solve

$$25\cdot x + 5\cdot 3x = 240$$

$$40x = 240 \Rightarrow x = \frac{240}{40}=6$$

The number of nickels is $3x = (3)(6) = 18$.

5. **(C)** We simplify the expression as follows:

$$\frac{x^2+18x+80}{x+8}=\frac{(x+8)(x+10)}{x+8}=x+10$$

6. **(D)** As x approaches -3 from the right-hand side, the values of $f(x)$ approach -4.

7. **(A)** As x approaches -3 from the left-hand side, the values of $f(x)$ approach 4.

8. **(B)** The left-hand and right-hand limits are not equal.

9. **(C)** The plane travels $325\cdot 2 = 650$ miles during the first 2 hours, $450\cdot 3 = 1,350$ miles during the next 3 hours, and 300 miles during the last hour. Therefore, we have:

$$\text{average speed} = \frac{\text{total distance}}{\text{total time}}=\frac{650+1350+300 \text{ miles}}{6 \text{ hrs}}\approx 383 \text{ mph}$$

10. **(A)** We use the Product Rule for logarithms as follows:

$$\log(8)+\log(6)=\log(8\cdot 6)=\log(48)$$

11. **(A)** We simplify the expression as follows:

$$\sqrt{48}+\sqrt{300}=\sqrt{16\cdot 3}+\sqrt{100\cdot 3}=4\sqrt{3}+10\sqrt{3}=14\sqrt{3}$$

12. **(A)** Mike can wash 1 car every 45 minutes $= 0.75$ hours. Thus, in 6 hours he can wash $\frac{6}{0.75}=8$ cars. His brother can wash 1 car every 90 minutes $= 1.5$ hours. Thus, in 6 hours he can wash $\frac{6}{1.5}=4$ cars. Working together, they can wash 12 cars ($8 + 4 = 12$ cars) in 6 hours.

13. **(A)** The probability of getting heads on a single toss is $\frac{1}{2}$. Each toss is independent, so the probability of getting heads on the fifth toss is $\frac{1}{2}$.

14. **(D)** There are six numbers divisible by 5 or 9 (5, 9, 15, 18, 20, and 30). There are nine numbers in the set. The desired probability is calculated as $\frac{6}{9} \approx 0.67 = 67\%$.

15. **(B)**

$$\left(\frac{1}{x}\right)^6 + \left(\frac{2}{x^2}\right)^3 = \frac{1^6}{x^6} + \frac{2^3}{\left(x^2\right)^3}$$

Rule: $\left(\frac{a}{b}\right)^n = \frac{a^n}{b^n}$

$$= \frac{1}{x^6} + \frac{8}{x^6}$$

Rule: $\left(a^n\right)^m = a^{n \cdot m}$

$$= \frac{9}{x^6}$$

16. **(A)** Note that $\log_5(125) = x$ is equivalent to the equation $5^x = 125$. This equation has the solution $x = 3$.

17. **(D)** We simplify the expression as follows:

$$8 - 3^2(2 - 6 + [8 - 2]) + 1 = 8 - 9(2 - 6 + [6]) + 1$$
$$= 8 - 9(-4 + 6) + 1$$
$$= 8 - 9(2) + 1$$
$$= 8 - 18 + 1$$
$$= -9$$

18. **(A)** We use the following conversions: 1 inch = 2.54 cm, 1 foot = 12 inches, and 1 yard = 3 feet.

$$(300 \text{ cm})\left(\frac{1 \text{ inch}}{2.54 \text{ cm}}\right)\left(\frac{1 \text{ foot}}{12 \text{ inches}}\right)\left(\frac{1 \text{ yard}}{3 \text{ feet}}\right) = \frac{300}{91.44} \approx 3.28 \text{ yards}$$

19. **(A)** We compute:

$$\frac{18 + 20 + 24 + 28 + 35 + 40 + 33 + 26 + 22}{9} = \frac{246}{9} = 27.33$$

20. **(C)** We list the values in increasing order: 18, 20, 22, 24, 26, 28, 33, 35, 40. The median value occurs at the middle position in the list; that is, the median = 26.

21. **(A)** We use the Fundamental Theorem of Calculus as follows:

$$\int_{1/e}^{e^3} \left(\frac{8}{x}\right) dx = 8\ln(x)\Big]_{1/e}^{e^3} = 8\left(\ln\left(e^3\right) - \ln(1/e)\right)$$
$$= 8\left(\ln\left(e^3\right) - \ln\left(e^{-1}\right)\right) = 8(3 + 1) = 32$$

22. **(A)** The probability that event A does not occur is given by:

$$1 - (\text{probability that event A does occur}) = 1 - \frac{3}{8} = \frac{5}{8}$$

23. **(C)** In 20 min. $\left(\frac{1}{3} \text{ hr.}\right)$, Parks has gone 10 mi. In another hour, he will have covered a total of 40 mi. $(10 + 30)$. Therefore, Susan must drive 40 mi. (for 1 hr.) to catch him.

24. **(C)** Note that $f' > 0$ when the graph has a positive slope, i.e., when the graph is increasing.

25. **(C)** The graph changes from decreasing to increasing at $x = 11.5$.

26. **(D)** The graph is concave down on the interval $(-\infty, 9)$.

27. **(B)** Note that $\lim_{x \to 9} \left(\frac{f(x) - f(9)}{x - 9}\right)$ equals the slope of the graph at the point where $x = 9$. We can approximate this slope by calculating the slope of the secant line that passes through the points $(8, 0)$ and $(11.5, -74.4)$:

$$\lim_{x \to 9}\left(\frac{f(x) - f(9)}{x - 9}\right) \approx \frac{-74.4 - 0}{11.5 - 8} \approx -21$$

28. **(A)** There are six ways that the sum of the numbers can equal 7, namely $1 + 6$, $2 + 5$, $3 + 4$, $6 + 1$, $5 + 2$, and $4 + 3$. Each die has six faces. This means that there are $(6)(6) = 36$ possible outcomes for tossing the two dice. Thus, the probability that the sum of the numbers equals 7 is given by $\frac{6}{36} = \frac{1}{6}$.

29. **(B)** We are choosing 5 elements from a 12-element set, without repetition, such that order matters. Thus, we are counting permutations. We use the formula:

$$_{12}P_5 = \frac{12!}{(12-5)!} = \frac{12!}{7!}$$

30. **(A)** Since the ratio of apples to oranges is 8:5, we solve with the following proportion:

$$\frac{8 \text{ apples}}{5 \text{ oranges}} = \frac{x \text{ apples}}{45 \text{ oranges}}$$

Note that $5 \cdot 9 = 45$. Thus, $8 \cdot 9 = x$. $x = 72$.

31. **(A)** Consider the following Venn diagram.

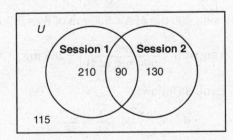

The total number of students $= 210 + 90 + 130 + 115 = 545$.

32. **(D)** Since the coefficient of the x^2 term is positive, P is a quadratic function whose graph is a parabola that opens up. This means that the function has its minimum value at the vertex of the parabola. The vertex of a quadratic function of the form $f(x) = ax^2 + bx + c$ occurs when $x = -\dfrac{b}{2a}$. Thus, the minimum value of $P(x) = 80x^2 - 320x + 500$ occurs when $x = -\dfrac{-320}{2(80)} = 2$. Therefore, P has a minimum value of $P(2) = 80(2)^2 - 320(2) + 500 = 180$.

33. **(A)** We use the conversion 1 kilogram $\approx$ 2.2 pounds as follows:

$$(78 \text{ kilograms})\left(\frac{2.2 \text{ pounds}}{1 \text{ kilogram}}\right) \approx 171.60 \text{ pounds}$$

34. **(D)** The vertex of a quadratic function of the form $f(x) = ax^2 + bx + c$ occurs when $x = -\dfrac{b}{2a}$. Thus, the vertex of $f(x) = -14x^2 + 560x - 1$ occurs when $x = -\dfrac{560}{2(-14)} = 20$. The y coordinate of the vertex is given by $f(20) = -14(20)^2 + 560(20) - 1 = 5599$. Therefore, the vertex is the point $(20, 5599)$.

35. **(A)** The truck must travel 60 miles in 45 minutes = 0.75 hour. We have the formula:

$$\text{speed} = \frac{\text{distance}}{\text{time}} = \frac{60 \text{ miles}}{0.75 \text{ hr}} = 80 \text{ mph}$$

36. **(A)** $^\circ C = \dfrac{5}{9}(50 - 32) = \dfrac{5}{9}(18) = 10$.

37. **(B)** We use the quadratic formula.

$$x = \frac{-b \pm \sqrt{b^2 - 4ac}}{2a} = \frac{-2 \pm \sqrt{2^2 - 4 \cdot 3 \cdot 5}}{2 \cdot 3} = \frac{-2 \pm \sqrt{-56}}{6}.$$

Since $\sqrt{-56}$ is not a real number, the equation has no real solutions.

38. **(B)** Note that $6^2 \cdot 6^3 = 6^{2+3} = 6^5 = 7{,}776$.

39. **(B)** The least common denominator for $\dfrac{8}{9}$ and $\dfrac{1}{2}$ is 18. Rewrite the fractions, using the least common denominator: $\dfrac{8 \cdot 2}{18} - \dfrac{1 \cdot 9}{18} = \dfrac{16}{18} - \dfrac{9}{18} = \dfrac{7}{18}$.

40. **(D)** We use the conversion 400 mg of A = 900 mg of B as follows:

$$(650 \text{ mg of B})\left(\frac{400 \text{ mg of A}}{900 \text{ mg of B}}\right) = 289 \text{ mg of A}$$

41. **(D)** We calculate the result as follows:

$$4^3 + 4^{-1} = 64 + \frac{1}{4} = \frac{257}{4}$$

42. **(A)** There are four numbers not divisible by either 2 or 3, that is, 1, 5, 7, 11.

Thus, the probability $= \dfrac{4}{12} = \dfrac{1}{3}$.

43. **(C)** 250 milligrams of aminophylline injection is equivalent to 200 milligrams of theophylline. Thus, aminophylline is 80% theophylline $\left(\frac{200}{250} = 80\%\right)$; therefore, 25 mg (1 mL) of aminophylline will contain only 20 mg of theophylline. Divide 320 mg by 20 mg/mL to obtain 16 mL.

44. **(B)** We plug into the given formula:

$$\text{CrCl} = \left(\frac{140 - 74}{72 \cdot 3.2}\right) \cdot (84) = \left(\frac{66}{72 \cdot 3.2}\right) \cdot (84) \approx 24$$

45. **(A)** Each point on the graph of $y = 5 \cdot f(x + 2) - 3$ is obtained by transforming the points on the graph of $y = f(x)$ as follows. Subtract 2 from each x-coordinate, multiply each y-coordinate by 5, and then subtract 3 from that y-coordinate.

46. **(B)**

> **STEP 1** An equation of the form $(x - h)^2 + (y - k)^2 = r^2$ is a circle with center (h,k) and radius r. The given circle has the equation $x^2 + y^2 = 25$.

> **STEP 2** The slope of any tangent line to this curve is given by the derivative, $\frac{dy}{dx}$.

Differentiating the given equation with respect to x yields:

$$\frac{d}{dx}\left(x^2 + y^2\right) = \frac{d}{dx}(25)$$

$$2x + 2y\,\frac{dy}{dx} = 0$$

$$\frac{dy}{dx} = -\frac{2x}{2y} = -\frac{x}{y}$$

> **STEP 3** At the point $(3, 4)$, the tangent slope is given by $\frac{dy}{dx} = -\frac{3}{4}$.

47. **(D)** The highest point on the graph has a y-coordinate equal to 750.

48. **(A)** The highest point on the graph occurs when the x-coordinate equals 4.

49. **(C)** We calculate the distance using the following formula:

$$\sqrt{\left(x_2 - x_1\right)^2 + \left(y_2 - y_1\right)^2} = \sqrt{\left(-2 - 3\right)^2 + \left(5 - 6\right)^2} = \sqrt{25 + 1} = \sqrt{26}$$

50. **(A)** If the house is 12 mi. from the park, at 12 mph Larry needed 1 hr. to make the trip. At only 3 mph, he needed 4 hr. to get back home. Thus, he traveled 24 mi. ($2 \cdot 12$ mi.) in 5 hr. ($1 + 4$ hr.). Divide 24 by 5 to get an average speed of 4.8 mph.

51. **(D)** Choice D represents an exponential relationship.

52. **(B)** We first need to rewrite the given equation in standard form by completing the square.

$$x^2 + 6x + y^2 - 10y - 3 = 0$$
$$x^2 + 6x + 9 + y^2 - 10y + 25 = 3 + 9 + 25$$
$$(x + 3)^2 + (y - 5)^2 = 37$$

An equation of the form $(x - h)^2 + (y - k)^2 = r^2$ is a circle with a radius equal to r. Therefore, we have $r = \sqrt{37}$.

53. **(B)** We calculate the mean as follows:

$$\text{mean} = \frac{10+11+9+7+5+6}{6} = 8$$

54. **(D)** The function $y = f(x)$ is increasing when its first derivative is positive, i.e., when the graph of the first derivative is above the x-axis. The correct answer is $[-3, 1] \cup [4, \infty]$.

55. **(D)** The function $y = f(x)$ is concave down when its second derivative is negative, i.e., when the graph of the first derivative has a negative slope.

56. **(A)** The particle is moving to the left when its velocity is negative, i.e., when the derivative of the position function is negative.

$$\frac{dp}{dt} = 3t^2 - 12t = 3t(t-4)$$

When $t < 0$, $\dfrac{dp}{dt} = 3t(t-4) = (-)(-) = +$

When $0 < t < 4$, $\dfrac{dp}{dt} = 3t(t-4) = (+)(-) = -$

When $t > 4$, $\dfrac{dp}{dt} = 3t(t-4) = (+)(+) = +$

57. **(A)** The original graph is shifted 2 units to the right.

58. **(D)** The original graph is shifted 2 units down.

59. **(B)** Since the tank is already $\frac{2}{3}$ full, the additional 8 gallons equals $\frac{1}{3}$ of the tank's capacity. Thus, $8 = \frac{1}{3}x \Rightarrow x = 24$.

60. **(D)** The clinic sees 55% of its daily patients after noon. Therefore, $(0.55)(40) = 22$ patients seen after noon.

61. **(D)** The projectile hits the ground when the height equals zero. Therefore, we solve the equation $-0.002x^2 + x = 0$.

$$-0.002x^2 + x = 0$$
$$x(-0.002x + 1) = 0$$

$$x = 0, \quad -0.002x + 1 = 0 \Rightarrow x = \frac{-1}{-0.002} = 500$$

62. **(C)** We apply the distance formula to points P and Q.

$$\sqrt{(x-0)^2 + (y-2)^2} = \sqrt{x^2 + (8 + x^2 - 2)^2} = \sqrt{x^2 + (6 - x^2)^2}$$

63. **(A)** The probability of obtaining a red ball would be 4 out of 12 (total number of balls in the bag). After being simplified, the answer is $\frac{1}{3}$.

64. **(B)** We use the Quotient Rule for Logarithms as follows:

$$\ln(100) - \ln(10) = \ln\left(\frac{100}{10}\right) = \ln(10)$$

65. **(A)** There are 9 possible ways not to choose a dime from a total of 15 coins. We use the formula: probability $= \frac{9}{15} = 0.60 = 60\%$.

66. **(A)** As x approaches 1 from the right, y approaches 1.5.

67. **(A)** As x approaches -1 from the right, y approaches positive infinity.

68. **(D)** As x approaches ∞, y approaches 0.

69. **(A)** Since $\lim_{x \to -1^+} f(x) = \infty$, $x = -1$ represents a vertical asymptote for the graph of $y = f(x)$.

70. **(B)** Since $\lim_{x \to \infty} f(x) = 0$, $y = 0$ represents a horizontal asymptote for the graph of $y = f(x)$.

71. **(B)**

(STEP 1) The slope of any tangent line to this curve is given by the derivative, $\frac{dy}{dx}$. Differentiating the given parabola equation with respect to x yields:

$$\frac{dy}{dx} = 2ax + b$$

(STEP 2) The desired tangent line, $y = 3x - 2$, has a slope equal to 3. We need $2ax + b = 3$. At the point $(1, 1)$, we have $2a + b = 3$.

(STEP 3) Since the point $(1, 1)$ is on the graph of the given parabola, we have:

$$y = ax^2 + bx$$
$$1 = a(1)^2 + b(1)$$
$$1 = a + b$$

(STEP 4) To find the values of a and b, we solve the system of equations:

$$2a + b = 3$$
$$a + b = 1$$

Subtracting the second equation from the first equation yields $a = 2$. Since $a + b = 1$, we have $2 + b = 1$, i.e., $b = -1$. The desired parabola equation is $y = 2x^2 - x$.

72. **(A)** We compute $\frac{f(3) - f(1)}{3 - 1} = \frac{9 - 1}{2} = 4$.

73. **(A)** Set up a proportion: $\dfrac{500 \text{ mg drug A}}{400 \text{ mg drug B}} = \dfrac{250 \text{ mg drug A}}{x \text{ mg}}$

Cross multiply and divide:

$$500x = 250 \cdot 400$$
$$500x = 100{,}000$$
$$x = 200 \text{ mg}$$

74. **(D)** We must exclude any values of x which cause $x^2 - 6 = 0$.

Since $x^2 - 6 = 0 \Rightarrow x = \pm\sqrt{6}$, we must exclude $x = -\sqrt{6}$, and $x = \sqrt{6}$.

75. **(B)** $\dfrac{\sqrt{36} \cdot \sqrt{16}}{\sqrt{9}} = \dfrac{6 \cdot 4}{3} = 8$.

76. **(A)** Apply the quadratic formula to $bx^2 + cx + a = 0$. The correct answer is

$x = \dfrac{-c \pm \sqrt{c^2 - 4ba}}{2b}$.

77. **(A)** Since the left-hand limit yields $\lim\limits_{x \to 2^-} f(x) = 3(2)^2 = 12$, but the right-hand limit

yields $\lim\limits_{x \to 2^+} f(x) = 1 - 5(2) = -9$, the overall limit $\lim\limits_{x \to 2} f(x)$ is undefined.

78. **(B)** We solve the equation as follows:

$$5(x + 2)(x - 1) = 5x^2 + 6x$$
$$5(x^2 + x - 2) = 5x^2 + 6x$$
$$5x^2 + 5x - 10 = 5x^2 + 6x$$
$$5x - 10 = 6x \Rightarrow -10 = x$$

79. **(D)** Compute $0.1004 + 0.2238 = 0.3242 = 32.42\%$.

80. **(B)** Compute $(0.0416)(6,400) = 266.24$, or approximately 266.

81. **(D)** There are six ways that the sum of the numbers can equal 7, namely $1 + 6$, $2 + 5$, $3 + 4$, $6 + 1$, $5 + 2$, and $4 + 3$. Each die has six faces. This means that there are $(6)(6) = 36$ possible outcomes for tossing the two dice. Thus, the probability that the sum of the numbers equals 7 is given by $\dfrac{6}{36} = \dfrac{1}{6}$. Therefore, the probability that the sum of the numbers does NOT equal 7 is given by $1 - \dfrac{1}{6} = \dfrac{5}{6}$.

82. **(D)** We use the Fundamental Theorem of Calculus to compute the definite

integral. Note that $\int \sin(2x)\,dx = -\dfrac{1}{2}\cos(2x)$.

$$\int_0^{\pi/4} \sin(2x)\,dx = \left[-\frac{1}{2}\cos(2x)\right]_{x=0}^{x=\frac{\pi}{4}}$$
$$= -\frac{1}{2}\cos\left(2\left(\frac{\pi}{4}\right)\right) - \left(-\frac{1}{2}\cos(2(0))\right)$$
$$= -\frac{1}{2}\cos\left(\frac{\pi}{2}\right) + \frac{1}{2}\cos(0) = 0 + \left(\frac{1}{2}\right)(1) = \frac{1}{2}$$

83. **(C)** To compute $F'(2)$, we must use the Chain Rule for derivatives, i.e.,
$\dfrac{d}{dx} g(h(x)) = g'(h(x)) \cdot h'(x)$.

$$\frac{dF}{dx}(2) = g'(h(2)) \cdot h'(2)$$
$$= g'(4) \cdot h'(2)$$
$$= 9 \cdot 8 = 72$$

84. **(A)** Since $x < 10$, this means that $x - 10 < 0$. Thus, $|x - 10| = -(x - 10)$. Therefore,

$$\frac{x^2 - 11x + 10}{|x - 10|} = \frac{(x - 10)(x - 1)}{-(x - 10)} = -(x - 1) = -x + 1$$

85. **(C)** With the understanding that the symbol $\cup$ means the set of elements either in A or B or in both, and $\cap$ means the set that contains all those elements that A and B have in common, we use the formula:

$$P(A \cup B) = P(A) + P(B) - P(A \cap B) = 0.26 + 0.42 - 0.12 = 0.56$$

86. **(A)** We use the following formula:

$$n(A \cup B) = n(A) + n(B) - n(A \cap B) = 20 + 11 - 5 = 26$$

87. **(A)** We calculate the slope using the formula $\frac{\Delta y}{\Delta x} = \frac{8 - 9}{-5 - 2} = \frac{1}{7}$.

88. **(A)** We solve the equation as follows:

$$\ln(w + 5x) = 3$$
$$e^{\ln(w + 5x)} = e^3$$
$$w + 5x = e^3$$
$$5x = e^3 - w \Rightarrow x = \frac{e^3 - w}{5}$$

89. **(B)** The Quotient Rule for logarithms states that $\log(M) - \log(N) = \log\left(\frac{M}{N}\right)$.

90. **(D)** A rational function will have a horizontal asymptote of $y = L$, provided $\lim_{x \to \pm\infty} f(x) = L$.

$$\lim_{x \to \pm\infty} f(x) = \lim_{x \to \pm\infty}\left(\frac{3x + 1}{5 - 4x}\right) \to \frac{3x}{-4x} \to -\frac{3}{4}$$

91. **(C)** The line with the equation $y = 4$ is horizontal. Therefore, we need the equation of the vertical line passing through the point $(5, -7)$. The answer is $x = 5$.

92. **(C)** We are choosing 5 elements from a 12-element set, without repetition, such that order does not matter. Thus, we are counting combinations. We use the formula:

$$_{12}C_5 = \frac{12!}{5!(12 - 5)!} = \frac{12!}{5!7!}$$

93. **(D)** To convert from °F to Kelvin, you must first convert the temperature from °F to °C. Therefore, the first step is to use $T_C = (T_F - 32)\left(\frac{5}{9}\right)$ to convert the temperature to Celsius. Then, to convert the Celsius temperature to Kelvin, add 273.15.

STEP 1

$$T_C = (T_F - 32)\left(\frac{5}{9}\right)$$
$$= (86 - 32)\left(\frac{5}{9}\right)$$
$$= (54)\left(\frac{5}{9}\right)$$
$$= 30°C$$

STEP 2

$$K = 30 + 273.15 \approx 303$$

94. **(D)** A logarithmic function is undefined unless the input value is strictly greater than zero. Thus, we solve $4x - 2 > 0$ and obtain $x > 0.5$.

95. **(D)** The total rental cost is given by the daily cost plus the mileage cost.

    Daily cost = ($25 per day)(6 days) = $150.

    Mileage cost = ($0.12 per mile)($x$ miles) = $0.12x$.

96. **(C)** The graph has symmetry with respect to the origin.

97. **(B)** The domain is given by the set of x-coordinates of the points on the graph.

98. **(D)** The range is given by the set of y-coordinates of the points on the graph.

99. **(B)** Since the red and blue crayons are in a $5 : 9$ ratio, we can set up the proportion $\dfrac{5 \text{ red}}{9 \text{ blue}} = \dfrac{20 \text{ red}}{x \text{ blue}}$. Now solve for x and then calculate $x - 20$.

    STEP 1

    $$\frac{5}{9} = \frac{20}{x}$$
    $$5x = (20)(9)$$
    $$5x = 180$$
    $$x = 36$$

    STEP 2 $36 - 20 = 16$ more blue crayons than red crayons.

100. **(D)** Note that $\dfrac{4}{11} - \dfrac{3}{8} = \dfrac{4 \cdot 8 - 3 \cdot 11}{11 \cdot 8} = \dfrac{32 - 33}{88} = -\dfrac{1}{88}$.

Critical Reading
Review and Practice

7

TIPS FOR THE CRITICAL READING SECTION

The critical reading section of the PCAT presents relatively short passages. The majority of the passages focus on physical/life/natural science topics; however, 40 percent of the passages will present social sciences/humanities topics. You are asked to read each passage carefully and then answer questions related to it. For each passage, there are generally 4–8 questions, with a total of 48 questions for the entire section. Keep in mind that the correct answer may be a direct statement taken from the reading passage. You will have 50 minutes to complete the critical reading section. Be careful to pace yourself to prevent running out of time.

Practice the reading passages and sample questions in this book. Some students prefer to read the passage first and then answer the questions, while others prefer to read the questions and then skim the passage to identify the answers. Use the practice passages and questions in this chapter to determine the strategy that works best for you. Do not be concerned with how many times you need to refer to the passage to answer the questions; just complete the section as quickly as possible, making sure you find the correct answer to every question.

Try to determine where your general strengths and weaknesses as a reader lie. Do you tend to get a quick grasp of the overall sense of a passage but miss the details? Or do you as a reader sometimes fail to see the forest for the trees? In other words, do you remember only the details and find yourself unable to state the basic meaning of the passage as a whole? In either case, take some time to improve your "weak" areas. Be patient with yourself as you practice. With adequate review, you should be able to work at your normal pace when you take the actual PCAT.

ANSWER SHEET
Critical Reading

1. (A) (B) (C) (D)
2. (A) (B) (C) (D)
3. (A) (B) (C) (D)
4. (A) (B) (C) (D)
5. (A) (B) (C) (D)
6. (A) (B) (C) (D)
7. (A) (B) (C) (D)
8. (A) (B) (C) (D)
9. (A) (B) (C) (D)
10. (A) (B) (C) (D)
11. (A) (B) (C) (D)
12. (A) (B) (C) (D)
13. (A) (B) (C) (D)

14. (A) (B) (C) (D)
15. (A) (B) (C) (D)
16. (A) (B) (C) (D)
17. (A) (B) (C) (D)
18. (A) (B) (C) (D)
19. (A) (B) (C) (D)
20. (A) (B) (C) (D)
21. (A) (B) (C) (D)
22. (A) (B) (C) (D)
23. (A) (B) (C) (D)
24. (A) (B) (C) (D)
25. (A) (B) (C) (D)
26. (A) (B) (C) (D)

27. (A) (B) (C) (D)
28. (A) (B) (C) (D)
29. (A) (B) (C) (D)
30. (A) (B) (C) (D)
31. (A) (B) (C) (D)
32. (A) (B) (C) (D)
33. (A) (B) (C) (D)
34. (A) (B) (C) (D)
35. (A) (B) (C) (D)
36. (A) (B) (C) (D)
37. (A) (B) (C) (D)
38. (A) (B) (C) (D)
39. (A) (B) (C) (D)

40. (A) (B) (C) (D)
41. (A) (B) (C) (D)
42. (A) (B) (C) (D)
43. (A) (B) (C) (D)
44. (A) (B) (C) (D)
45. (A) (B) (C) (D)
46. (A) (B) (C) (D)
47. (A) (B) (C) (D)
48. (A) (B) (C) (D)
49. (A) (B) (C) (D)
50. (A) (B) (C) (D)

50 Questions

PASSAGE 1

As evictions and lowered crop prices squeezed tens of thousands of farmers from the land after 1934, they ran headlong into the pattern of economic distress that had dominated the nonagricultural economy since the start of the decade. If anything, the cities and towns had suffered more than rural areas as the Depression tightened its grip on the commercial life of the region in the first half of the thirties. Depression-era unemployment data are sketchy and not always reliable, but the available estimates indicate that the Southwest contended with higher percentages of unemployment than other predominately rural sections of the country. The federal government's Committee on Economic Security estimated Arkansas's rate of nonagricultural unemployment to be the third highest in the nation (39.2 percent) during the nadir year of 1933. Oklahoma, Texas, and Missouri, with rates varying between 29 and 32 percent, exceeded nearly all other states in the South or on the northern plains. We have no data on the four recovery years which followed, but the 1937 federal unemployment census, taken just as the nation's economy entered another decline, found 22 percent of all available Southwestern workers either unemployed or engaged on work relief projects. Another 10 percent were considered partly unemployed. Conditions improved somewhat during the last two and a half years of the decade. When census takers visited homes in 1940, the unemployment rate in the Western South was down to 14.3 percent, but the level still remained higher than most rural states.

With the partial exception of Missouri, the Southwestern states had few resources with which to assist the jobless and needy. Local and state relief funds were quickly exhausted as unemployment soared and tax revenues fell in the first years of the Depression, and usually offered little more than emergency groceries to those in need. Private charities like the Red Cross also helped, but in general the level of assistance available prior to 1933 was minimal. The establishment of the Federal Emergency Relief Administration shortly after Franklin Roosevelt assumed the presidency improved matters considerably. Through 1934 and 1935, federal relief funds sustained more than two and a half million Southwesterners, almost 20 percent of the region's population, on a continuing basis. In some areas the relief burden was much larger. During certain drought months in 1934, up to 90 percent of the population of particular eastern Oklahoma counties collected relief payments.

Excerpted from *American Exodus: The Dust Bowl Migration and Okie Culture in California*, by James N. Gregory. New York: Oxford University Press, 1989.

1. The Great Depression began in the year _____ during the presidency of _____.

   (A) 1933; Franklin Roosevelt
   (B) 1933; Herbert Hoover
   (C) 1929; Herbert Hoover
   (D) 1929; Franklin Roosevelt

2. The first paragraph mentions the "nadir year of 1933." In this case, "nadir" refers to

   (A) the lowest point ("rock-bottom").
   (B) the highest point ("peak").
   (C) the mid-point.
   (D) a point of stability.

3. What would be the most appropriate title for this passage?

   (A) Effects of the Great Depression on the Southwestern United States
   (B) Federal Response to the Great Depression
   (C) Migration Patterns During the Great Depression
   (D) Nonagricultural Unemployment During the Great Depression

4. In the mid-1930s, approximately what percent of individuals in the Southwest received federal relief?

   (A) 90
   (B) 10
   (C) 40
   (D) 20

PASSAGE 2

To the average physician, Lyme disease is suspected when a patient arrives at a clinic or hospital complaining of a strange bull's-eye rash, known as erythema migrans, or EM, together with one or more flulike symptoms, such as fever, chills, muscle aches, or lethargy. The physician will take a blood sample for laboratory confirmation, but will feel quite confident to make a diagnosis of Lyme disease after noting the telltale combination of symptoms, as well as the circumstances surrounding the infection. The patient will undoubtedly have been bitten by the black-legged tick *Ixodes scaplaris*, formerly called the deer tick, or a close relative, which transferred to him or her the *B. burgdorferi* bacterium. Most likely, the physician will prescribe an oral course of antibiotics and will duly report the case to the county or state health department, which will include it in the morbidity statistics for Lyme disease.

Accurate diagnosis and effective treatment of Lyme disease are not always so straightforward, particularly in regions of the country newly invaded by the epidemic. In these regions, health care professionals and the public need to be educated about the confusing and generalized symptoms, the generally poor, but growing, accuracy of lab tests, and the efficacy of various antibiotic treatments. If Lyme disease is left untreated for some time, *B. burgdorferi* may persist in the patient's tissues and can migrate to the central and peripheral nervous systems or to joints and cause more severe late-stage symptoms, which include arthritis and neurological disorders, such as dizziness, memory loss, and disorientation. Vaccines that protect against Lyme disease are now being field tested by pharmaceutical companies, but none has yet been approved by the Food and Drug Administration for public use. Even if an effective vaccine were certified and marketed, the primary means that individuals have of protecting themselves against the disease is avoiding the tick in the first place.

Excerpted from "The Ecology of Lyme-Disease Risk," by Richard S. Ostfeld, *The American Scientist*, Vol. 85, p. 338, reprinted by permission of *American Scientist*, magazine of Sigma Xi, The Scientific Research Society.

5. When a patient reports to a clinic or hospital with symptoms of Lyme disease, he or she has undoubtedly been bitten by

   (A) the black-legged tick *Ixodes scaplaris.*
   (B) a tick-bearing wild mammal.
   (C) *B. burgdorferi.*
   (D) None of the above; Lyme disease is generally believed to be spread by an airborne pathogen.

6. An appropriate title for this passage would be

   (A) Diagnosis of Lyme Disease.
   (B) Diagnosis, Treatment, and Challenges of Lyme Disease.
   (C) Developing Vaccinations to Protect Against Lyme Disease.
   (D) Complications of Lyme Disease.

7. Lyme disease may affect the human body's

   (A) gastrointestinal system.
   (B) cardiovascular system.
   (C) reproductive system.
   (D) musculoskeletal system.

8. In addition to noting the telltale combination of symptoms in a patient with Lyme disease, a physician is likely to

   (A) seek laboratory confirmation of the diagnosis.
   (B) prescribe an analgesic to alleviate symptoms.
   (C) recommend bed rest for a brief duration.
   (D) hospitalize the patient for treatment.

9. If Lyme disease is left untreated for some time,

   (A) health care professionals and the public will not be educated about its confusing and generalized symptoms.
   (B) the accuracy of diagnostic lab tests may be poor.
   (C) the disease may progress, with symptoms increasing in severity.
   (D) antibiotic treatments will no longer be effective.

PASSAGE 3

In the past two decades, people living in the northeastern, north-central, and western United States have unwittingly entered a dangerous enzootic cycle—a cycle of disease that typically is restricted to wildlife. Wild mammals and birds host a wide variety of disease agents, with effects ranging from mild symptoms to mortality, but in most cases the pathogen affects only one or a few host species and never causes disease in humans. However, as a result of a complicated sequence of events, people have become frequent accidental hosts for ticks and the disease agents they carry, including a corkscrew-shaped bacterium called *Borrelia burgdorferi*, the agent of Lyme disease. As of 1995, cases of Lyme disease had been reported in 48 of the 50 states and appear to be increasing, both in numbers of people affected and in geographic distribution.

Where does this disease come from, why has it emerged so rapidly, and what can people do to reduce their risk of exposure? It is possible to address these questions not from a medical point of view, but rather from an ecological one. All living organisms—from the *B. burgdorferi* bacterium and the ticks it infects to the mice and deer on which the ticks feed—form an ecological relationship with their habitats. Understanding the complex interactions between plant and animal species within those habitats may help people to predict the places where they are most likely to encounter disease-bearing ticks and become infected. Thus armed, individuals may ultimately be able to protect themselves from Lyme disease.

Currently, to prevent Lyme disease people wear protective clothing when they are in wooded areas and perform "tick checks" after leaving the woods. One underemphasized means to avoid exposure to Lyme disease, however, is avoiding the most heavily tick-infested habitats at the times of year when ticks are most abundant or dangerous. Recent research has suggested that such habitats can be predicted, often well in advance. Ultimately, it is the hope of ecologists studying this problem that we can use our expertise in pinpointing these habitats to warn the public away from areas that are likely to contain an abundance of disease-carrying ticks.

Excerpted from "The Ecology of Lyme-Disease Risk," by Richard S. Ostfeld, *The American Scientist*, Vol. 85, p. 338, reprinted by permission of *American Scientist*, magazine of Sigma Xi, The Scientific Research Society.

10. What is the primary message or theme of the first paragraph of the passage?

(A) Diseases found in mammals and birds are never found in humans.
(B) Lyme disease has been diagnosed throughout almost all states in the United States and is expected to increase.
(C) Humans living in the United States are immune to pathogens carried by ticks, and therefore are not contributors to the spread of Lyme disease.
(D) Humans living in the United States have become hosts for ticks and disease agents, contributing to the spread of pathogens such as *Borrelia burgdorferi*.

11. The aim of understanding Lyme disease from an ecological as well as a medical point of view is

   (A) to help preserve the mice and deer on which the ticks feed.
   (B) to help people predict the places where they are most likely to encounter disease-bearing ticks and become infected.
   (C) to develop a vaccine against the disease.
   (D) to further our understanding of the relationship between ticks and their habitats.

12. Prevention of Lyme disease

   (A) is the purview of medical professionals and ecologists.
   (B) does not have an ecological component.
   (C) may be accomplished through the use of herbal remedies.
   (D) requires proactive consideration of factors both before and after exploring the woods.

13. As of 1995, Lyme disease had been reported in 48 of the 50 states and

   (A) had been eradicated in the two remaining states.
   (B) appeared to be increasing in the number of people affected and in geographic distribution.
   (C) appeared to be decreasing in the number of people affected.
   (D) appeared to be increasing in the geographic distribution within those 48 states.

14. One underemphasized means to avoid exposure to Lyme disease is

   (A) wearing protective clothing.
   (B) avoiding the most heavily tick-infested areas at certain times of the year.
   (C) using insect repellent.
   (D) remembering to get vaccinated before going into areas that are known to be heavily tick-infested.

PASSAGE 4

Unlike an electron, a single red blood cell cannot go through two openings at once. Indeed, it is generally true that the physicist seeking to understand the circulation of the blood can ignore most of the perplexities of twentieth-century physics. Given the scale of the circulatory system and the speed of blood flow, neither quantum mechanics nor relativity applies. Instead the flow of blood through the heart and the vascular tree can be adequately described by the familiar mechanics of Newton and Galileo.

If the circulation of the blood obeys the laws of classical mechanics, however, this does not mean that it is simple. An early experimental model of the vascular tree was a system of glass tubes filled with water. But unlike water, blood is not an "ideal" fluid. Instead it is a suspension of cells that, under certain circumstances, can behave in non-Newtonian ways. Moreover, flow through the vascular tree is pulsatile rather than steady; blood vessels taper and are elastic rather than rigid; and flow in any part of the densely interconnected system is affected by flow in neighboring regions. When these factors and the fantastic geometrical complexity of the labyrinthine vascular system are taken into account, the equations of blood flow, while remaining classical in inspiration, quickly become too complex to be solved explicitly.

Confronted with a system of overwhelming complexity, scientists typically resort to the intelligent simplification, that is, to a model. The first mathematical model of the human circulation was the *windkessel*, or compression chamber, model developed by Otto Frank in 1899 to explain how pulsatile flow from the heart is converted into steadier flow in the peripheral circulation. Sophisticated analytical models, the descendants of the *windkessel* model, still provide insight into the functioning of the circulatory system. But they are increasingly supplemented by numerical models, which exploit the power of the computer to arrive at accurate approximations of values that satisfy systems of equations that would otherwise be unsolvable. The computer can also be used to produce stunning images that allow otherwise cryptic measurements or calculations to be grasped intuitively.

———————

Excerpted from "The Biophysics of Stroke," by George J. Hademenos, *The American Scientist*, Vol. 85, p. 226, reprinted by permission of *American Scientist*, magazine of Sigma Xi, The Scientific Research Society.

15. Quantum physics and relativity may be ignored by the physicist seeking to understand the circulation of the blood because

    (A) electrons cannot go through two openings at once in the vascular tree.
    (B) the mechanics of Newton and Galileo do not apply.
    (C) the scale of the circulatory system and the speed of blood flow can be adequately described by the mechanics of Newton and Galileo.
    (D) blood is an "ideal" fluid.

16. An early experimental model of the vascular tree

    (A) revealed that blood cannot behave in non-Newtonian ways.
    (B) consisted of a system of glass tubes filled with water.
    (C) was developed by Galileo.
    (D) yielded equations that, although complex, could be solved quickly and explicitly.

17. When scientists are confronted with a system of overwhelming complexity, they typically

    (A) give up.
    (B) resort to intelligent simplification, that is, to a model.
    (C) adjust their most arbitrary assumptions accordingly.
    (D) abandon the mechanics of Galileo and Newton.

18. Otto Frank developed the *windkessel* model in 1899 for the purpose of

    (A) explaining how pulsatile flow from the heart is converted into steadier flow in the peripheral circulation.
    (B) improving on previous mathematical models.
    (C) converting the flow of blood from the heart into steadier flow in the peripheral circulation of human subjects.
    (D) augmenting the mechanics of Galileo and Newton.

19. In the twentieth century,

    (A) quantum physics and relativity gave us some useful insights into the functioning of the circulatory system.
    (B) the *windkessel* model was still in use.
    (C) computers did not prove as useful as physicists had hoped since many systems of equations remain unsolvable.
    (D) computers were used to produce images that allowed cryptic measurements or calculations to be grasped intuitively.

PASSAGE 5

An important method that anthropologists use to learn about ways of thinking is to consider how people explain and deal with misfortunes that happen to them. On such occasions, people draw on ideas that they have been socialized to share but which may or may not be apparent in everyday conversation as they may be taken for granted. These ideas are often related to religion, a spirit world, or a system of classification that draws on ideas about supernatural powers that some specialist people are believed to control. For others, or even for the same people in different situations, answers are found in *science*, and again most people would turn to specialists—doctors or engineers perhaps—for help in solving particular problems. In all cases, they are drawing on a *cosmology*, a system of ideas about the world, how it is classified, how it works, and how they fit into that world.

    An influential study on this subject was published in a book named *Witchcraft, Oracles and Magic among the Azande* by E.E. Evans-Pritchard, whose fieldwork in the Southern Sudan enabled him to discover and explain a rather different system of logic to the one he started out with. The Azande people draw on ideas of witchcraft to explain unfortunate things that happen in their lives. For them, witchcraft is not something frightening, as it might be for people in Britain, but simply an annoying everyday occurrence. It was, therefore, brought frequently to the attention of the anthropologist learning their language, and Evans-Pritchard explained that the logic behind this use of the term provides a complete explanation for unfortunate events, such as crop failure, accidental injury, or illness.

This doesn't mean that the Azande are unaware of 'natural' explanations. If a person falls over a root in the path, they know that the root caused them to trip; if their crops fail because of a lack of rain, they know that they needed water to thrive; if members of a family fall sick after eating something unusual, they know that it may have been bad. What witchcraft explains in all these cases is why that bad thing happened to those particular people at that particular time: why the person who tripped walked that way, why the rain fell elsewhere and missed the crops, and why the ones who fell sick happened to eat that food on that day. To explain such things in terms of having been bewitched takes an explanation that others may simply wonder about to a complete logical conclusion, he argued.

Excerpted from *Anthropology*, by Joy Hendry and Simon Underdown. Oxford, England: Oneworld Publications, 2012.

20. *Cosmology* refers to _____.

   (A) the attitudes and beliefs thought to be unique to a given culture
   (B) ideas about the world as an ordered system and the place of humans in the world
   (C) the study of material culture
   (D) comparative analysis of cultural patterns to explain variation among societies

21. For the Azande, witchcraft is

   (A) a rare occurrence.
   (B) a story-telling tradition.
   (C) an everyday occurrence.
   (D) a frightening prospect.

22. Which of the following statements accurately reflects the Azande belief system, as described in the passage?

   (A) Witchcraft is used only to explain malicious acts such as murder.
   (B) Witchcraft does not explain why an event occurred, only who was affected.
   (C) Natural events such as a drought or illness are the result of witchcraft.
   (D) Witchcraft is performed to punish individuals who violate community norms.

23. Where did Evans-Pritchard conduct his fieldwork with the Azande?

   (A) Africa
   (B) Asia
   (C) Europe
   (D) South America

24. According to the passage, why are anthropologists interested in how people explain misfortune?

    (A)   To learn about ways of coping

    (B)   To learn about social rituals

    (C)   To learn about religious ceremonies

    (D)   To learn about ways of thinking

25. According to Evans-Pritchard, for the Azande

    (A)   witchcraft offers a complete explanation of unfortunate events.

    (B)   witchcraft offers a partial explanation of unfortunate events.

    (C)   witchcraft offers protection from the influence of non-Azande cultures.

    (D)   witchcraft offers a means of communication with non-Azande individuals.

PASSAGE 6

Allergic drug reactions account for 5% to 20% of all observed adverse drug reactions. Adverse drug reactions have been reported to occur in as many as 30% of hospitalized patients, and 3% of all hospitalizations are a result of adverse drug reactions. In a computerized surveillance study of over 36,000 hospitalized patients, 731 adverse events were identified. Of those, 1% were categorized as severe, life-threatening, and allergic in nature. The potential morbidity and mortality associated with allergic drug reactions is great even though these outcomes occur infrequently.

In order to appropriately diagnose and treat a patient experiencing an allergic reaction, it is necessary to be able to differentiate allergic reactions from other closely related adverse drug reactions. One method of classification divides adverse reactions into those that are "predictable, usually dose-dependent, and related to the pharmacologic actions of the drug," and those that are "unpredictable, often dose-independent, and related to the individual's immunologic response or to genetic differences in susceptible patients." Under this classification scheme, drug allergy or drug hypersensitivity is an unpredictable adverse drug reaction that is immunologically mediated.

Excerpted with permission from "Chapter 6, Anaphylaxis and Drug Allergies," page 6-1, *Applied Therapeutics: The Clinical Use of Drugs, Sixth Edition*, edited by Lloyd Yee Young and Mary Anne Koda-Kimble, published by Applied Therapeutics, Inc., Vancouver, Washington, © 1995.

26. Which of the following is necessary to appropriately diagnose and treat a patient experiencing an allergic reaction to a drug?

    (A) A way to differentiate allergic reactions from other adverse drug reactions
    (B) Determination that the reaction is dose-dependent and related to the pharmacological actions of the drug
    (C) Access to appropriate statistics, such as computerized surveillance studies
    (D) Hospitalization

27. If an adverse reaction is not predictable, dose-independent, and related to the pharmacologic actions of the drug, then it is likely to be

    (A) adverse but not allergic.
    (B) unrelated to genetic differences in patients.
    (C) related to the individual's immunologic response.
    (D) unrelated to the individual's immunologic response.

28. Allergic drug reactions account for as many as what percent of all observed adverse drug reactions?

    (A) 1% to 5%
    (B) 5% to 20%
    (C) 30%
    (D) 1%

29. Of 731 adverse drug events identified in a surveillance study of over 36,000 patients, 1% were characterized as

    (A) dose-dependent.
    (B) allergic but not severe or life-threatening.
    (C) severe, life-threatening, and allergic in nature.
    (D) adverse but not allergic.

PASSAGE 7

Art history in its modern form originated in Germany in the nineteenth century. People had thought about the art of the past before, of course, but they did so in a way which we would now say was unhistorical: namely, they looked, not for what makes particular works significant in their own right, but how far these works realized what were thought to be universal aesthetic norms. Art theory was taught in the European academies which had been established in the seventeenth and eighteenth centuries for the training of artists, and included discussion of the art of the past; but individual artists and schools (that is, works of art grouped according to their country of origin) were judged according to whether they had achieved a representation of ideal beauty.

   The Italian artist, Giorgio Vasari (1511–1574) is often called the first art historian. His *The Lives of the Artists*, first published in 1550, provided an influential model for the understanding of past art. Vasari's art history was not historical in the modern sense, however. In his view, art's development over time was cyclical, and he discussed the achievement of individual artists with respect to their place in this cyclical process. According to Vasari, art achieved its first high point in the golden age of ancient Greek art, declined in the fourth and fifth centuries A.D., was revived by Giotto in the thirteenth century, improved by Masaccio, Piero della Francesca and Mantegna in the fifteenth, and brought to new heights by Leonardo, Raphael and Michelangelo in Vasari's own time. But while Vasari saw art change during each cycle, approaching ever nearer to an aesthetic ideal, he did not understand these changes as a result of particular historical or social conditions at work at the time when each artist lived. A historical understanding of art in the modern sense did not start to develop until the end of the eighteenth century; until that time, history was thought to be extrinsic to art in the way that earthquakes are extrinsic to it. Art's value lay in striving to achieve timeless aesthetic norms, norms that were elaborated systematically by such French art theorists as André Félibien (1619–1695) and Roger de Piles (1635–1709) in the late seventeenth and early eighteenth centuries. When the University of Göttingen in Germany founded the first chair in art history in 1813, this was not the dawn of art history as we now know it. The man appointed, Johann Dominicus Fiorillo, was a drawing master and his lectures followed the tradition of academic art theory.

_____

Excerpted from *Art History: A Critical Introduction to Its Methods*, by Michael Hatt and Charlotte Klonk. New York: Manchester University Press, 2006.

30. Vasari believed art developed as part of

   (A)   historical conditions.
   (B)   a linear process.
   (C)   a cyclical process.
   (D)   social conditions.

31. In what European country did the modern form of art history emerge?

   (A)   Italy
   (B)   Greece
   (C)   Germany
   (D)   France

32. What was the nationality of the individual known as the first art historian?

   (A)   Italian
   (B)   Greek
   (C)   German
   (D)   French

33. According to the passage, Vasari believed that new heights of artistic achievement were reached by artists who lived during what historical era?

   (A)   Enlightenment
   (B)   Romantic
   (C)   Antiquity
   (D)   Renaissance

34. Prior to the advent of modern art history, schools of art referred to

    (A) works of art grouped according to country of origin.
    (B) academies established to teach art theory.
    (C) works of art grouped by aesthetic and technique.
    (D) academies established to train young artists.

PASSAGE 8

Sulfasalazine, the most frequently prescribed drug for inflammatory bowel disease therapy, has been used commonly for 50 years for the induction of disease remission in patients with mild acute exacerbations of ulcerative colitis. Initial uncontrolled observations of its efficacy indicated that 80% to 90% of patients improved with the use of this agent. The first placebo-controlled trial using objective parameters of efficacy demonstrated that 80% of the treated group improved as compared to 35% receiving the placebo. These data were confirmed subsequently, although improvement may not occur until after four weeks of therapy. Sulfasalazine, 250 to 500 mg four times a day, often is considered the drug of choice in ulcerative colitis exacerbation because its efficacy has been demonstrated and because it has less severe adverse effects than corticosteroids. However, controlled trials have shown that corticosteroids may be more prompt in onset of action than sulfasalazine, alone or in combination with corticosteroid, for the treatment of severe acute ulcerative colitis. While comparative efficacy trials are lacking, the combination of sulfasalazine and prednisone does not appear to be detrimental and often has been used in hope of alleviating patients' symptoms.

_____

Excerpted with permission from "Chapter 24, Inflammatory Bowel Disease," page 24-3, *Applied Therapeutics: The Clinical Use of Drugs, Sixth Edition,* edited by Lloyd Yee Young and Mary Anne Koda-Kimble, published by Applied Therapeutics, Inc., Vancouver, Washington, © 1995.

35. The most frequently prescribed drug for inflammatory bowel disease therapy is

    (A) prednisone.
    (B) sulfasalazine.
    (C) estrogen.
    (D) aspirin.

36. What percentage of the patients in the uncontrolled observation did NOT improve with sulfasalazine therapy?

    (A) 35% to 50%
    (B) 5% to 10%
    (C) 10% to 20%
    (D) 80% to 90%

37. What percentage of the patients in the placebo group in the placebo-controlled trial did NOT improve?

    (A) 35%
    (B) 45%
    (C) 55%
    (D) 65%

38. According to the passage, how many times per day is sulfasalazine given?

    (A) Four
    (B) Five
    (C) Six
    (D) Eight

39. The combination of sulfasalazine and prednisone

    (A) appears to be dangerous.
    (B) offers hope.
    (C) shows no benefit.
    (D) is not recommended.

PASSAGE 9

Angina pectoris can be defined as a sense of discomfort arising in the myocardium as a result of myocardial ischemia in the absence of infarction. Although angina usually implies severe chest pain or discomfort, its presentation is variable. At one extreme, angina may occur predictably with strenuous exercise; at the other, angina may develop unexpectedly with little or no exertion.

Patients who have a reproducible pattern of angina that is associated with a certain level of physical activity have chronic stable angina or exertional angina. In contrast, patients with unstable angina are experiencing new angina or a change in their angina intensity, frequency, or duration. Both chronic stable angina and unstable angina often reflect underlying atherosclerotic narrowing of coronary arteries. Classic Prinzmetal's variant angina, or vasospastic angina, occurs in patients without coronary heart disease and is due to a spasm of the coronary artery that decreases myocardial blood flow. When coronary vasospasm occurs at the site of a fixed atherosclerotic plaque, mixed angina can result.

Silent myocardial ischemia, which is a transient change in myocardial perfusion, function, or electrical activity, can be detected on an electrocardiogram (ECG) in most angina patients. The patient, however, does not experience chest pain or other signs of angina [e.g., jaw pain, shortness of breath] during these episodes. Silent myocardial ischemia also can occur in patients with no angina history.

Excerpted with permission from "Chapter 13, Ischematic Heart Disease: Anginal Syndromes," pages 13-1 to 13-2, *Applied Therapeutics: The Clinical Use of Drugs, Sixth Edition*, edited by Lloyd Yee Young and Mary Anne Koda-Kimble, published by Applied Therapeutics, Inc., Vancouver, Washington, © 1995.

40. The term angina usually refers to

    (A) headache.
    (B) chest pain.
    (C) athlete's foot.
    (D) sore throat.

41. Angina associated with physical activity is

    (A) Prinzmetal's angina.
    (B) variant angina.
    (C) vasocolonic angina.
    (D) stable angina.

42. Which type of angina occurs in patients without coronary heart disease?

    (A) Variant angina
    (B) Exertional angina
    (C) Prinzmetal's variant angina
    (D) Unstable angina

43. Silent myocardial ischemia

    (A) is atherosclerotic plaque.
    (B) has no consequences.
    (C) is a permanent change in myocardial perfusion, function, or electrical activity.
    (D) is a transient change in myocardial perfusion, function, or electrical activity.

44. Of the titles below, which would best describe the passage?

    (A) Angina—the Silent Killer
    (B) The Different Types of Angina
    (C) Chest Pain
    (D) Treating Chest Pain

PASSAGE 10

With the lifting of trade restrictions on the Mississippi River following the 1803 Louisiana Purchase, the New Orleans economy entered a period of unprecedented prosperity that would last over half a century. The population of the city had already doubled by the time, less than a decade later, that the first steamboat—aptly named the *New Orleans*—was put into service on the Mississippi, facilitating upstream navigation and further enhancing New Orleans's position as a major hub of commerce. The effect of this shift can be measured by the staggering growth in downriver cargo received at the port: between 1801 and 1807, an average of $5 million worth of goods came downstream each year, but in 1851 alone almost $200 million worth of freight was measured. Shipments of cotton constituted almost half of these receipts, but many other goods—grain, sugar, molasses, tobacco, manufactured items, and much more—as well as people passed through this New Orleans hub, creating a prosperous, cosmopolitan environment that few cities in the New World could match.

This localized economic boom, built on the contingencies of geography, began to subside in the years following the Civil War. The city's position on the wrong side of the Mason-Dixon line was only one small part of the problem. Even more pressing was an inexorable shift in the nation's infrastructure. During the closing decades of the nineteenth century, the railroad gradually replaced the steamboat as the major transportation industry in America. Trading hubs grew up elsewhere, and New Orleans's position at the gateway of the major inland water system waned in importance. Economic woes were further aggravated by chronic political corruption. The result: by 1874, the state of Louisiana was insolvent, unable to pay either principal or the accumulated interest on its $53 million debt. Investment capital, to the extent that it stayed within the region, gravitated to natural resources and oil fields, with attendant wealth moving outside New Orleans to other parts of Louisiana and beyond the state line to Texas. The boisterous histories of New Orleans jazz often obscure this underlying truth: by the time of the birth of jazz, New Orleans was already a city in decline.

The city's population had increased more than fourfold during the half-century from 1825 to 1875, but in 1878, 2 percent of the city's inhabitants perished in a devastating yellow fever epidemic. The risk of pestilence was always present in nineteenth-century New Orleans, especially during the long, hot summer months. The city sits below sea level, and its damp, warm climate combined with dismal local sanitation—the city had no sewage system until 1892, long after most North American cities had adopted modern methods of fluid waste disposal—made the Crescent City an ideal breeding ground for mosquitoes, roaches, and other assorted vermin. New Orleans bassist Pops Foster recalled conditions being so poor that he was required to wear mosquito nets during some performances. After the 1878 epidemic, population growth resumed at a sluggish 1 percent annual rate, but the number of foreign-born members of the population actually declined, as new immigrants sought more flourishing economics and healthier surroundings.

Excerpted from *The History of Jazz*, by Ted Gioia. New York: Oxford University Press, 2011.

45. An epidemic of what disease killed 2 percent of the population of New Orleans in 1878?

(A) Typhus
(B) Cholera
(C) Smallpox
(D) Yellow Fever

46. According to the passage, New Orleans lagged behind other cities in the U.S. in installing

(A) a public transportation system.
(B) a sewage system.
(C) a public health system.
(D) a tax collection system.

47. Which of the following factors played a primary role in the economic decline of New Orleans?

(A) The invention of the steamboat
(B) The expansion of the railroad
(C) The influx of immigrants
(D) The corruption of bankers who controlled investment capital

48. What would be the most appropriate title for this passage?

(A) Prosperity and Pestilence in New Orleans
(B) The Steamboat's Golden Age
(C) Population Shifts in New Orleans in the 19th Century
(D) The Economy of the South After the Civil War

49. What lesson can be learned regarding the economic shifts experienced by New Orleans?

(A) The corruption of state politicians has minimal effect on the local economy.
(B) Changes to the national transportation infrastructure have little impact on the local economy.
(C) Changes to the national transportation infrastructure may significantly impact the local economy.
(D) Being a gateway to a major inland water system guarantees ongoing economic prosperity, despite changes in the national transportation infrastructure.

50. Which of the following goods was the most profitable shipment that passed through New Orleans in the early decades of the 1800s?

(A) Grain
(B) Cotton
(C) Sugar
(B) Molasses

ANSWER KEY
Critical Reading

1.	**C**	14.	**B**	27.	**C**	40.	**B**
2.	**A**	15.	**C**	28.	**B**	41.	**D**
3.	**A**	16.	**B**	29.	**C**	42.	**C**
4.	**D**	17.	**B**	30.	**C**	43.	**D**
5.	**A**	18.	**A**	31.	**C**	44.	**B**
6.	**B**	19.	**D**	32.	**A**	45.	**D**
7.	**D**	20.	**B**	33.	**D**	46.	**B**
8.	**A**	21.	**C**	34.	**A**	47.	**B**
9.	**C**	22.	**C**	35.	**B**	48.	**A**
10.	**D**	23.	**A**	36.	**C**	49.	**C**
11.	**B**	24.	**D**	37.	**D**	50.	**B**
12.	**D**	25.	**A**	38.	**A**		
13.	**B**	26.	**A**	39.	**B**		

ANSWERS EXPLAINED

The numbers in the margins of the reprinted passages indicate the statements in which the answer to the questions can be found.

PASSAGE 1

As evictions and lowered crop prices squeezed tens of thousands of farmers from the land after 1934, they ran headlong into the pattern of economic distress that had dominated the nonagricultural economy since the start of the decade. If anything, the cities and towns had suffered more than rural areas as the Depression tightened its grip on the commercial life of the region in the first half of the thirties. Depression-era unemployment data are sketchy and not always reliable, but the available estimates indicate that the Southwest contended with higher percentages of unemployment than other predominately rural sections of the country. The federal government's Committee on Economic Security estimated Arkansas's rate of nonagricultural unemployment to be

2 the third highest in the nation (39.2 percent) during the nadir year of 1933. Oklahoma, Texas, and Missouri, with rates varying between 29 and 32 percent, exceeded nearly all other states in the South or on the northern plains. We have no data on the four recovery years which followed, but the 1937 federal unemployment census, taken just as the nation's economy entered another decline, found 22 percent of all available Southwestern workers either unemployed or engaged on work relief projects. Another 10 percent were considered partly unemployed. Conditions improved somewhat during the last two and a half years of the decade. When census takers visited homes in 1940, the unemployment rate in the Western South was down to 14.3 percent, but the level still remained higher than most rural states.

With the partial exception of Missouri, the Southwestern states had few resources with which to assist the jobless and needy. Local and state relief funds were quickly exhausted as unemployment soared and tax revenues fell in the first years of the Depression, and usually offered little more than emergency groceries to those in need.

1 Private charities like the Red Cross also helped, but in general the level of assistance available prior to 1933 was minimal. The establishment of the Federal Emergency Relief Administration shortly after Franklin Roosevelt assumed the presidency improved

4 matters considerably. Through 1934 and 1935, federal relief funds sustained more than two and a half million Southwesterners, almost 20 percent of the region's population, on a continuing basis. In some areas the relief burden was much larger. During certain drought months in 1934, up to 90 percent of the population of particular eastern Oklahoma counties collected relief payments.

1. **(C)** According to the passage, little assistance was available to those affected by the Depression before 1933, suggesting that the Depression began before 1933. This eliminates choices A and B. The passage also states that availability of assistance in 1933 and in the following years improved after Franklin Roosevelt became president. This eliminates choice D. Choice C is therefore correct—the Great Depression began in 1929 during the presidency of Herbert Hoover. Franklin Roosevelt succeeded Hoover, becoming president in 1933.

2. **(A)** "Nadir" is defined as the lowest point. In the "nadir year of 1933," the United States hit its lowest point during the Great Depression. The years 1932 and 1933 are generally considered the worst years of the Depression, due to the steep fall of the gross national product and the dramatic rise in unemployment.

3. **(A)** The passage addresses the impact of the Great Depression on the Southwestern United States. Although some aspects of the federal response to the Depression (choice B) and nonagricultural unemployment rates (choice D) are mentioned, neither is the primary focus of the passage. Migration patterns (choice C) during the Depression are not mentioned.

4. **(D)** As per the second paragraph of the passage, almost 20 percent of the Southwest region's population received federal relief funds in the mid-1930s.

PASSAGE 2

To the average physician, Lyme disease is suspected when a patient arrives at a clinic or hospital complaining of a strange bull's-eye rash, known as erythema migrans, or EM, together with one or more flulike symptoms, such as fever, chills, muscle aches, or
8 lethargy. The doctor will take a blood sample for laboratory confirmation, but will feel quite confident to make a diagnosis of Lyme disease after noting the telltale combina-
5 tion of symptoms, as well as the circumstances surrounding the infection. The patient will undoubtedly have been bitten by the black-legged tick *Ixodes scaplaris*, formerly called the deer tick, or a close relative, which transferred to him or her the *B. burgdorferi* bacterium. Most likely, the physician will prescribe an oral course of antibiotics and will duly report the case to the county or state health department, which will include it in the morbidity statistics for Lyme disease.

Accurate diagnosis and effective treatment of Lyme disease are not always so straightforward, particularly in regions of the country newly invaded by the epidemic. In these regions, health care professionals and the public need to be educated about the confusing and generalized symptoms, the generally poor, but growing, accuracy of lab
7 tests, and the efficacy of various antibiotic treatments. If Lyme disease is left untreated for some time, *B. burgdorferi* may persist in the patient's tissues and can migrate to the
9 central and peripheral nervous system or to joints and cause more severe late-stage symptoms, which include arthritis and neurological disorders, such as dizziness, memory loss and disorientation. Vaccines that protect against Lyme disease are now being field tested by pharmaceutical companies, but none has yet been approved by the Food and Drug Administration for public use. Even if an effective vaccine were certified and marketed, the primary means that individuals have of protecting themselves against the disease is avoiding the tick in the first place.

5. **(A)** For the pathogen *B. burgdorferi* to pass from tick to human, the human must be bitten by the tick—in this case, the black-legged tick, *Ixodes scaplaris*. A tick-bearing mammal (choice B) might provide the tick, but not the bite. The microbe *B. burgdorferi* is not capable of biting, so choice C cannot be correct. Choice D is irrelevant (Lyme disease is not airborne).

6. **(B)** Because the passage discusses both the diagnosis of and strategies to treat Lyme disease, as well as the challenges in addressing Lyme disease, such as lack of public awareness, choice B represents the most appropriate title. Choice A addresses only one part of the passage, a similar problem with choices C and D.

7. **(D)** As noted in the second paragraph of the passage, Lyme disease can migrate to joints, which belong to the musculoskeletal system.

8. **(A)** As stated in the passage, the physician will take a blood sample to get laboratory confirmation of the diagnosis. Choices B, C, and D are not true.

9. **(C)** Choice A is not addressed in the paragraph. Choice B is false since leaving the disease untreated is not mentioned in the passage as having any effect on lab tests. Choice D is neither stated nor implied in the passage. The result of leaving Lyme disease untreated is clearly described in choice C.

PASSAGE 3

In the past two decades, people living in the northeastern, north-central, and western United States have unwittingly entered a dangerous enzootic cycle—a cycle of disease that typically is restricted to wildlife. Wild mammals and birds host a wide variety of disease agents, with effects ranging from mild symptoms to mortality, but in most cases the pathogen affects only one or a few host species and never causes disease in humans.
10 However, as a result of a complicated sequence of events, people have become frequent accidental hosts for ticks and the disease agents they carry, including a corkscrew-
13 shaped bacterium called *Borrelia burgdorferi*, the agent of Lyme disease. As of 1995, cases of Lyme disease had been reported in 48 of the 50 states and appear to be increasing, both in numbers of people affected and in geographic distribution.

Where does this disease come from, why has it emerged so rapidly, and what can people do to reduce their risk of exposure? It is possible to address these questions not from a medical point of view, but rather from an ecological one. All living organisms— from the *B. burgdorferi* bacterium and the ticks it infects to the mice and deer on which
11 the ticks feed—form an ecological relationship with their habitats. Understanding the complex interactions between plant and animal species within those habitats may help people to predict the places where they are most likely to encounter disease-bearing ticks and become infected. Thus armed, individuals may ultimately be able to protect themselves from Lyme disease.
12   Currently, to prevent Lyme disease people wear protective clothing when they are in
14 wooded areas and perform "tick checks" after leaving the woods. One underemphasized means to avoid exposure to Lyme disease, however, is avoiding the most heavily tick-infested habitats at the times of year when ticks are most abundant or dangerous. Recent research has suggested that such habitats can be predicted, often well in advance. Ultimately, it is the hope of ecologists studying this problem that we can use our expertise in pinpointing these habitats to warn the public away from areas that are likely to contain an abundance of disease-carrying ticks.

10. **(D)** The first paragraph clearly describes how humans have accidentally become hosts to ticks and pathogens such as *Borrelia burgdorferi*. While choice B is a true statement, it is not the primary focus of the paragraph. Choices A and C are not true.

11. **(B)** While choices A and D might well be sound ecological goals in other circumstances, when it comes to Lyme disease, ecologists are motivated by a desire to help people predict and avoid the places where they are likely to become infected (choice B). Although choice C is an important medical consideration, the development of a vaccine is not the province of ecologists.

12. **(D)** As stated in the last paragraph of the passage, preventative steps in remaining Lyme disease–free include wearing protective clothing (a step taken prior to exploring the woods) and performing physical "tick checks" after leaving the woods. The remaining answer choices are not true.

13. **(B)** Choice B is a true statement taken directly from the passage. Choices A, C, and D are false.

14. **(B)** Choice B is a true statement taken directly from the passage. Choice A is mentioned as an often-used, rather than an underemployed, protective measure. Choices C and D are irrelevant.

PASSAGE 4

Unlike an electron, a single red blood cell cannot go through two openings at once.
15 Indeed, it is generally true that the physicist seeking to understand the circulation of the blood can ignore most of the perplexities of twentieth-century physics. Given the scale of the circulatory system and the speed of blood flow, neither quantum mechanics nor relativity applies. Instead the flow of blood through the heart and the vascular tree can be adequately described by the familiar mechanics of Newton and Galileo.

If the circulation of the blood obeys the laws of classical mechanics, however, this
16 does not mean that it is simple. An early experimental model of the vascular tree was a system of glass tubes filled with water. But unlike water, blood is not an "ideal" fluid. Instead it is a suspension of cells that, under certain circumstances, can behave in non-Newtonian ways. Moreover, flow through the vascular tree is pulsatile rather than steady; blood vessels taper and are elastic rather than rigid; and flow in any part of the densely interconnected system is affected by flow in neighboring regions. When these factors and the fantastic geometrical complexity of the labyrinthine vascular system are taken into account, the equations of blood flow, while remaining classical in inspiration, quickly become too complex to be solved explicitly.

17 Confronted with a system of overwhelming complexity, scientists typically resort to the intelligent simplification, that is, to a model. The first mathematical model of the
18 human circulation was the *windkessel*, or compression chamber, model developed by Otto Frank in 1899 to explain how pulsatile flow from the heart is converted into steadier flow in the peripheral circulation. Sophisticated analytical models, the descendants of the *windkessel* model, still provide insight into the functioning of the circulatory system. But they are increasingly supplemented by numerical models, which exploit the power of the computer to arrive at accurate approximations of values that

19 satisfy systems of equations that would otherwise be unsolvable. The computer can also be used to produce stunning images that allow otherwise cryptic measurements or calculations to be grasped intuitively.

15. **(C)** The passage states that the mechanics of Newton and Galileo are adequate for describing the circulatory system and blood flow. Choice A is irrelevant; choices B and D contradict information given in the passage.

16. **(B)** As described in the passage, an early experimental model was a system of glass tubes filled with water (choice B). Choice A is irrelevant, choice C is false, and choice D is both false and absurd.

17. **(B)** According to the passage, scientists are likely to turn to a model when confronted with a system of overwhelming complexity (choice B). Choices A and D are decidedly untrue. Choice D actually contradicts information given in the passage.

18. **(A)** As stated in the passage, Frank developed his *windkessel* model of the circulatory system to explain how pulsatile flow from the heart is converted into steadier flow in the peripheral circulation (choice A). Since he made use of the model, not human subjects, the answer cannot be choice C (which is a nonsense statement anyway). His was the first mathematical model, so choice B cannot be correct. Frank was not attempting to augment the mechanics of Galileo and Newton (choice D).

19. **(D)** As the passage indicates, quantum physics and relativity are not relevant to the study of the circulatory system, so choice A cannot be the correct answer. Nor is choice B correct, since the *windkessel* dates back to 1899 and was no longer in use. Choice C contradicts information stated in the passage. Only choice D actually occurs as a statement in the passage.

PASSAGE 5

24 An important method that anthropologists use to learn about ways of thinking is to consider how people explain and deal with misfortunes that happen to them. On such occasions, people draw on ideas that they have been socialized to share but which may or may not be apparent in everyday conversation as they may be taken for granted. These ideas are often related to religion, a spirit world, or a system of classification that draws on ideas about supernatural powers that some specialist people are believed to control. For others, or even for the same people in different situations, answers are found in *science*, and again most people would turn to specialists—doctors or engineers perhaps—for help in solving particular problems. In all cases, they are drawing on a
20 *cosmology*, a system of ideas about the world, how it is classified, how it works, and how they fit into that world.

An influential study on this subject was published in a book named *Witchcraft, Oracles and Magic among the Azande* by E.E. Evans-Pritchard, whose fieldwork in
23 the Southern Sudan enabled him to discover and explain a rather different system of logic to the one he started out with. The Azande people draw on ideas of witchcraft to
21 explain unfortunate things that happen in their lives. For them, witchcraft is not something frightening, as it might be for people in Britain, but simply an annoying everyday

occurrence. It was, therefore, brought frequently to the attention of the anthropologist

25 learning their language, and Evans-Pritchard explained that the logic behind this use of the term provides a complete explanation for unfortunate events, such as crop failure, accidental injury, or illness.

This doesn't mean that the Azande are unaware of 'natural' explanations. If a person falls over a root in the path, they know that the root caused them to trip; if their crops fail because of a lack of rain, they know that they needed water to thrive; if members of a family fall sick after eating something unusual, they know that it may have been bad. What witchcraft explains in all these cases is why that bad thing happened to those particular people at that particular time: why the person who tripped walked that way, why the rain fell elsewhere and missed the crops, and why the ones who fell sick happened to eat that food on that day. To explain such things in terms of having been bewitched takes an explanation that others may simply wonder about to a complete logical conclusion, he argued.

20. **(B)** As defined in the first paragraph, *cosmology* is defined as a system of ideas about the world, which most closely matches the definition provided in choice B. Choices A, C, and D are the definitions of other anthropological terms (i.e., core values, archeology, ethnography).

21. **(C)** As stated in the second paragraph, witchcraft is an everyday occurrence for the Azande.

22. **(C)** The passage notes that the Azande believe natural events occur as a result of witchcraft (choice C). Witchcraft explains why a bad thing happened to particular people at that particular time (which contradicts choice B). The passage does not address malicious acts (choice A) or punishment (choice D).

23. **(A)** Evans-Pritchard conducted his fieldwork in the African country of Sudan.

24. **(D)** According to the first sentence of the passage, anthropologists are interested in how people explain misfortune to learn about ways of thinking.

25. **(A)** According to the last sentence of the second paragraph, for the Azande, witchcraft offers a complete explanation for unfortunate events.

PASSAGE 6

28 Allergic drug reactions account for 5% to 20% of all observed adverse drug reactions. Adverse drug reactions have been reported to occur in as many as 30% of hospitalized patients, and 3% of all hospitalizations are a result of adverse drug reactions. In a computerized surveillance study of over 36,000 hospitalized patients, 731 adverse events

29 were identified. Of those, 1% were categorized as severe, life-threatening, and allergic in nature. The potential morbidity and mortality associated with allergic drug reactions is great even though these outcomes occur infrequently.

26   In order to appropriately diagnose and treat a patient experiencing an allergic reaction, it is necessary to be able to differentiate allergic reactions from other closely related adverse drug reactions. One method of classification divides adverse reactions

into those that are "predictable, usually dose-dependent, and related to the pharmaco-

27 logic actions of the drug," and those that are "unpredictable, often dose-independent, and are related to the individual's immunologic response or to genetic differences in susceptible patients." Under this classification scheme, drug allergy or drug hypersensitivity is an unpredictable adverse drug reaction that is immunologically mediated.

26. **(A)** As the passage states, allergic reactions must be differentiated from other closely related adverse drug reactions (choice A). Choice B describes reactions that are typically adverse but not allergic, and choice C is irrelevant to diagnosing and treating allergic drug reactions appropriately. While some allergic reactions may require hospitalization (choice D), this is not necessary to diagnose appropriately and treat all allergic reactions to drugs.

27. **(C)** Choice C appears in the passage. Choices A, B, and D are not true.

28. **(B)** According to the passage, 5% to 20% of all observed adverse drug reactions represent allergic drug reactions.

29. **(C)** That 1% of the 731 adverse drug events were characterized as severe, life-threatening, and allergic in nature is stated in the passage (choice C). Choice B is only partially true, since the allergic reactions identified were of a severe and life-threatening nature. Both choices A and D refer to adverse reactions that are not classified as allergic.

PASSAGE 7

31 Art history in its modern form originated in Germany in the nineteenth century. People had thought about the art of the past before, of course, but they did so in a way which we would now say was unhistorical: namely, they looked, not for what makes particular works significant in their own right, but how far these works realized what were thought to be universal aesthetic norms. Art theory was taught in the European academies which had been established in the seventeenth and eighteenth centuries for the training of artists, and included discussion of the art of the past; but individual artists and

34 schools (that is, works of art grouped according to their country of origin) were judged according to whether they had achieved a representation of ideal beauty.

32   The Italian artist, Giorgio Vasari (1511–1574) is often called the first art historian. His *The Lives of the Artists*, first published in 1550, provided an influential model for the understanding of past art. Vasari's art history was not historical in the modern sense,

30 however. In his view, art's development over time was cyclical, and he discussed the achievement of individual artists with respect to their place in this cyclical process. According to Vasari, art achieved its first high point in the golden age of ancient Greek art, declined in the fourth and fifth centuries A.D., was revived by Giotto in the thirteenth century, improved by Masaccio, Piero della Francesca and Mantegna in the fifteenth,

33 and brought to new heights by Leonardo, Raphael and Michelangelo in Vasari's own time. But while Vasari saw art change during each cycle, approaching ever nearer to an aesthetic ideal, he did not understand these changes as a result of particular historical or social conditions at work at the time when each artist lived. A historical understanding of art in the modern sense did not start to develop until the end of the eighteenth

century; until that time, history was thought to be extrinsic to art in the way that earthquakes are extrinsic to it. Art's value lay in striving to achieve timeless aesthetic norms, norms that were elaborated systematically by such French art theorists as André Félibien (1619–1695) and Roger de Piles (1635–1709) in the late seventeenth and early eighteenth centuries. When the University of Göttingen in Germany founded the first chair in art history in 1813, this was not the dawn of art history as we now know it. The man appointed, Johann Dominicus Fiorillo, was a drawing master and his lectures followed the tradition of academic art theory.

30. **(C)** As stated in the second paragraph, Vasari believed art's development is cyclical over time.

31. **(C)** As stated in the first paragraph, the modern form of art history emerged from Germany.

32. **(A)** Giorgio Vasari, who is considered to be the first art historian, was Italian.

33. **(D)** New heights were reached by Leonardo, Michelangelo, and Raphael, artists who lived during the Renaissance.

34. **(A)** As per the first paragraph, schools of art referred to works of art grouped by their country of origin.

PASSAGE 8

35 Sulfasalazine, the most frequently prescribed drug for inflammatory bowel disease therapy, has been used commonly for 50 years for the induction of disease remission

36 in patients with mild acute exacerbations of ulcerative colitis. Initial uncontrolled observations of its efficacy indicated that 80% to 90% of patients improved with the use

37 of this agent. The first placebo-controlled trial using objective parameters of efficacy demonstrated that 80% of the treated group improved as compared to 35% receiving the placebo. These data were confirmed subsequently, although improvement may

38 not occur until after four weeks of therapy. Sulfasalazine, 250 to 500 mg four times a day, often is considered the drug of choice in ulcerative colitis exacerbation because its efficacy has been demonstrated and because it has less severe adverse effects than corticosteroids. However, controlled trials have shown that corticosteroids may be more prompt in onset of action than sulfasalazine, alone or in combination with corticosteroid, for the treatment of severe acute ulcerative colitis. While comparative

39 efficacy trials are lacking, the combination of sulfasalazine and prednisone does not appear to be detrimental and often has been used in hope of alleviating patients' symptoms.

35. **(B)** Although prednisone (choice A) is used to treat inflammatory bowel disease, the first sentence of the passage clearly states that the most frequently prescribed drug for inflammatory bowel disease therapy is sulfasalazine.

36. **(C)** The passage states that 80% to 90% of patients improved during the initial uncontrolled observations, leaving 10% to 20% who did not improve.

37. **(D)** The passage states that 35% of patients in the placebo group improved, leaving 65% who did not improve.

38. **(A)** Sulfasalazine is given four times per day at doses of 250–500 mg.

39. **(B)** The passage clearly states that the combination of sulfasalazine and prednisone does not appear to be detrimental (dangerous, choice A) and often has been used in hope of alleviating patients' symptoms (choice B).

PASSAGE 9

Angina pectoris can be defined as a sense of discomfort arising in the myocardium as
40 a result of myocardial ischemia in the absence of infarction. Although angina usually implies severe chest pain or discomfort, its presentation is variable. At one extreme, angina may occur predictably with strenuous exercise; at the other, angina may develop unexpectedly with little or no exertion.

41   Patients who have a reproducible pattern of angina that is associated with a certain level of physical activity have chronic stable angina or exertional angina. In contrast, patients with unstable angina are experiencing new angina or a change in their angina intensity, frequency, or duration. Both chronic stable angina and unstable angina often
42 reflect underlying atherosclerotic narrowing of coronary arteries. Classic Prinzmetal's variant angina, or vasospastic angina, occurs in patients without coronary heart disease and is due to a spasm of the coronary artery that decreases myocardial blood flow. When coronary vasospasm occurs at the site of a fixed atherosclerotic plaque, mixed angina can result.

43   Silent myocardial ischemia, which is a transient change in myocardial perfusion, function, or electrical activity, can be detected on an electrocardiogram (ECG) in most angina patients. The patient, however, does not experience chest pain or other signs of angina [e.g., jaw pain, shortness of breath] during these episodes. Silent myocardial ischemia also can occur in patients with no angina history.

40. **(B)** Although a headache (choice A) may accompany chest pain (choice B), angina usually implies severe chest pain. Choice C is absurd in the context of the passage. Choice D is not true.

41. **(D)** Prinzmetal's and variant angina (choices A and B) are due to a spasm of the coronary artery. There is no such disorder as vasocolonic angina (choice C). Angina that is associated with a certain level of physical activity is called stable angina or exertional angina (choice D).

42. **(C)** The passage states that Prinzmetal's variant angina occurs in patients without coronary heart disease. Choices A, B, and D are untrue.

43. **(D)** The passage states that silent myocardial ischemia is a transient change in myocardial perfusion, function, or electrical activity; therefore, choice D is correct, while choice C is incorrect. Silent myocardial ischemia is not atherosclerotic plaque (choice A), although atherosclerotic plaque may cause ischemia. Myocardial ischemia can cause serious damage (consequences, choice B).

44. **(B)** Since the passage does not discuss the mortality rates associated with angina or the treatment of chest pain, choices A and D are incorrect. Chest pain (choice C) is too broad a title for this passage. Choice B, The Different Types of Angina, best describes the focus of this passage.

PASSAGE 10

With the lifting of trade restrictions on the Mississippi River following the 1803 Louisiana Purchase, the New Orleans economy entered a period of unprecedented prosperity that would last over half a century. The population of the city had already doubled by the time, less than a decade later, that the first steamboat—aptly named the *New Orleans*—was put into service on the Mississippi, facilitating upstream navigation and further enhancing New Orleans's position as a major hub of commerce. The effect of this shift can be measured by the staggering growth in downriver cargo received at the port: between 1801 and 1807, an average of $5 million worth of goods came downstream each year, but in 1851 alone almost $200 million worth of freight was measured.

50 Shipments of cotton constituted almost half of these receipts, but many other goods— grain, sugar, molasses, tobacco, manufactured items, and much more—as well as people passed through this New Orleans hub, creating a prosperous, cosmopolitan environment that few cities in the New World could match.

This localized economic boom, built on the contingencies of geography, began to subside in the years following the Civil War. The city's position on the wrong side of the Mason-Dixon line was only one small part of the problem. Even more pressing was an

47 inexorable shift in the nation's infrastructure. During the closing decades of the nineteenth century, the railroad gradually replaced the steamboat as the major transportation industry in America. Trading hubs grew up elsewhere, and New Orleans's position at the gateway of the major inland water system waned in importance. Economic woes were further aggravated by chronic political corruption. The result: by 1874, the state of Louisiana was insolvent, unable to pay either principal or the accumulated interest on its $53 million debt. Investment capital, to the extent that it stayed within the region, gravitated to natural resources and oil fields, with attendant wealth moving outside New Orleans to other parts of Louisiana and beyond the state line to Texas. The boisterous histories of New Orleans jazz often obscure this underlying truth: by the time of the birth of jazz, New Orleans was already a city in decline.

The city's population had increased more than fourfold during the half-century from

45 1825 to 1875, but in 1878, 2 percent of the city's inhabitants perished in a devastating yellow fever epidemic. The risk of pestilence was always present in nineteenth-century New Orleans, especially during the long, hot summer months. The city sits below sea

46 level, and its damp, warm climate combined with dismal local sanitation—the city had no sewage system until 1892, long after most North American cities had adopted modern methods of fluid waste disposal—made the Crescent City an ideal breeding ground for mosquitoes, roaches, and other assorted vermin. New Orleans bassist Pops Foster recalled conditions being so poor that he was required to wear mosquito nets during some performances. After the 1878 epidemic, population growth resumed at a sluggish 1 percent annual rate, but the number of foreign-born members of the population actually declined, as new immigrants sought more flourishing economics and healthier surroundings.

45. **(D)** An epidemic of yellow fever killed 2 percent of the population of New Orleans in 1878.

46. **(B)** New Orleans lagged behind other cities in the U.S. in installing a sewage system.

47. **(B)** As explained in the second paragraph, the railroad gradually replaced the steamboat as the primary transportation industry in the country, which negatively impacted the economy of New Orleans (choice B). The invention of the steamboat (choice A) positively affected the New Orleans economy, and the influx of immigrants (choice C) was a sign of a healthy economy. Therefore, neither choice A nor choice C correctly answered the question. Choice D was not addressed in the passage.

48. **(A)** The passage described the economic prosperity and decline experienced by New Orleans during the 1800s, as well as sanitation issues faced by the city (pestilence); thus, choice A is the most appropriate title for the passage. The passage was not primarily focused on the steamboat (choice B) or population changes in New Orleans (choice C). The passage also did not address economics in the post–Civil War South (choice D).

49. **(C)** The passage largely attributed the economic decline of New Orleans to changes in the nation's transportation infrastructure (specifically, the shift from the steamboat to the railroad); thus, choice C is the correct choice, while choices B and D are not true. In contrast to choice A, corrupt state politicians had a negative impact on the economy.

50. **(B)** The passage states that almost half of the freight receipts were for shipments of cotton (choice B), indicating that this good was more profitable than grain (choice A), sugar (choice C), or molasses (choice D).

The PCAT
Writing Section

8

PCAT WRITING SECTION

The writing section of the PCAT presents a topic that requires you to write a short literary composition as a "problem-solving" essay. The problem-solving essay topic is presented in the form of a statement that poses a problem to be solved. The writing topic or prompt may be based on health issues, science issues, or social/cultural/political issues. The essay should present and coherently explain your suggested solution to the problem presented in the statement, as well as possible alternatives to the primary solution being presented. The writing section is scored according to two writing rubrics: "Conventions of Language" and "Problem Solving."

You will not be able to use a dictionary or any other reference material(s). You will have 30 minutes to complete the essay. You should allow yourself enough time to determine what your response to the topic will be (brainstorm), to organize and write your essay (you may find that writing a quick outline may help with this), and to edit and proofread your response. The greatest portion of the 30-minute time allotment should be spent writing the essay; remember to pace yourself and to keep track of time. As with the other sections of the PCAT, the essay will be written on the computer using the computer-based platform provided at the testing center. The PCAT website (*www.pcatweb.info*) offers writing practice tests that will be useful when preparing for the PCAT.

TIP

Be sure to present and coherently explain your suggested solution to the problem.

PCAT WRITING SECTION SCORES

On the PCAT score report, you will receive a score for the writing test as well as the mean of all writing scores for the same test administration period. The score on the writing test will utilize a six-point scale, ranging from 1 = "Inadequate" to 6 = "Superior." The six score possibilities for each rubric are characterized on the next page, as outlined on the PCAT website (*www.pcatweb.info*).

The writing score will be included on the score report received by the candidate and sent to those institutions chosen by the candidate. However, the score is not incorporated into the composite scaled or percentile scores of the PCAT. Some schools do not use the PCAT writing score at all in their admission processes. Please confirm with the school you are interested in as to what they do with the PCAT writing score as it relates to your candidacy evaluation.

Writing Section Score	Conventions of Language Description
One—"Inadequate"	Application of the conventions of language is limited.
Two—"Marginal"	Several mistakes distract from the essay response that is being presented, and the ability to fully understand the points of the essay may be diminished.
Three—"Satisfactory"	There are several mistakes in structure that may interfere with the ease of the essay's interpretation, but the basic structural pattern (beginning, middle, end) is intact.
Four—"Effective"	While there are mistakes in structure that may interfere with the essay's flow, the general meaning is not compromised.
Five—"Proficient"	Overall, the writer correctly applies the conventions of language. There may be some errors, but they do not interfere with understanding the points intended or the flow of the essay.
Six—"Superior"	Few, if any, errors are made and the writer exhibits good technique in presentation of the essay components.

Writing Section Score	Problem-Solving Description
One—"Inadequate"	The relationship between the problem and the solution is not clear, support is unconvincing, and the organization is problematic.
Two—"Marginal"	Although the solution is related to the problem, the structure of the essay detracts from the flow of ideas, the essay lacks a logical argument, and the solution is not clear.
Three—"Satisfactory"	The essay's solution is adequately related to the problem, but is too general in presentation to be persuasive, and organization may be weak.
Four—"Effective"	The essay's solution is clear, but is too general in presentation, and organization may be weak so as to lessen the effectiveness of the argument.
Five—"Proficient"	The essay shows a clear relationship between problem and solution. However, while support is appropriate and logical, it lacks depth.
Six—"Superior"	The essay presents a clear, well-reasoned relationship between problem and solution with convincing support and a powerful argument. Organization has logical flow.

PCAT ESSAY WRITING TIPS

There are many existing guides and tutorials that discuss the construction of an effective essay. For additional guidance on how to write a persuasive essay, refer to

www.hamilton.edu/writing/writing-resources/persuasive-essays

Please note that this website is not specific to the PCAT. You must keep in mind the 30-minute time limit for the PCAT writing section. Below are several tips you can use to help you compose an essay.

- The introduction paragraph is the first paragraph of your essay. In your introduction, include some background information and the problem to be solved based on the topic. Use a clear thesis statement to present the topic and inform the reader as to what the essay will be about.

- Follow your introduction with one or more supporting paragraphs to make up the main body of your essay. It is important to develop each point in your essay in a properly structured paragraph. Make sure there is a link between your thesis and the supporting paragraphs. Present applicable and appropriate references based on academic studies or personal experiences.

- Use clear and simple structure for your sentences. Avoid the use of clichés, slang, jargon, and abstract terms that tend to fill space but provide no specific points in your essay. Elaborate on your ideas, leading the reader to your conclusions. You are to present a solution or build a case in support of your viewpoint.

- Use a clear writing style. Avoid redundant words, long sentences, and vague information. Do not use 35 words when five words will efficiently and effectively present your information. Write concisely and cover the topic presented.

- Use appropriate grammar, punctuation, usage, and style. Avoid abbreviations and acronyms when possible.

- Finish with a conclusion, either as a statement or a closing paragraph after the main body of your essay. It is important that your conclusion logically follows the points you have developed in the supporting paragraphs of the essay.

- Always proofread your essay. Glaring or frequent spelling or grammatical errors could be construed as poor writing.

PRACTICE ESSAY QUESTIONS

(Please note, the actual PCAT exam will have only one question/writing section.)

Directions: Write a well-constructed essay addressing the statement below.

According to the Centers for Disease Control and Prevention, obesity has doubled in children and tripled in adolescents over the past three decades, resulting in increased risk for cardiovascular disease and diabetes, among other disease states. Discuss a solution to the problem of childhood obesity and its associated health risks.

Directions: Write a well-constructed essay addressing the statement below.

According to the American Public Health Association (APHA), tobacco use contributes to six million deaths worldwide on an annual basis. One in three cancer deaths is attributable to tobacco use. The APHA also notes that nine out of every ten smokers begins using tobacco by age 18. Discuss strategies to address the problem of tobacco use, particularly among adolescents.

PRACTICE TESTS

Practice Test 1

9

This sample PCAT is not a copy of an actual PCAT, but it has been designed to closely represent the types of questions that may be included in an actual exam. As in the actual PCAT, this test has five separate sections—Biological Processes, Chemical Processes, Quantitative Reasoning, Critical Reading, and Writing. The actual PCAT may have additional experimental questions that are being tested for use on future exams. Because the experimental questions do not count toward your actual PCAT score, there are no equivalent questions included in this sample PCAT. It is important to do your best on every question since you will not be able to distinguish the experimental questions.

You may find it best to proceed with this practice exam as if you were taking the actual PCAT by adhering to the time allowed for each section in the table below. Your overall strategy should be to answer every question in the time allotted, while getting as many correct answers as possible. Do not leave any questions unanswered, as there will be no penalty for guessing on the actual PCAT. Your score on this sample PCAT will give you a good idea of the subject areas you need to study further. By timing yourself on the sample PCAT, you will also learn whether you need to increase your speed or slow down when you take the actual PCAT.

After completing the sample PCAT, you may grade your exam by using the answer key. Regardless of your score on the sample PCAT, it will benefit you to review all the explanatory answers at the end of the sample PCAT. If your answer to a question was incorrect, the explanation may help you understand where you went wrong. If your answer was correct, the explanation may broaden your understanding of the topic area being tested.

Before starting the exam, please refresh your memory on the test-taking strategies discussed earlier in this book. Good luck on the examination.

Section	Time Allowed*
1. Biological Processes	40 minutes
2. Chemical Processes	40 minutes
3. Quantitative Reasoning	45 minutes
4. Critical Reading	50 minutes
5. Writing (Essay)	30 minutes

*Please note: The order of the subjects (test sections) may vary from test to test.

ANSWER SHEET
Practice Test 1

BIOLOGICAL PROCESSES (1–48)

1. Ⓐ Ⓑ Ⓒ Ⓓ   13. Ⓐ Ⓑ Ⓒ Ⓓ   25. Ⓐ Ⓑ Ⓒ Ⓓ   37. Ⓐ Ⓑ Ⓒ Ⓓ
2. Ⓐ Ⓑ Ⓒ Ⓓ   14. Ⓐ Ⓑ Ⓒ Ⓓ   26. Ⓐ Ⓑ Ⓒ Ⓓ   38. Ⓐ Ⓑ Ⓒ Ⓓ
3. Ⓐ Ⓑ Ⓒ Ⓓ   15. Ⓐ Ⓑ Ⓒ Ⓓ   27. Ⓐ Ⓑ Ⓒ Ⓓ   39. Ⓐ Ⓑ Ⓒ Ⓓ
4. Ⓐ Ⓑ Ⓒ Ⓓ   16. Ⓐ Ⓑ Ⓒ Ⓓ   28. Ⓐ Ⓑ Ⓒ Ⓓ   40. Ⓐ Ⓑ Ⓒ Ⓓ
5. Ⓐ Ⓑ Ⓒ Ⓓ   17. Ⓐ Ⓑ Ⓒ Ⓓ   29. Ⓐ Ⓑ Ⓒ Ⓓ   41. Ⓐ Ⓑ Ⓒ Ⓓ
6. Ⓐ Ⓑ Ⓒ Ⓓ   18. Ⓐ Ⓑ Ⓒ Ⓓ   30. Ⓐ Ⓑ Ⓒ Ⓓ   42. Ⓐ Ⓑ Ⓒ Ⓓ
7. Ⓐ Ⓑ Ⓒ Ⓓ   19. Ⓐ Ⓑ Ⓒ Ⓓ   31. Ⓐ Ⓑ Ⓒ Ⓓ   43. Ⓐ Ⓑ Ⓒ Ⓓ
8. Ⓐ Ⓑ Ⓒ Ⓓ   20. Ⓐ Ⓑ Ⓒ Ⓓ   32. Ⓐ Ⓑ Ⓒ Ⓓ   44. Ⓐ Ⓑ Ⓒ Ⓓ
9. Ⓐ Ⓑ Ⓒ Ⓓ   21. Ⓐ Ⓑ Ⓒ Ⓓ   33. Ⓐ Ⓑ Ⓒ Ⓓ   45. Ⓐ Ⓑ Ⓒ Ⓓ
10. Ⓐ Ⓑ Ⓒ Ⓓ   22. Ⓐ Ⓑ Ⓒ Ⓓ   34. Ⓐ Ⓑ Ⓒ Ⓓ   46. Ⓐ Ⓑ Ⓒ Ⓓ
11. Ⓐ Ⓑ Ⓒ Ⓓ   23. Ⓐ Ⓑ Ⓒ Ⓓ   35. Ⓐ Ⓑ Ⓒ Ⓓ   47. Ⓐ Ⓑ Ⓒ Ⓓ
12. Ⓐ Ⓑ Ⓒ Ⓓ   24. Ⓐ Ⓑ Ⓒ Ⓓ   36. Ⓐ Ⓑ Ⓒ Ⓓ   48. Ⓐ Ⓑ Ⓒ Ⓓ

CHEMICAL PROCESSES (49–96)

49. Ⓐ Ⓑ Ⓒ Ⓓ   61. Ⓐ Ⓑ Ⓒ Ⓓ   73. Ⓐ Ⓑ Ⓒ Ⓓ   85. Ⓐ Ⓑ Ⓒ Ⓓ
50. Ⓐ Ⓑ Ⓒ Ⓓ   62. Ⓐ Ⓑ Ⓒ Ⓓ   74. Ⓐ Ⓑ Ⓒ Ⓓ   86. Ⓐ Ⓑ Ⓒ Ⓓ
51. Ⓐ Ⓑ Ⓒ Ⓓ   63. Ⓐ Ⓑ Ⓒ Ⓓ   75. Ⓐ Ⓑ Ⓒ Ⓓ   87. Ⓐ Ⓑ Ⓒ Ⓓ
52. Ⓐ Ⓑ Ⓒ Ⓓ   64. Ⓐ Ⓑ Ⓒ Ⓓ   76. Ⓐ Ⓑ Ⓒ Ⓓ   88. Ⓐ Ⓑ Ⓒ Ⓓ
53. Ⓐ Ⓑ Ⓒ Ⓓ   65. Ⓐ Ⓑ Ⓒ Ⓓ   77. Ⓐ Ⓑ Ⓒ Ⓓ   89. Ⓐ Ⓑ Ⓒ Ⓓ
54. Ⓐ Ⓑ Ⓒ Ⓓ   66. Ⓐ Ⓑ Ⓒ Ⓓ   78. Ⓐ Ⓑ Ⓒ Ⓓ   90. Ⓐ Ⓑ Ⓒ Ⓓ
55. Ⓐ Ⓑ Ⓒ Ⓓ   67. Ⓐ Ⓑ Ⓒ Ⓓ   79. Ⓐ Ⓑ Ⓒ Ⓓ   91. Ⓐ Ⓑ Ⓒ Ⓓ
56. Ⓐ Ⓑ Ⓒ Ⓓ   68. Ⓐ Ⓑ Ⓒ Ⓓ   80. Ⓐ Ⓑ Ⓒ Ⓓ   92. Ⓐ Ⓑ Ⓒ Ⓓ
57. Ⓐ Ⓑ Ⓒ Ⓓ   69. Ⓐ Ⓑ Ⓒ Ⓓ   81. Ⓐ Ⓑ Ⓒ Ⓓ   93. Ⓐ Ⓑ Ⓒ Ⓓ
58. Ⓐ Ⓑ Ⓒ Ⓓ   70. Ⓐ Ⓑ Ⓒ Ⓓ   82. Ⓐ Ⓑ Ⓒ Ⓓ   94. Ⓐ Ⓑ Ⓒ Ⓓ
59. Ⓐ Ⓑ Ⓒ Ⓓ   71. Ⓐ Ⓑ Ⓒ Ⓓ   83. Ⓐ Ⓑ Ⓒ Ⓓ   95. Ⓐ Ⓑ Ⓒ Ⓓ
60. Ⓐ Ⓑ Ⓒ Ⓓ   72. Ⓐ Ⓑ Ⓒ Ⓓ   84. Ⓐ Ⓑ Ⓒ Ⓓ   96. Ⓐ Ⓑ Ⓒ Ⓓ

QUANTITATIVE REASONING (97–144)

97. Ⓐ Ⓑ Ⓒ Ⓓ   109. Ⓐ Ⓑ Ⓒ Ⓓ   121. Ⓐ Ⓑ Ⓒ Ⓓ   133. Ⓐ Ⓑ Ⓒ Ⓓ
98. Ⓐ Ⓑ Ⓒ Ⓓ   110. Ⓐ Ⓑ Ⓒ Ⓓ   122. Ⓐ Ⓑ Ⓒ Ⓓ   134. Ⓐ Ⓑ Ⓒ Ⓓ
99. Ⓐ Ⓑ Ⓒ Ⓓ   111. Ⓐ Ⓑ Ⓒ Ⓓ   123. Ⓐ Ⓑ Ⓒ Ⓓ   135. Ⓐ Ⓑ Ⓒ Ⓓ
100. Ⓐ Ⓑ Ⓒ Ⓓ   112. Ⓐ Ⓑ Ⓒ Ⓓ   124. Ⓐ Ⓑ Ⓒ Ⓓ   136. Ⓐ Ⓑ Ⓒ Ⓓ
101. Ⓐ Ⓑ Ⓒ Ⓓ   113. Ⓐ Ⓑ Ⓒ Ⓓ   125. Ⓐ Ⓑ Ⓒ Ⓓ   137. Ⓐ Ⓑ Ⓒ Ⓓ
102. Ⓐ Ⓑ Ⓒ Ⓓ   114. Ⓐ Ⓑ Ⓒ Ⓓ   126. Ⓐ Ⓑ Ⓒ Ⓓ   138. Ⓐ Ⓑ Ⓒ Ⓓ
103. Ⓐ Ⓑ Ⓒ Ⓓ   115. Ⓐ Ⓑ Ⓒ Ⓓ   127. Ⓐ Ⓑ Ⓒ Ⓓ   139. Ⓐ Ⓑ Ⓒ Ⓓ
104. Ⓐ Ⓑ Ⓒ Ⓓ   116. Ⓐ Ⓑ Ⓒ Ⓓ   128. Ⓐ Ⓑ Ⓒ Ⓓ   140. Ⓐ Ⓑ Ⓒ Ⓓ
105. Ⓐ Ⓑ Ⓒ Ⓓ   117. Ⓐ Ⓑ Ⓒ Ⓓ   129. Ⓐ Ⓑ Ⓒ Ⓓ   141. Ⓐ Ⓑ Ⓒ Ⓓ
106. Ⓐ Ⓑ Ⓒ Ⓓ   118. Ⓐ Ⓑ Ⓒ Ⓓ   130. Ⓐ Ⓑ Ⓒ Ⓓ   142. Ⓐ Ⓑ Ⓒ Ⓓ
107. Ⓐ Ⓑ Ⓒ Ⓓ   119. Ⓐ Ⓑ Ⓒ Ⓓ   131. Ⓐ Ⓑ Ⓒ Ⓓ   143. Ⓐ Ⓑ Ⓒ Ⓓ
108. Ⓐ Ⓑ Ⓒ Ⓓ   120. Ⓐ Ⓑ Ⓒ Ⓓ   132. Ⓐ Ⓑ Ⓒ Ⓓ   144. Ⓐ Ⓑ Ⓒ Ⓓ

CRITICAL READING (145–192)

145. Ⓐ Ⓑ Ⓒ Ⓓ   157. Ⓐ Ⓑ Ⓒ Ⓓ   169. Ⓐ Ⓑ Ⓒ Ⓓ   181. Ⓐ Ⓑ Ⓒ Ⓓ
146. Ⓐ Ⓑ Ⓒ Ⓓ   158. Ⓐ Ⓑ Ⓒ Ⓓ   170. Ⓐ Ⓑ Ⓒ Ⓓ   182. Ⓐ Ⓑ Ⓒ Ⓓ
147. Ⓐ Ⓑ Ⓒ Ⓓ   159. Ⓐ Ⓑ Ⓒ Ⓓ   171. Ⓐ Ⓑ Ⓒ Ⓓ   183. Ⓐ Ⓑ Ⓒ Ⓓ
148. Ⓐ Ⓑ Ⓒ Ⓓ   160. Ⓐ Ⓑ Ⓒ Ⓓ   172. Ⓐ Ⓑ Ⓒ Ⓓ   184. Ⓐ Ⓑ Ⓒ Ⓓ
149. Ⓐ Ⓑ Ⓒ Ⓓ   161. Ⓐ Ⓑ Ⓒ Ⓓ   173. Ⓐ Ⓑ Ⓒ Ⓓ   185. Ⓐ Ⓑ Ⓒ Ⓓ
150. Ⓐ Ⓑ Ⓒ Ⓓ   162. Ⓐ Ⓑ Ⓒ Ⓓ   174. Ⓐ Ⓑ Ⓒ Ⓓ   186. Ⓐ Ⓑ Ⓒ Ⓓ
151. Ⓐ Ⓑ Ⓒ Ⓓ   163. Ⓐ Ⓑ Ⓒ Ⓓ   175. Ⓐ Ⓑ Ⓒ Ⓓ   187. Ⓐ Ⓑ Ⓒ Ⓓ
152. Ⓐ Ⓑ Ⓒ Ⓓ   164. Ⓐ Ⓑ Ⓒ Ⓓ   176. Ⓐ Ⓑ Ⓒ Ⓓ   188. Ⓐ Ⓑ Ⓒ Ⓓ
153. Ⓐ Ⓑ Ⓒ Ⓓ   165. Ⓐ Ⓑ Ⓒ Ⓓ   177. Ⓐ Ⓑ Ⓒ Ⓓ   189. Ⓐ Ⓑ Ⓒ Ⓓ
154. Ⓐ Ⓑ Ⓒ Ⓓ   166. Ⓐ Ⓑ Ⓒ Ⓓ   178. Ⓐ Ⓑ Ⓒ Ⓓ   190. Ⓐ Ⓑ Ⓒ Ⓓ
155. Ⓐ Ⓑ Ⓒ Ⓓ   167. Ⓐ Ⓑ Ⓒ Ⓓ   179. Ⓐ Ⓑ Ⓒ Ⓓ   191. Ⓐ Ⓑ Ⓒ Ⓓ
156. Ⓐ Ⓑ Ⓒ Ⓓ   168. Ⓐ Ⓑ Ⓒ Ⓓ   180. Ⓐ Ⓑ Ⓒ Ⓓ   192. Ⓐ Ⓑ Ⓒ Ⓓ

WRITING

For the essay portion of the test, you may compose your response on page 251 or on a separate sheet of paper.

BIOLOGICAL PROCESSES

48 QUESTIONS (#1–#48)
TIME: 40 MINUTES

Directions: Choose the **best** answer to each of the following questions.

QUESTIONS 1 THROUGH 4 REFER TO THE FOLLOWING PASSAGE:

A woman visits an emergency clinic complaining of a nagging cough. An X-ray of her lungs shows heavy density obstructing her alveoli. She is given a medicine to treat the infection. After one week, a follow-up X-ray shows no changes, and her cough remains persistent. After two additional medications are tried, each for one week, a fourth medicine then clears up the infection, and her cough is gone.

Below is a table of the four medications prescribed to the woman. The name and order in which she took each medication is listed. The mechanism of action describes what the drug targets in a cell.

	Name	Mechanism of Action	Effective (Y/N)
1st	Penicillin	Targets peptidoglycan production	No
2nd	Ciprofloxacin	Targets prokaryote DNA replication	No
3rd	Streptomycin	Targets 30S ribosome subunit	No
4th	Amphotericin B	Targets ergosterol in plasma membrane	Yes

1. The first drug, penicillin, targets peptidoglycan production. What category of biomolecule is peptidoglycan?

   (A) Polysaccharide
   (B) Polypeptide
   (C) Nucleic acid
   (D) Fat

2. Which medication targets the process of cell division of bacteria?

   (A) Penicillin
   (B) Ciprofloxacin
   (C) Streptomycin
   (D) Amphotericin B

3. Which medication targets the process of protein production of bacteria?

   (A) Penicillin
   (B) Ciprofloxacin
   (C) Streptomycin
   (D) Amphotericin B

4. Based on the mode of action of each drug tried, what type of organism likely caused her infection?

   (A) Archaea
   (B) Gram positive bacteria
   (C) Gram negative bacteria
   (D) Fungus

QUESTIONS 5 THROUGH 8 REFER TO THE FOLLOWING PASSAGE:

The first cells to evolve on Earth were the prokaryotes. In general, these single-celled organisms contain a cell membrane, cell wall, ribosomes, and one circular chromosome. Over time, the more complex eukaryotic cells arose. These cells share many similarities to their prokaryotic ancestors, but they evolved to become a larger size than prokaryotes and developed membrane-bound organelles as well as multiple chromosomes.

The figure below depicts an animal cell (left) and a bacterial cell (right).

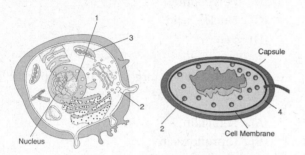

5. Number 1 is pointing to what structure?

   (A) Nucleolus
   (B) Golgi apparatus
   (C) Endoplasmic reticulum
   (D) Mitochondria

6. Number 2 is pointing to structures that are shared between both eukaryotic and prokaryotic cells. What is that structure?

   (A) DNA
   (B) Ribosomes
   (C) Carbohydrates
   (D) Vesicles

7. Number 3 is pointing to what structure?

   (A) Lysosome
   (B) Golgi apparatus
   (C) Nucleus
   (D) Mitochondria

8. Number 4 is pointing to what structure?

   (A) Cell wall
   (B) Golgi apparatus
   (C) Smooth endoplasmic reticulum
   (D) Rough endoplasmic reticulum

_____

9. DNA replication results in

   (A) two DNA molecules, one with two newly synthesized strands and one with two parental strands.
   (B) two DNA molecules, each with two newly synthesized strands.
   (C) two DNA molecules, each of which has one parental strand and one newly synthesized strand.
   (D) two DNA molecules, each of which has strands of unknown origins.

10. A microorganism that obtains its carbon, as well as its energy, from organic compounds is called

   (A) an autotroph.
   (B) a heterotroph.
   (C) a heterozygote.
   (D) a homozygote.

11. If "A" represents a dominant trait and "a" represents a recessive trait, which of the following crosses would be expected to result in 25% of the offspring as "aa"?

   (A) Aa × aa
   (B) AA × aa
   (C) Aa × Aa
   (D) Aa × AA

12. Which of the following structures respond(s) to dim light for black-and-white vision?

   (A) Cones
   (B) Rods
   (C) Iris
   (D) Cornea

13. Normal red blood cells have an average life span of

   (A) 30 days.
   (B) 60 days.
   (C) 120 days.
   (D) 180 days.

14. ATP is a molecule that stores energy in the form of a

   (A) hydrogen bond.
   (B) phosphate bond.
   (C) nitrogen bond.
   (D) carbon bond.

15. Which of the following is a monomer?

   (A) Starch
   (B) Peptidoglycan
   (C) Glucose
   (D) Chitin

16. Kinesin and dynein transport vesicles throughout the cell. What category of protein are kinesin and dynein?

   (A) Motor proteins
   (B) Structural proteins
   (C) Storage proteins
   (D) Receptor proteins

17. In the cell cycle, what phase occurs just prior to cytokinesis?

   (A) Telophase
   (B) Metaphase
   (C) Prophase
   (D) Anaphase

18. Genes that are capable of relocating from one part of the genome to another are called

   (A) mesosomes.
   (B) transposons.
   (C) plasmids.
   (D) fimbriae.

19. _____ are gram-positive, spore-forming bacilli. The major diseases associated with these bacteria are caused by exotoxins.

   (A) E. coli
   (B) Eubacterium
   (C) Clostridium
   (D) Lactobacillus

QUESTIONS 20 THROUGH 23 REFER TO THE FOLLOWING PASSAGE:

Many diseases can be passed from parent to offspring through chromosomal inheritance. An example of a genetically-inherited disease is sickle-celled anemia (SCA). SCA is caused by a mutation in the β-hemoglobin gene on chromosome 11. The resulting abnormal protein causes red blood cells to misform. The resulting disease leads to reduced energy, issues with development, and frequent infections, among other symptoms. Below are four family trees of genetically-inherited diseases. Males are squares, and females are circles. White indicates a healthy individual and black indicates a diseased individual.

A.

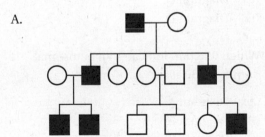

B.

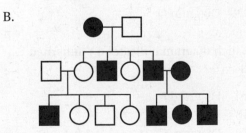

C.

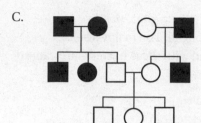

D.

20. Which diagram indicates an autosomal recessive disease?

    (A) Diagram A
    (B) Diagram B
    (C) Diagram C
    (D) Diagram D

21. Which diagram indicates an X-linked recessive disease?

    (A) Diagram A
    (B) Diagram B
    (C) Diagram C
    (D) Diagram D

22. Which diagram indicates an autosomal dominant disease?

    (A) Diagram A
    (B) Diagram B
    (C) Diagram C
    (D) Diagram D

23. Which diagram indicates a Y-inherited disease?

    (A) Diagram A
    (B) Diagram B
    (C) Diagram C
    (D) Diagram D

24. What structure connects the middle ear to the throat?

    (A) Auricle
    (B) Eustachian tube
    (C) Tympanic membrane
    (D) Cochlea

25. A resistance to which hormone causes type 2 diabetes?

    (A) Glucose
    (B) Cortisol
    (C) Insulin
    (D) Testosterone

26. Which of the following enzymes connects Okazaki fragments on the lagging strand during DNA replication in eukaryotic cells?

    (A) DNA ligase
    (B) DNA helicase
    (C) DNA polymerase I
    (D) DNA polymerase III

27. Microorganisms that lack cell walls are known as _____; they do not synthesize the precursors of peptidoglycan.

    (A) photosynthetic bacteria
    (B) archaea
    (C) mycoplasmas
    (D) plasmids

28. What organ filters blood from the digestive tract and returns the blood to the heart via hepatic veins?

    (A) Pancreas
    (B) Gallbladder
    (C) Kidneys
    (D) Liver

29. The superficial protective layer of the skin is the

    (A) dermis.
    (B) hypodermis.
    (C) epidermis.
    (D) exodermis.

30. What does the term *evolution* mean?

   (A) The characteristics of a population change through time.
   (B) The characteristics of a species become more complex over time.
   (C) The characteristics of an individual change through the course of its life in response to natural selection.
   (D) The strongest individuals produce the most offspring.

31. The adrenal glands produce which two hormones?

   (A) Melatonin and serotonin
   (B) Adrenalin and noradrenaline
   (C) Insulin and glucagon
   (D) Estrogen and testosterone

QUESTIONS 32 THROUGH 35 REFER TO THE FOLLOWING PASSAGE:

During an action potential event in a neuron, sodium and potassium channels are opened. The movement of these ions across the cell membrane causes a depolarization. As the axon of the neuron is depolarized, the action potential eventually reaches the terminus of the axon, and neurotransmitters are released.

The sodium potassium protein pump is important in helping neurons return to a resting state after a neuron has undergone an action potential. The pump moves three sodium ions out of a neuron while two potassium ions are moved inside the neuron. ATP is utilized by the pump during this process. The relative concentration in mM of each ion in a mammalian neuron at rest and during an action potential is shown in the table below.

Ion	Intracellular ion concentration	Extracellular ion concentration
Na^+	15 mM	135 mM
K^+	150 mM	5.5 mM

32. Which of the following best describes the direction of the movement of the sodium and potassium in the sodium-potassium pump?

   (A) Uniport
   (B) Symport
   (C) Antiport
   (D) Coupled transport

33. Which of the following best describes the movement of the sodium ions out of the neuron?

   (A) Active transport
   (B) Passive transport
   (C) Simple diffusion
   (D) Facilitated diffusion

34. Which of the following best describes the movement of the potassium ions into the neuron?

   (A) Active transport
   (B) Passive transport
   (C) Simple diffusion
   (D) Facilitated diffusion

35. During an action potential, the movement of ions across the membrane will have an effect on what type of nearby channel proteins?

   (A) Ligand-gated channel proteins
   (B) Mechanical-gated channel proteins
   (C) Voltage-gated channel proteins
   (D) Non-gated channel proteins

36. In aerobic cellular respiration, most of the ATP is synthesized during

   (A) the Krebs cycle.
   (B) electron transport.
   (C) electron oxidation.
   (D) the citric acid cycle.

37. A normal cell spends approximately 90% of its time in

    (A) prophase.
    (B) metaphase.
    (C) interphase.
    (D) anaphase.

38. In the human respiratory system, there is a net diffusion of carbon dioxide from

    (A) hemoglobin to mitochondria.
    (B) alveoli to blood.
    (C) blood to the air in the alveoli.
    (D) air to blood in bronchi.

39. Which of the following is a water-soluble vitamin?

    (A) Vitamin A
    (B) Vitamin E
    (C) Vitamin C
    (D) Vitamin D

QUESTIONS 40 THROUGH 43 REFER TO THE FOLLOWING PASSAGE:

The animal brain is the control center of the body of an organism. It is composed of soft, spongy tissue. This delicate organ is protected from damage by the cranial bone that makes up the skull. Below that bone is a thick layer of cells called the meninges.

   A professional football player named Matt suffers a head injury when he is tackled. He is knocked unconscious for two minutes. After he wakes up, Matt is clearly confused, and as he talks to his coach, his words make no sense. A physician is called immediately and told of Matt's symptoms. The physician orders a CT (computed tomography) scan of Matt's brain to look for cranial bleeding or swelling.

40. Based on Matt's language issue, which area of the brain would you hypothesize has bleeding or swelling?

    (A) The occipital lobe
    (B) The hippocampus
    (C) The cerebellum
    (D) The temporal lobe

41. After 24 hours in the hospital, Matt recovers his ability to speak. He is able to tell his doctor that he has had blurred vision since the accident. What area of the brain may have also been damaged during his injury?

    (A) The spinal cord
    (B) The cerebellum
    (C) The temporal lobe
    (D) The occipital lobe

42. After 48 hours in the hospital, Matt no longer has blurred vision and claims to feel fine. However, he does not remember anything about the day the accident happened. His physician fears that Matt may have short term memory loss. What area of the brain may be damaged if Matt is experiencing memory loss?

    (A) The medulla oblongata
    (B) The temporal lobe
    (C) The cerebellum
    (D) The hippocampus

43. Before Matt can leave the hospital, his physician orders a full physical. All of his vitals appear normal, and his physician is ready to discharge him. As Matt gets out of his hospital bed and prepares to leave, he notices that his left leg is dragging, and he has a staggering gait (ataxia) when he walks. What area of his brain may also be injured?

    (A) The medulla oblongata
    (B) The spinal cord
    (C) The occipital lobe
    (D) The cerebellum

44. Why is it difficult to develop a vaccine against viruses with high mutation rates like HIV?

    (A) The vaccines tend to be unstable and deteriorate over time.
    (B) The virus proteins are only recognized by killer T cells.
    (C) New viral mutations constantly change the viral proteins.
    (D) The virions contain so many different proteins that the immune system is overwhelmed.

45. Which of the following cell types would engulf and digest bacteria?

    (A) Killer T cells
    (B) B cells
    (C) Natural killer cells
    (D) Macrophages

46. The genomes of viruses may contain

    (A) double-stranded DNA only.
    (B) single-stranded RNA only.
    (C) double-stranded DNA or double-stranded RNA.
    (D) double-stranded DNA, single-stranded DNA, single-stranded RNA, or double-stranded RNA.

47. A bacteriophage

    (A) is a virus that infects bacteria.
    (B) is a fungus.
    (C) does not contain DNA or RNA.
    (D) is a bacterium that infects fungi.

48. In general, enzyme activity is influenced by temperature, enzyme concentration, substrate concentration, and

    (A) water.
    (B) pH.
    (C) oxygen concentration.
    (D) carbon dioxide concentration.

STOP

End of Biological Processes section. If you have any time left, you may go over your work in this section only.

CHEMICAL PROCESSES

48 QUESTIONS (#49–#96)
TIME: 40 MINUTES

The periodic table is provided below, if needed.

H																	He
Li	Be											B	C	N	O	F	Ne
Na	Mg											Al	Si	P	S	Cl	Ar
K	Ca	Sc	Ti	V	Cr	Mn	Fe	Co	Ni	Cu	Zn	Ga	Ge	As	Se	Br	Kr
Rb	Sr	Y	Zr	Nb	Mo	Tc	Ru	Rh	Pd	Ag	Cd	In	Sn	Sb	Te	I	Xe
Cs	Ba	La	Hf	Ta	W	Re	Os	Ir	Pt	Au	Hg	Tl	Pb	Bi	Po	At	Rn
Fr	Ra	Ac	Rf	Ha	Sg	Ns	Hs	Mt									

Ce	Pr	Nd	Pm	Sm	Eu	Gd	Tb	Dy	Ho	Er	Tm	Yb	Lu
Th	Pa	U	Np	Pu	Am	Cm	Bk	Cf	Es	Fm	Md	No	Lr

> **Directions:** Choose the **best** answer to each of the following questions.

QUESTIONS 49 THROUGH 52 REFER TO THE FOLLOWING PASSAGE:

Prior to cell division (mitosis), the genetic material must be duplicated such that the DNA in each daughter cell is identical to that of the mother cell. Mitosis is part of the cell cycle and is called the M stage. Other parts of the cell cycle are two gaps (G1 and G2) and the S phase during which the cell's DNA is synthesized. During DNA synthesis, the polymerization of nucleotides is catalyzed by DNA polymerases. Details on the enzymes' requirements and functions are known, and in addition to the polymerization activity, they have an exonuclease or proofreading activity. Thus, errors in DNA synthesis are largely avoided. Since DNA is the permanent copy of genetic material in the cell and is used as a pattern for protein synthesis throughout the cell's life, fidelity in the process is required.

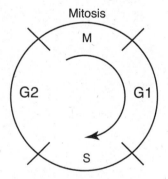

The Cell Cycle

DNA synthesis phase

49. What is the name of the process by which new DNA molecules are synthesized?

(A) Transcription
(B) Translation
(C) Replication
(D) Translocation

50. The monomers used by DNA polymerase include

   (A) ribonucleotides.
   (B) adenosine diphosphate.
   (C) deoxyuridine triphosphate.
   (D) deoxyguanidine triphosphate.

51. The reaction catalyzed by DNA polymerase connects a phosphate to what functional group on the carbohydrate of the nucleotide?

   (A) An acetal
   (B) A secondary alcohol
   (C) An amine
   (D) A primary alcohol

52. A three base sequence in DNA corresponds to the incorporation of

   (A) a monosaccharide in a polysaccharide.
   (B) an amino acid in the mRNA.
   (C) a nucleotide in tRNA
   (D) an amino acid in a protein.

QUESTIONS 53 THROUGH 56 REFER TO THE FOLLOWING PASSAGE:

The statins are a class of drugs used in patients with high blood cholesterol (hypercholesterolemia). For many years, atorvastatin (Lipitor) was the number one selling drug in the U.S. Hypercholesterolemia has been associated with an increased risk of myocardial infarction, stroke, and atherosclerosis. Appropriate dietary choices and increased exercise can lower serum cholesterol (a steroid) and is usually the first recommendation to patients diagnosed with hypercholesterolemia. If drug therapy is needed, a statin may be prescribed. Statins inhibit the first committed step in steroid biosynthesis and thus decrease the amount of cholesterol found in the blood. Since the primary site of cholesterol biosynthesis is the liver, liver function tests are recommended while taking a statin.

The structure of atorvastatin is given below.

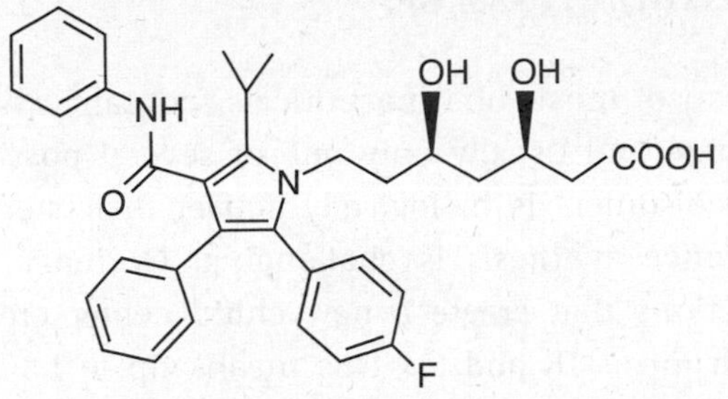

53. Cholesterol is biosynthesized as well as absorbed from dietary fats and is necessary for

   (A) hormone production.
   (B) hemoglobin production.
   (C) DNA synthesis.
   (D) the prevention of cardiovascular disease.

54. Which functional group is NOT found in atorvastatin?

   (A) An alkyne
   (B) An arene
   (C) A secondary alcohol
   (D) An amide

55. Atorvastatin contains a carboxylic acid functional group. Which of the following methods can be used to produce a carboxylic acid?

   (A) Hydrolysis of a nitrile
   (B) Oxidation of a ketone
   (C) Hydrolysis of an epoxide
   (D) Halogenation of an alkene

56. Which of the following bands would NOT be expected in the infrared (IR) spectrum of atorvastatin?

   (A) 3300 cm^{-1}
   (B) 2100 cm^{-1}
   (C) 1700 cm^{-1}
   (D) 3000 cm^{-1}

Because most pharmaceuticals contain chiral centers and usually only one of several possible stereoisomers is biologically active, their stereo-selective synthesis is challenging. Ordinary lab reactions that create a new chiral center create both forms (R and S). This means up to half of the product is likely biologically inert, repre-senting a waste of resources. For example, when (S)-2-chlorobutane is made by the addition of HCl to 2-butene, a racemic mixture (50% R and 50% S) results.

2-butene

Efforts to selectively synthesize a single stereoisomer include the use of a chiral auxiliary (chiral groups temporarily installed to enhance the rate of formation of one stereoisomer) and enzymes (biological catalysts which often selectively produce a single stereoisomer). Careful planning in a synthetic scheme is necessary to maximize the yield of the desired product.

57. Which synthetic scheme below would maximize the yield of m-nitrotoluene from benzene?

(A) Nitration with nitric acid and sulfuric acid followed by methylation via a Friedel-Craft alkylation

(B) Chlorination with chlorine and iron (III) chloride followed by nitration with nitric acid and sulfuric acid

(C) Methylation via Friedel-Craft acylation followed by nitration with ammonia

(D) Nitration with ammonia and aluminum chloride followed by methylation via a Grignard reaction

58. The reduction of (S)-methyl 2-bromopropa-noic acid to (S)-2-bromo-1-propanol maintains optical purity since the reaction does not occur at the chiral center. Which reagent would accomplish this conversion?

(A) $KMnO_4$
(B) $LiAlH_4$
(C) $NaBH_4$
(D) H_2

59. Which of the following methods would NOT produce the reactant in question 58?

(A) The reaction of a carboxylic acid with an alcohol

(B) The reaction of a carboxylic acid halide with an alcohol

(C) The reaction of a carboxylic acid anhydride with an alcohol

(D) The reaction of an amide with an alcohol

60. Two molecules that are stereoisomers but are not nonsuperimposable mirror images are called

(A) diastereomers.
(B) meso forms.
(C) enantiomers.
(D) constitutional isomers.

QUESTIONS 61 THROUGH 65 REFER TO THE
FOLLOWING PASSAGE:

The three-dimensional shape of a protein is intimately linked to its biological activity. Extreme changes in temperature or pH can disrupt the protein's secondary and tertiary structure and result in a loss of biological activity. Normal physiologic pH is 7.4, and the side chains of several amino acids are essentially completely ionized at that pH. If the pKa of the functional group in the side chain is more than two units above or below 7.4, the side chain is assumed to be completely ionized.

The ionization of side chains is important in forming "salt bridges" in proteins. Salt bridges are the attraction between oppositely charged functional groups in protein side chains. Changes in the pH can thus affect the percent ionization and destroy salt bridges that may be necessary for biological function. Ionized side chains of proteins are also often involved in the active site binding of substrates and the mechanism of enzyme catalysis.

61. The side chain of which of the following amino acids is expected to be completely ionized at physiologic pH?

    (A) Alanine
    (B) Glutamic acid
    (C) Valine
    (D) Glycine

62. The amino acid sequence in proteins is the protein's

    (A) primary structure.
    (B) secondary structure.
    (C) tertiary structure.
    (D) quaternary structure.

63. What type of intermolecular force is responsible for the formation of an alpha helix in a protein?

    (A) Hydrogen bonding between the side chains of amino acids
    (B) Hydrogen bonding between peptide bonds
    (C) London forces
    (D) Dipole-dipole interactions between the side chains of amino acids

64. Biologically, buffers are necessary to prevent pH changes that may be deleterious. Which of the following is a buffer solution?

    (A) H_2SO_4 and Na_2SO_4
    (B) H_2SO_4
    (C) CH_3COOH
    (D) CH_3COOH and CH_3COONa

65. Peptide bonds connect amino acids making proteins. What type of functional group is a peptide bond?

    (A) An ester
    (B) A carboxylic acid anhydride
    (C) An amide
    (D) An amine

QUESTIONS 66 THROUGH 69 REFER TO THE FOLLOWING PASSAGE:

According to the FBI, copper theft has become a public safety concern as well as an issue of national security. Copper is found in many easily accessible structures like electrical substations, cell towers, phone lines, construction sites, and vacant homes. Copper, like many of the other elemental metals, is able to conduct heat and electricity. It is also malleable and ductile. In fact, one reason it is used in electrical wiring is because it is highly ductile while remaining flexible.

The theft of copper can result in disruptions in the flow of electricity and communication. There have been cases where tornado warning systems have malfunctioned due to wiring theft. The primary reason theft of copper occurs is money. Previously, thieves were able to sell stolen copper to scrap metal buyers but many now only buy copper from licensed contractors. The price of copper worldwide climbed over the past 10 years, fueled by the demand in developing countries.

66. The specific heat of copper is 0.385 J/g°C. If 15.0 J of heat is absorbed by a 5.0 g sample of copper at 25°C, what will be the approximate new temperature of the copper?

    (A) 55°C
    (B) 47°C
    (C) 33°C
    (D) 15°C

67. The element with an atomic number of 29 and an atomic mass of 65 contains

    (A) 29 neutrons.
    (B) 65 protons.
    (C) 36 neutrons.
    (D) 29 electrons.

68. Different isotopes of copper will have a different number of

    (A) electrons.
    (B) neutrons.
    (C) protons.
    (D) ions.

69. What is the molarity of a solution prepared by dissolving 37.5 g of $Cu(NO_3)_2$ in enough water to make 500.0 mL of solution?
    (Cu = 63.5 amu, N = 14 amu, O = 16 amu)

    (A) 0.20 M
    (B) 0.60 M
    (C) 0.30 M
    (D) 0.40 M

___

QUESTIONS 70 THROUGH 73 REFER TO THE FOLLOWING PASSAGE:

Helium, the gas in floating party balloons, is critical to the operation of several medical machines and scientific instruments. Liquid helium is very cold. You may have seen a video of someone using liquid nitrogen to freeze a flower or a tennis ball. At 1 atm of pressure, nitrogen boils at –196°C but He boils at –270°C or 4 Kelvin! The high magnetic field produced by a superconducting magnet requires low temperatures, so without liquid helium these machines and instruments will be useless.

The only U.S. supplier of this gas is the federal government, and its stores are almost depleted. Academic Nuclear Magnetic Resonance (NMR) facilities as well as Magnetic Resonance Imaging (MRI) centers are finding it difficult to obtain the gas required for operation. It's not that the world is running out of helium—there are significant underground stores across the globe. Interruptions in its "mining," however, have resulted in the supply shortages. The shortages have had a positive impact though. Currently, investigations into helium recycling and potential alternatives for MRI and NMR are underway.

70. What is the density in grams per liter of helium gas, He, if the pressure is 1.00 atmosphere and the temperature is 35°C?
    $(R = 0.082/L \cdot atm/K \cdot mole)(He = 4\ amu)$

    (A) 0.16 g/L
    (B) 0.87 g/L
    (C) 1.66 g/L
    (D) 2.35 g/L

71. A sample of gas contains approximately 56 grams of nitrogen, N_2, and 32 grams of helium, He. What is the partial pressure, in atmospheres, of nitrogen if the total pressure of the gas sample is 1.6 atmospheres?
    (He = 4 amu, N = 14 amu)

    (A) 0.68 atm
    (B) 0.80 atm
    (C) 0.15 atm
    (D) 0.32 atm

72. The conversion of a liquid into a gas is called _____, and it is usually _____ at room temperature.

    (A) evaporation; endothermic
    (B) evaporation; exothermic
    (C) condensation; endothermic
    (D) condensation; exothermic

73. The solubility of gases in liquids increases with

    (A) increased temperature.
    (B) decreased pressure.
    (C) increased agitation.
    (D) increased pressure.

74. In the following reaction:

$$CS_2 + 3O_2 \rightarrow CO_2 + 2SO_2$$

38.0 grams of CS_2 (carbon disufide) are reacted with excess O_2 to produce 32.0 grams of SO_2. What is the percent yield of this reaction? (S = 32 amu, O = 16 amu, C = 12 amu, H = 1 amu)

(A) 50
(B) 25
(C) 38
(D) 13

75. How many milliliters of 4.0 M NaOH solution must be used to prepare 100 milliliters of 2.0 M solution?

(A) 50
(B) 13
(C) 800
(D) 200

76. Which of the following wavelengths of light will have the highest frequency?

(A) 0.300 m
(B) 2.75 mm
(C) 630 nm
(D) 0.69 km

77. A chloride ion and a sulfide ion

(A) have the same charge.
(B) have the same number of valence electrons.
(C) have the same number of protons.
(D) are diatomic ions.

78. Which of the following is a basic oxide?

(A) CO_2
(B) K_2O
(C) SO_2
(D) P_2O_5

79. Hydrogen bonding can exist between molecules of all the following EXCEPT

(A) H_2O
(B) CH_4
(C) CH_3OH
(D) NH_3

80. The following reactions have equilibrium constants as indicated below:

$$A + B \leftrightarrow C + D \quad K^1$$
$$E + F \leftrightarrow G + H \quad K^2$$

The reactions are added to give the following overall reaction. What will be the overall equilibrium constant for the new equation?

$$A + B + E + F \leftrightarrow C + D + G + H$$

(A) $K^1 + K^2$
(B) $(K^1)(K^2)$
(C) K^1/K^2
(D) K^2/K^1

81. In which of the following are the acids listed correctly in decreasing order of strength (i.e., the strongest acid is first and the weakest acid last)?

(A) HF > HCl > HBr > HI
(B) HI > HBr > HCl > HF
(C) HBr > HCl > HI > HF
(D) HCl > HBr > HI > HF

82. The following reaction:

$$^{90}_{38}Sr \rightarrow {}^{90}_{39}Y + {}^{0}_{-1}e$$

represents

(A) nuclear fission.
(B) gamma emission.
(C) beta decay.
(D) alpha decay.

83. Which of the following is a statement of the First Law of Thermodynamics?

    (A) Entropy for a crystalline substance is zero at absolute zero temperature.
    (B) Energy can be converted from one form to another but is neither created nor destroyed.
    (C) Entropy increases in spontaneous reactions and remains the same in equilibrium systems.
    (D) The Gibbs Free Energy is a measure of the spontaneity of a reaction.

84. Consider the substitution reaction of (R)-2-methyl-2-iodobutane with hydrosulfide ion (HS⁻). If the reactant is levorotatory, what do you expect to be true of the optical activity of the substitution product?

    (A) The product is expected to be optically inactive.
    (B) The product is expected to be levorotatory.
    (C) The product is expected to be dextrorotatory.
    (D) It impossible to predict whether or not the product will be optically active.

85. Which statement is true concerning aqueous solutions of Acid A ($K_a = 6 \times 10^{-8}$) and Acid B ($K_a = 3 \times 10^{-5}$)?

    (A) Acid A is stronger than Acid B.
    (B) The pH of the Acid B solution is less than that of Acid A.
    (C) Both solutions are neutral.
    (D) The pKa of Acid B is greater than the pKa of Acid A.

86. The reaction of Br_2 with C_2H_4 to produce $C_2H_4Br_2$ is an example of

    (A) a nucleophilic substitution reaction.
    (B) a free radical reaction.
    (C) an electrophilic addition reaction.
    (D) an elimination reaction.

87. Which statement describes carbohydrates?

    (A) They are used as monomers in protein synthesis.
    (B) They are oxidized to produce usable chemical energy.
    (C) They are composed of polymers of phosphates.
    (D) They are not commonly found inside cells.

88. Which of the following statements about benzene is INCORRECT?

    (A) The benzene molecule has 120° bond angles.
    (B) All bonds in benzene are equivalent in length.
    (C) Hybridization of the carbon atoms is sp^2.
    (D) The benzene molecule is planar.

89. The following compound is

$$CH_3CH_2CHCH_2COOH$$
$$\overset{|}{CH_3}$$

    (A) 3-methylpentanoic acid.
    (B) 2-methylpentanoic acid.
    (C) 2-methylbutanoic acid.
    (D) 3-methylbutanoic acid.

90. What is the name of the following molecule?

    (A) (S)-isopentanol
    (B) (S)-3-methyl-2-butanol
    (C) (R)-3-methyl-2-butanol
    (D) (R)-2-methyl-3-butanol

91. What is the percentage of hydrogen, H, present in ammonium sulfate, $(NH_4)_2SO_4$? (S = 32 amu, O = 16 amu, N = 14 amu, H = 1 amu)

(A) 11
(B) 6
(C) 3
(D) 4

92. The following reaction creates two chiral centers.

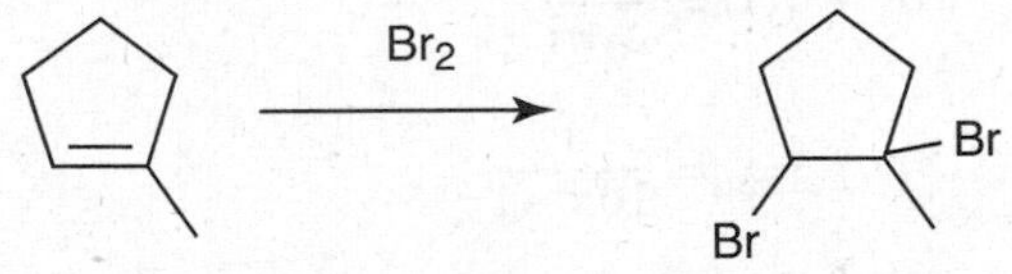

The mechanism of the reaction involves the anti addition of the Br_2 molecule to the alkene. Which statement is true concerning the product?

(A) The product is a 50:50 mixture of enantiomers.
(B) The product is a meso form.
(C) The product is a 50:50 mixture of diastereomers.
(D) The product is a non-50:50 mixture of diastereomers.

93. How many grams of sodium hydroxide (FW 40) are needed to neutralize 2.2 mL of pentanoic acid (FW 102, density = 0.93 g/mL) by the equation

$$CH_3(CH_2)_3COOH + NaOH \rightarrow$$
$$H_2O + CH_3(CH_2)_3COONa$$

(A) 0.80 g
(B) 2.04 g
(C) 0.02 g
(D) 0.051 g

94. What is the final volume in milliliters of a solution prepared by dissolving 18 grams of sugar, $C_6H_{12}O_6$, in sufficient water to produce a 0.5 M solution? (O = 16 amu, C = 12 amu, H = 1 amu)

(A) 36
(B) 100
(C) 200
(D) 52

95. The reaction of a neutron with a uranium-235 nucleus to generate a strontium atom, a xenon atom, and three neutrons as shown in the equation below is known as

$$^{235}_{92}U + ^{1}_{0}n \rightarrow ^{90}_{38}Sr + ^{143}_{54}Xe + 3^{1}_{0}n$$

(A) radioactive decay.
(B) nuclear fusion.
(C) carbon-14 dating.
(D) nuclear fission.

96. If two moles of acetic acid are generated from the cleavage of an organic molecule by ozonolysis followed by reductive work up, what is the name of the organic molecule?

(A) 1-butyne
(B) 2-butyne
(C) 2-butene
(D) cyclobutyne

STOP

End of Chemical Processes section. If you have any time left, you may go over your work in this section only.

Directions: Choose the **best** answer to each of the following questions.

97. $\sqrt{32} + \sqrt{18} =$

    (A) $6\sqrt{2}$

    (B) $8\sqrt{2}$

    (C) $7\sqrt{2}$

    (D) $9\sqrt{2}$

98. Lisa's gas tank is $\frac{3}{5}$ full. She completely filled the tank by putting in an additional 6 gallons. What is the capacity of the gas tank?

    (A) 20 gallons
    (B) 15 gallons
    (C) 25 gallons
    (D) 10 gallons

99. $\lim\limits_{x \to \infty} \left(\dfrac{7x^5 + 2x^3 - 5x + 50}{13x^2 - 2x^5} \right)$

    (A) $-\dfrac{7}{2}$

    (B) ∞

    (C) $\dfrac{7}{2}$

    (D) $\dfrac{7}{13}$

100. Determine the inverse function for

    $f(x) = \dfrac{x+1}{10x}$.

    (A) $f^{-1}(x) = \dfrac{10x}{x+1}$

    (B) $f^{-1}(x) = \dfrac{1}{10x-1}$

    (C) $f^{-1}(x) = \dfrac{1}{10x+1}$

    (D) $f^{-1}(x) = \dfrac{x-1}{10x}$

101. $5^2 + 5^3 =$

    (A) 3,125
    (B) 1,000
    (C) 150
    (D) 25

102. A crate of fruit contains 14 apples, 8 bananas, and 4 lemons. What is the probability that a randomly chosen piece of fruit is NOT a banana?

    (A) $\dfrac{9}{13}$

    (B) $\dfrac{4}{13}$

    (C) $\dfrac{1}{8}$

    (D) $\dfrac{7}{8}$

103. Students in a certain chemistry class must take two midterms, each worth 24% of the course grade, and a cumulative final exam that is worth 52% of the course grade. Suppose your average on the midterms is 84%. What is the lowest possible percentage score you can earn on the final exam in order to have a course average greater than 88%? Round your answer to the nearest whole number.

    (A) 92%
    (B) 93%
    (C) 94%
    (D) 95%

104. Find the **radius** of a circle with the equation $x^2 + y^2 - 12x + 14y + 9 = 0$.

    (A) $\sqrt{76}$

    (B) 76

    (C) 85

    (D) $\sqrt{85}$

105. Find the exact value of the shaded area.

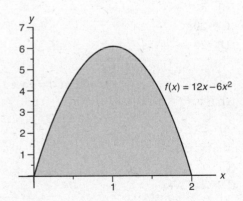

$f(x) = 12x - 6x^2$

    (A) 2
    (B) 6
    (C) 4
    (D) 8

106. How many numbers between 1 and 500, inclusive, are **NOT** divisible by 3 or by 5?

    (A) 467
    (B) 567
    (C) 367
    (D) 267

107. Evaluate the integral $\int_{1}^{2}(5x^4)\,dx$.

    (A) 32
    (B) 140
    (C) 180
    (D) 31

108. A box contains 8 balls, numbered 1 through 8. One ball is removed at random from the box and then replaced. This process is repeated three more times. The numbers on the balls removed from the box are written down in the order in which they are removed, forming a four-digit number. How many different four-digit numbers can be obtained in this way?

    (A) 4,096
    (B) 1,680
    (C) 5,040
    (D) 3,360

109. Simplify the expression $\dfrac{x^2 - 11x + 24}{x - 8}$.

    (A) $x + 3$
    (B) $x - 14$
    (C) $x - 3$
    (D) $x + 14$

110. Find all real solutions for the quadratic equation $6x^2 + x + 1 = 0$.

    (A) $x = \dfrac{-1 \pm \sqrt{23}}{12}$

    (B) No real solutions

    (C) $x = \dfrac{-1 \pm \sqrt{-23}}{12}$

    (D) $x = \dfrac{1 \pm \sqrt{23}}{12}$

111. The graph of a function $y = f(x)$ contains the point (3, 1). Determine which point must be on the graph of $y = 5f(x + 2) - 3$.

    (A) (1, 2)
    (B) (5, 2)
    (C) (1, –10)
    (D) (5, –10)

112. If $x^{\ln(x)} = e^4$, then

    (A) $x = 2, x = -2$
    (B) $x = e^2, x = e^{-2}$
    (C) $x = e, x = e$
    (D) $x = 1, x = -1$

113. $\lim\limits_{x \to 4}\left(\dfrac{x^2 - 10x + 24}{4 - x}\right) =$

    (A) Undefined
    (B) 2
    (C) –2
    (D) 1

114. What is the mean of the following numbers: 8, 35, 8, 9, 5, 10, 7, 3, 12?

    (A) 8
    (B) 10.77
    (C) 15.24
    (D) 9

115. A rental car company charges $30 per day, plus 14 cents per mile. Express the total rental cost of a 7-day rental as a function of the number of miles driven, x.

    (A) $C(x) = 30 + 14x$
    (B) $C(x) = 30 + 0.14x$
    (C) $C(x) = 210 + 14x$
    (D) $C(x) = 210 + 0.14x$

116. A fair coin is tossed ten times. What is the probability that the outcome will be heads for all ten tosses?

    (A) $\dfrac{1}{512}$

    (B) $\dfrac{1}{10}$

    (C) $\dfrac{1}{1024}$

    (D) $\dfrac{1}{5}$

117. Find the instantaneous rate of change for the function $f(t) = 5e^{4t-8}$ at the moment when $t = 2$.

    (A) $5e$
    (B) 5
    (C) $20e$
    (D) 20

118. Given $f(x) = x^2 + 2x - 1$, and $g(x) = 2x + 1$, what is $(f + g)(x)$?

    (A) $2x^2 + 4x$
    (B) $x^2 - 4x$
    (C) $x^2 + 4x$
    (D) $2x^2 - 4x$

119. The equation $4(x + 3)(x - 2) = 4x^2 + x$ has solution

    (A) $x = -8$
    (B) $x = 8$
    (C) $x = -2$
    (D) $x = 2$

120. If a die is rolled, what is the probability that the number will be odd?

   (A) 50%
   (B) 100%
   (C) 25%
   (D) 0%

121. $\dfrac{5}{9} - \dfrac{3}{10} =$

   (A) $\dfrac{77}{90}$

   (B) $-\dfrac{23}{90}$

   (C) $-\dfrac{77}{90}$

   (D) $\dfrac{23}{90}$

122. It takes your sister 30 minutes to walk to school, and it takes you 40 minutes. Suppose your sister leaves the house 6 minutes after you leave. How many minutes will it take for her to catch up to you?

   (A) 20 minutes
   (B) 18 minutes
   (C) 16 minutes
   (D) 22 minutes

123. A pair of fair six-sided dice is thrown. What is the probability that the sum of the numbers shown is NOT equal to 5?

   (A) $\dfrac{1}{6}$

   (B) $\dfrac{1}{9}$

   (C) $\dfrac{1}{3}$

   (D) $\dfrac{8}{9}$

124. Evaluate $\int (x+2)\,dx$.

   (A) $\dfrac{1}{2}x^2 + 2x + C$

   (B) $\dfrac{1}{x^2} + C$

   (C) $x + C$

   (D) $\dfrac{x}{C}$

QUESTIONS 125 AND 126 ARE BASED ON THE GRAPH BELOW:

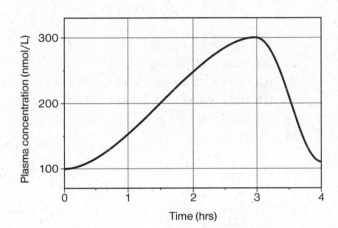

125. What is the maximum plasma concentration?

   (A) 100 nmol/L
   (B) 150 nmol/L
   (C) 200 nmol/L
   (D) 300 nmol/L

126. When does the maximum plasma concentration occur?

   (A) At 3 hours
   (B) At 1 hour
   (C) At 4 hours
   (D) At 2 hours

127. Determine the value(s) of q, if any, for which $10x^2 + \pi x + q = 0$ has a double root.

(A) $q = \dfrac{\pi^2}{40}$

(B) $q = \dfrac{40}{\pi^2}$

(C) $q > \dfrac{\pi^2}{40}$

(D) $q > \dfrac{40}{\pi^2}$

128. Find the domain of the given function.

$$f(x) = \frac{x-4}{x^2 + 9x + 18}$$

(A) $\{x \mid x \neq -6, x \neq -3\}$
(B) $\{x \mid x = -6, x = -3\}$
(C) $\{x \mid x \neq -6, x \neq -3, x \neq 4\}$
(D) $\{x \mid x = -6, x = -3, x = 4\}$

129. $9^3 \cdot 9^{-1} =$

(A) $\dfrac{1}{729}$

(B) 81

(C) -81

(D) $\dfrac{1}{81}$

130. Five people are chosen at random from a group of 3 boys and 5 girls. What is the probability that 3 girls and 1 boy are chosen?

(A) $\dfrac{4}{7}$

(B) $\dfrac{1}{2}$

(C) $\dfrac{3}{4}$

(D) $\dfrac{3}{7}$

131. Find the vertex for the given function.

$$f(x) = 9x^2 + 18x - 7$$

(A) $(-1,0)$
(B) $(-1,-16)$
(C) $(1,20)$
(D) $(1,0)$

132. Determine the slope of the tangent line to the graph of the function $f(x) = \dfrac{x}{x+1}$ at the point whose x-coordinate equals 0.

(A) 1
(B) -1
(C) 0
(D) 2

133. If $\ln(p - 4x) = 2$, then

(A) $x = \dfrac{e^2 - p}{-4}$

(B) $x = \dfrac{e^2 - p}{4}$

(C) $x = \dfrac{2e - p}{-4}$

(D) $x = \dfrac{2e - p}{4}$

134. A box contains apples and oranges in a ratio of $3 : 7$. If the box contains 9 apples, how many oranges does the box contain?

(A) 13
(B) 21
(C) 10
(D) 18

135. Portions of a segment are removed in stages according to the following pattern. At each stage, the existing segments are divided into thirds, and then the middle third is removed.

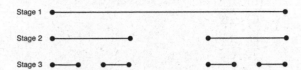

Stage 1
Stage 2
Stage 3

The total segment length that remains at Stage 3 is what fraction of the original segment length at Stage 1?

(A) $\dfrac{4}{9}$

(B) $\dfrac{5}{9}$

(C) $\dfrac{2}{3}$

(D) $\dfrac{1}{3}$

136. In an employee survey, 300 employees indicated they would attend Workshop I, and 120 employees indicated they would attend Workshop II. If 65 employees plan to attend both workshops and 260 indicated they could not attend either workshop, how many employees participated in the survey?

(A) 615
(B) 745
(C) 550
(D) Not enough information

137. Given the following graph of the function $y = f(x)$, evaluate the limit.

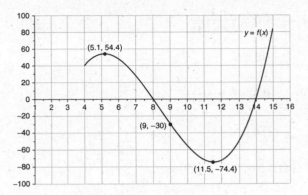

$$\lim_{x \to 5.1}\left(\frac{f(x) - f(5.1)}{x - 5.1}\right) =$$

(A) 54.4
(B) 5.1
(C) 0
(D) Not enough information

138. Determine the domain of the function $f(x) = \ln(2x - 7)$.

(A) $(-\infty, \infty)$
(B) $[-\infty, \infty]$
(C) $[3.5, \infty)$
(D) $(3.5, \infty)$

139. Find the extreme value of the given function and state whether that value represents a maximum or a minimum value for the function.

$$P(x) = 35x^2 + 420x - 50$$

(A) –1,310, maximum
(B) –1,310, minimum
(C) –6, maximum
(D) –6, minimum

140. Simplify the expression $\dfrac{\dfrac{1}{x+h} - \dfrac{1}{x}}{h}$.

(A) $\dfrac{1}{(x+h)x}$

(B) 1

(C) $-\dfrac{1}{(x+h)x}$

(D) -1

141. $\log(75) - \log(3) =$

(A) $\dfrac{1}{25}$

(B) $\log(25)$

(C) $\dfrac{\log(75)}{3}$

(D) $\log(72)$

142. A truck is 48 miles from its destination at 5:00 P.M. At what speed must the truck travel to arrive by 5:45 P.M.?

(A) 64 mph

(B) 60 mph

(C) 70 mph

(D) 74 mph

143. Determine the radius of a circle with the equation $(x-4)^2 + (y+3)^2 = 36$.

(A) 36

(B) 6

(C) ±6

(D) ±36

144. Solve the equation $\dfrac{2x}{x-5} + \dfrac{x}{x+3} = 3$.

(A) $x = \dfrac{45}{7}$

(B) $x = -\dfrac{7}{45}$

(C) $x = \dfrac{7}{45}$

(D) $x = -\dfrac{45}{7}$

STOP

End of Quantitative Reasoning section. If you have any time left, you may go over your work in this section only.

CRITICAL READING

48 QUESTIONS (#145–#192)

TIME: 50 MINUTES

Directions: Read each of the following passages, and choose the one **best** answer to each of the questions that follow each passage.

Passage 1

Bronchial asthma is a common disease of children and adults. Although the clinical manifestations of asthma have been known since antiquity, it is a disease that still defies precise definition. The word *asthma* is of Greek origin and means "panting." More than 2,000 years ago, Hippocrates used the word *asthma* to describe episodic shortness of breath; however, the first detailed clinical description of the asthmatic patient was made by Aretaeus in the second century. Since that time *asthma* has been used to describe any disorder with episodic shortness of breath or dyspnea; thus, the terms *cardiac asthma* and *bronchial asthma* have been used to delineate the etiologies of the dyspnea. These terms are now obsolete and *asthma* refers to a disorder of the respiratory system characterized by episodes of difficulty in breathing. An Expert Panel of the National Institutes of Health National Asthma Education Program (NAEP) has defined asthma as a lung disease characterized by (1) airway obstruction that is reversible (but not completely so in some patients) either spontaneously or with treatment; (2) airway inflammation; and (3) increased airway responsiveness to a variety of stimuli. This descriptive definition for asthma is attributed to our lack of knowledge of the precise pathogenic defect that results in the clinical syndrome we recognize as asthma. The current definition does allow for the important heterogeneity of the clinical presentation of asthma. New technologies have added substantially to our understanding of the interrelationships of immunology, biochemistry, and physiology to the clinical presentation of asthma, and further research may yet uncover a specific genetic defect associated with asthma. Until such time, asthma will continue to defy exact definition.

An estimated 10 million persons in the United States have asthma (about 5% of the population). The reported prevalence increased 29% from 1980 to 1987 to 40.1 per 1000 population. African-Americans have a 19% higher incidence of asthma than whites and are twice as likely to be hospitalized. The estimated cost of asthma in the United States in 1990 was $6.2 billion. The largest single direct medical expenditure was for inpatient hospital services (emergency care), reaching almost $1.5 billion, followed by prescription medications ($1.1 billion). The costs of medication increased 54% between 1985 and 1990. In total, 43% of the economic impact was associated with emergency room use, hospitalization, and death. Asthma accounted for 1% of all ambulatory care visits according to the National Ambulatory Medical Care Survey and results in more than 450,000 hospitalizations per year.

_____

Excerpted with permission from *Pharmacotherapy, A Pathophysiological Approach*, Third Edition, by Joseph T. DiPiro, et al., page 553. Stamford, CT: Appleton & Lange, 1996.

145. Bronchial asthma is best described as a

    (A) precisely defined disease commonly occurring in both children and adults.

    (B) common disease in children and adults that defies precise definition.

    (C) common disease found only in children that defies precise description.

    (D) precisely defined disease rarely occurring in children and adults.

146. The etiologies of the episodic shortness of breath were once divided into two terms:

(A) antiquity and panting.
(B) reversible and spontaneous.
(C) inpatient and outpatient.
(D) bronchial asthma and cardiac asthma.

147. According to the NAEP, one way to characterize asthma is by

(A) the homogeneity of its clinical presentation.
(B) inflamed airways.
(C) a decrease in airway responsiveness.
(D) airway obstruction that is always completely reversible.

148. What was the cost of asthma in the United States in 1990, not including the cost of prescription medications?

(A) $1.5 billion
(B) $6.2 billion
(C) $5.1 billion
(D) $1.1 billion

149. The passage suggests that in the future researchers are likely to understand more about

(A) new technologies to treat asthma.
(B) wheezing and episodes of shortness of breath.
(C) a specific genetic defect associated with asthma.
(D) the interrelationship of immunology, biochemistry, and physiology.

150. Asthma results in more than _____ hospitalizations per year.

(A) 6.2 billion
(B) 29% of
(C) 10 million
(D) 450,000

151. The estimated number of persons in the United States who have asthma is

(A) 100 million.
(B) 2.5 million.
(C) fewer than 2%.
(D) 10 million.

152. Today, the term *asthma* refers to

(A) panting.
(B) dyspnea of cardiac etiology.
(C) dyspnea of bronchial etiology.
(D) a disorder of the respiratory system characterized by episodes of difficulty in breathing.

153. The word *asthma* has a Greek origin and was used by

(A) Aretaeus.
(B) an Expert Panel of the National Institutes of Health.
(C) Hippocrates.
(D) the National Ambulatory Medical Care Survey.

154. The passage contains which of the following?

(A) A description of pharmacists' role in asthma treatment
(B) Facts about the prevalence of asthma in the United States
(C) An explanation of the worldwide increase in the prevalence of asthma
(D) An in-depth treatment plan for asthma

Passage 2

When Italy emerged into the light of history about 700 BC, it was already inhabited by various peoples of different cultures and languages. Most natives of the country lived in villages or small towns, supported themselves by agriculture or animal husbandry (Italia means "Calf Land"), and spoke an Italic dialect belonging to the Indo-European family of languages. Oscan and Umbrian were closely related Italic dialects spoken by the inhabitants of the Apennines. The other two Italic dialects, Latin and Venetic, were likewise closely related to each other and were spoken, respectively, by the Latins of Latium (a plain of west-central Italy) and the people of northeastern Italy (near modern Venice). Apulians (Iapyges) and Messapians inhabited the southeastern coast. Their language resembled the speech of the Illyrians on the other side of the Adriatic. During the fifth century BC the Po valley of northern Italy (Cisalpine Gaul) was occupied by Gallic tribes who spoke Celtic and who had migrated across the Alps from continental Europe. The Etruscans were the first highly civilized people of Italy and were the only inhabitants who did not speak an Indo-European language. By 700 BC several Greek colonies were established along the southern coast. Both Greeks and Phoenicians were actively engaged in trade.

Modern historical analysis is making rapid progress in showing how Rome's early development occurred in a multicultural environment and was particularly influenced by the higher civilizations of the Etruscans to the north and the Greeks to the south. Roman religion was indebted to the beliefs and practices of the Etruscans. The Romans borrowed and adapted the alphabet from the Etruscans, who in turn had borrowed and adapted it from the Greek colonies of Italy. Senior officials of the Roman Republic derived their insignia from the Etruscans: curule chair, purple-bordered toga (*toga praetexta*) and bundle of rods (*fasces*). Gladiatorial combats and the military triumph were other customs adopted from the Etruscans. Rome lay 12 miles (19.3 km) inland from the sea on the Tiber River, the border between Latium and Etruria. Because the site commanded a convenient river crossing and lay on a land route from the Apennines to the sea, it formed the meeting point of three distinct peoples: Latins, Etruscans, and Sabines. Although Latin in speech and culture, the Roman population must have been somewhat diverse from earliest times, a circumstance that may help to account for the openness of Roman society in historical times.

_____

Excerpted from *Ancient Rome: From Romulus and Remus to the Visigoth Invasion*, edited by Kathleen Kuiper. New York: Britannica Educational Publishing, 2011.

155. According to the passage, the Romans adopted the speech of which of the following civilizations?

  (A) The Apulians
  (B) The Messapians
  (C) The Latins
  (D) The Umbrians

156. According to the passage, Roman religion was based on the beliefs of which of the following civilizations?

  (A) The Etruscans
  (B) The Greeks
  (C) The Latins
  (D) The Apulians

157. In the early history of Italy, communities were largely

  (A) agrarian.
  (B) urban.
  (C) nomadic.
  (D) trade-based.

158. The Romans adapted the Etruscan _____, which was originally adapted from Italy's _____ colonies.

  (A) religion, Phoenecian
  (B) gladiatorial combat, Greek
  (C) alphabet, Greek
  (D) government insignias, Phoenecian

159. What is the primary theme of the first paragraph of the passage?

(A) Geography of ancient Italy
(B) Migration and cultures of ancient Italy's inhabitants
(C) Economy of ancient Italy
(D) Inhabitants of ancient Italy and their languages

160. Which of the following is NOT an Italic dialect?

(A) Latin
(B) Oscan
(C) Umbrian
(D) Etruscan

161. According to the passage, the location of Rome

(A) contributed to its isolationism.
(B) resulted in a somewhat diverse population.
(C) made it vulnerable to invaders.
(D) created conflict between Latium and Etruria.

Passage 3

Gastroesophageal reflux disease (GERD) is a common medical disorder seen by health care practitioners of all specialties. It is generally chronic in nature, and long-term therapy may be required. While the mortality associated with GERD is very low (1 death per 100,000 patients), the quality of life experienced by the patient can be greatly diminished.

GERD refers to any symptomatic clinical condition or histologic alteration that results from episodes of gastroesophageal reflux. Gastroesophageal reflux refers to the retrograde movement of gastric contents from the stomach into the esophagus. Many people experience some degree of reflux, especially after eating, which may be considered a benign physiologic process. When the esophagus is repeatedly exposed to refluxed material for prolonged periods of time, inflammation of the esopha-

gus (i.e., reflux esophagitis) can occur. It is important to realize that gastroesophageal reflux must precede the development of GERD or reflux esophagitis. In severe cases, reflux may lead to a multitude of serious complications including esophageal strictures, esophageal ulcers, motility disorders, perforation, hemorrhage, aspiration, and Barrett's esophagus. While mild disease is often managed with lifestyle changes and antacids, more intensive therapeutic intervention with histamine (H_2) antagonists, sucralfate, prokinetic agents, or proton pump inhibitors is generally required for patients with more severe disease. In general, response to pharmacologic intervention is dependent on the efficacy of the agent, dosage regimen employed, duration of therapy, and severity of the disease. Following discontinuation of therapy, relapse is common and long-term maintenance therapy may be required. Historically, surgical intervention has been reserved for patients in whom conventional treatment modalities fail. However, the recent development of laparoscopic antireflux surgical procedures has led to a reevaluation of the role of surgery in the long-term management of GERD. Some clinicians have suggested that laparoscopic antireflux surgery may be a cost-effective alternative to long-term maintenance therapy in young patients. However, long-term comparative trials evaluating the cost effectiveness of the various treatment modalities are warranted.

The pathogenesis of gastroesophageal reflux is related to the complex balance between defense mechanisms and aggressive factors. Understanding both the normal protective mechanisms and the aggressive factors that may contribute to or promote gastroesophageal reflux helps one to design rational therapeutic treatment regimens. Gastric acid, pepsin, bile acids, and pancreatic enzymes are considered aggressive factors and may promote esophageal damage upon reflux into the esophagus. Thus, the composition (potency) and volume of the refluxate are aggressive factors that may lead to esophageal injury. Conversely, normal protective mechanisms include anatomic factors, the lower esophageal sphincter pressure, esophageal clearing, mucosal resistance, and gastric emptying. Rational therapeutic regimens in the treatment of gastroesophageal reflux are designed to maximize normal defense mechanisms and/or attenuate the aggressive factors.

————

Excerpted with permission from *Pharmacotherapy, A Pathophysiological Approach*, Third Edition, by Joseph T. DiPiro, et al., page 675. Stamford, CT: Appleton & Lange, 1996.

162. The mortality rate associated with GERD is

   (A) 1 death in 1,000 patients
   (B) 1 death in 10,000 patients
   (C) 1 death in 100,000 patients
   (D) 1 death in 1,000,000 patients

163. One possible complication of reflux is

   (A) perforation.
   (B) mucosal resistance.
   (C) gastric emptying.
   (D) lower esophageal sphincter pressure.

164. Reflux esophagitis is

   (A) a rational therapeutic treatment regimen.
   (B) a surgical intervention.
   (C) the inflammation of the esophagus due to repeated exposure to refluxed gastric contents for prolonged periods of time.
   (D) a normal defense mechanism.

165. After therapy is discontinued

   (A) no further intervention is needed.
   (B) brief periods of medication therapy will be needed periodically throughout the patient's life.
   (C) long-term maintenance may be required to prevent relapse following the discontinuation of therapy.
   (D) GERD is considered cured and no relapses are expected.

166. In GERD patients, response to pharmacologic intervention is dependent on

   (A) physical exercise.
   (B) efficacy of the agent.
   (C) intramuscular administration of drugs.
   (D) limiting duration of therapy.

167. Long-term comparative trials evaluating the cost effectiveness of various treatment modalities for GERD are

   (A) warranted.
   (B) not feasible.
   (C) premature.
   (D) aggressive.

168. Some clinicians have suggested that a cost-effective alternative therapy for GERD may be

   (A) histamine antagonists.
   (B) prokinetic agents.
   (C) laparoscopic antireflux surgery.
   (D) proton pump inhibitors.

169. Aggressive factors that may promote esophageal damage upon reflux into the esophagus are

   (A) gastric acid and pancreatic enzymes.
   (B) bile acids and esophageal clearing.
   (C) lower esophageal sphincter pressure and gastric emptying.
   (D) lipids and plaques.

Passage 4

Many people in the United States are diagnosed with diabetes mellitus. Type 2 diabetes is the most common type of diabetes and it is associated with a significant amount of morbidities and mortalities. Type 2 diabetes is classified as an endocrine disorder characterized by defects in insulin secretion as well as in insulin action. In type 2 diabetes patients, a defect also exists in insulin receptor binding. These defects lead to increased serum glucose concentrations or hyperglycemia.

Sulfonylureas are one of the most popular classes of agents used to treat type 2 diabetes. One of the newest agents to treat type 2 diabetes is acarbose, an oral alpha-glucosidase inhibitor. Acarbose interferes with the hydrolysis of dietary disaccharides and complex carbohydrates, thereby delaying absorption of glucose and other monosaccharides. Acarbose is available for oral administration only. To be most effective, it should be taken at the beginning of a meal. The recommended starting dose is 25 mg three times daily and doses as high as 200 mg three times a day have been safely used. The most common adverse experiences associated with the use of acarbose are abdominal cramps, flatulence, diarrhea, and abdominal distension. Most of the adverse effects are due to the unabsorbed carbohydrates undergoing fermentation in the colon. Acarbose has also been associated with decreased intestinal absorption of iron, thereby possibly leading to anemia. The occurrence of hypoglycemia when using acarbose in combination with other agents used to lower serum glucose is great. Glucose should be administered to treat hypoglycemia in patients taking acarbose because sucrose may not be adequately hydrolyzed and absorbed. The effectiveness of this agent to lower serum glucose concentrations in patients with type 2 diabetes has been clearly demonstrated in clinical trials. Acarbose provides another option for treating type 2 diabetes.

170. Which of the following does NOT describe the term *type 2 diabetes*?

(A) Endocrine in nature
(B) Hyperglycemia
(C) May be due to a defect in insulin receptor binding
(D) Results in iron deficiencies

171. Which of the following is the most common type of agent used to treat type 2 diabetes?

(A) A sulfonylurea agent
(B) Glucose
(C) Sucrose
(D) Fructose

172. To be most effective, when should acarbose be taken?

(A) At the beginning of a meal
(B) At bedtime
(C) At the end of a meal
(D) At noon

173. According to the passage, which of the following is the most common side effect associated with the use of acarbose?

(A) Hyperglycemia
(B) Anemia
(C) Gastrointestinal discomfort
(D) Rash

174. Which of the following is the best agent to treat hypoglycemia in patients taking acarbose?

(A) A sulfonylurea agent
(B) Glucose
(C) Sucrose
(D) Fructose

175. According to the passage, which of the following has NOT been associated with the use of acarbose?

(A) Low serum glucose concentrations
(B) Gastrointestinal discomfort
(C) Decreased iron absorption
(D) Obstruction of the urinary tract

176. Which of the following used in combination with acarbose increases the risk of experiencing hypoglycemia?

(A) A sulfonylurea agent
(B) Glucose
(C) Iron
(D) Increased caloric intake

177. Which of the following is the best title for this passage?

(A) Diabetes in the United States
(B) Agents Used to Treat Type 2 Diabetes
(C) The Use of Acarbose in the Treatment of Type 2 Diabetes
(D) Adverse Effects of Acarbose

Passage 5

At the first session of the Confederation Congress, it was decided that nine states constituted a quorum, with two delegates necessary for a state to qualify as present. But on multiple occasions throughout the spring and summer of 1781, no official business could be done because five or more state delegations were either absent altogether or only partially represented. Part of the problem lay with the state legislatures, which were slow to select their delegates; part of the problem was that the leading candidates refused to serve, preferring to perform their public duties at the state level. John Witherspoon of New Jersey became the most frequent and vocal critic of this sorry situation, waiting around with nothing to do because his erstwhile colleagues had failed to show up, but the attendance problem accurately reflected the political priorities of the most prominent American leaders. In truth, it would be misleading to say that local and state concerns trumped the national interest, because in most minds no such thing as the national interest even existed.

A second source of systemic malfunction was the coordination of foreign policy. All business came before the full Congress, an unwieldy arrangement at best, rendered more maddeningly chaotic because the membership of state delegations kept changing. When Arthur Lee joined the Virginia delegation, for example, his inveterate suspicion of Benjamin Franklin's ties to the French Court—Lee, it soon became clear, was suspicious of everyone, especially non-Virginians—split the Virginia vote on almost every foreign policy issue, essentially negating the largest state's voice.

_____

Excerpted from *The Quartet: Orchestrating the Second American Revolution, 1783–1789*, by Joseph J. Ellis. New York: Alfred A. Knopf, 2015.

178. The formal definition of a "quorum" is

(A) the minimum number of people who must be present at a meeting for decisions to be made.
(B) majority rules, wherein the majority of a group must be present at a meeting for decisions to be made.
(C) all members of a group must be present for decisions to be made.
(D) a presiding body of officials who make decisions on behalf of a nation.

179. What is the primary theme of this passage?

(A) The antics of Arthur Lee
(B) Barriers to conducting business in the Confederation Congress
(C) Critiquing the priorities of state legislatures
(D) Political priorities in the Confederation Congress

180. The Confederation Congress was formed during what significant historical event in American history?

   (A)   The Revolutionary War
   (B)   The Civil War
   (C)   The Spanish-American War
   (D)   The Great War

181. Concerns at which level took precedence in the minds of political leaders at the time of the Confederation Congress?

   (A)   Foreign
   (B)   National
   (C)   Congressional
   (D)   State

182. What was a key obstacle faced by state legislatures when appointing delegates to the Confederation Congress?

   (A)   Lack of travel funds for delegates
   (B)   Distrust of delegates from other states
   (C)   Disinterest in the aims of the Confederation Congress
   (D)   Leading candidates refused to serve

183. In the Confederation Congress, a quorum was established when

   (A)   the delegations of nine states were present, with each state having at least one delegate.
   (B)   the delegations of nine states were present, with each state having all delegates.
   (C)   the delegations of nine states were present, with each state having at least two delegates.
   (D)   the delegations of all states were present, with each state having at least two delegates.

184. According to the passage, what was the source of John Witherspoon's frustration?

   (A)   The requirement that all foreign policy business be conducted before the full Congress
   (B)   Poor attendance of his fellow delegates at Confederation Congress sessions
   (C)   The consistent splitting of Virginia's vote on foreign policy issues
   (D)   The requirements for establishing a quorum, as defined by the Confederation Congress

Passage 6

Although phenytoin may be used to treat cardiac arrhythmias, migraines, and trigeminal neuralgia, the primary use of phenytoin is to treat seizure disorders. Phenytoin, one of the most important agents used to manage seizures, works similarly to other hydantoin-derivative anticonvulsants. It decreases seizure activity by stabilizing neuronal membranes and by increasing efflux or decreasing influx of sodium ions across cell membranes in the motor cortex during generation of nerve impulses. Phenytoin is commercially available as oral suspension, tablets, and capsules. It is also available as an injection. The dosage of phenytoin varies according to the frequency of seizures, the type of seizures, and the patient's tolerance for phenytoin. Therefore, it is extremely important to monitor the patient for seizure activity as well as to monitor phenytoin serum concentrations. Phenytoin has a narrow therapeutic window and monitoring of serum concentrations is necessary. Therapeutic serum concentrations of phenytoin are usually 10–20 mcg per mL (millimeter) and depend on the assay method used. Serum concentrations above 20 mcg per mL often result in toxicity. Adverse reactions associated with dose-related toxicities include blurred vision, lethargy, rash, fever, slurred speech, nystagmus, and confusion. In some patients, seizure control is not achieved when plasma concentrations are within the therapeutic concentration range and therefore clinical response of the patient is more meaningful than plasma concentrations.

Generally, therapeutic steady state serum concentrations are achieved within 30 days of therapy with an oral dosage of 300 mg daily in adults. Following an intravenous administration of 1000–1500 mg, at a rate not exceeding 50 mg per minute, therapeutic concentrations can be attained within 2 hours. Rapid administration of intravenous phenytoin may result in adverse effects such as decreased blood pressure and other cardiac complications. The use of phenytoin has been associated with osteomalacia, thrombocytopenia, and gastrointestinal upset.

185. According to the passage, which of the following is treated with phenytoin?

   (A) Trigeminal neuralgia
   (B) Arthritis
   (C) Osteomalacia
   (D) Nystagmus

186. The primary use of phenytoin is to treat

   (A) cardiac arrhythmias.
   (B) migraines.
   (C) seizure disorders.
   (D) arthritis.

187. Which of the following best represents the mechanism of action of phenytoin in treating seizures?

   (A) Increases neuronal activity
   (B) Excites peripheral impulses to excite neuronal activity
   (C) Stabilizes neuronal membranes and decreases seizure activity by decreasing the entrance of sodium ions across the cell membranes in the motor cortex during the generation of nerve impulses
   (D) Stabilizes neuronal membranes and decreases seizure activity by increasing the entrance of sodium ions across the cell membranes in the motor cortex during the generation of nerve impulses

188. Which of the following does NOT affect the dosage of phenytoin?

   (A) Phenytoin serum concentration
   (B) Number of seizures experienced
   (C) Adverse events experienced
   (D) Puncture sites available

189. Which of the following best explains the meaning of the sentence "Phenytoin has a narrow therapeutic window and monitoring of serum concentrations is necessary"?

   (A) There is a small difference in the serum concentrations known to produce seizures and the serum concentrations known to produce adverse experiences. Therefore, serum concentrations should be monitored.
   (B) There is no difference in the serum concentrations known to produce desirable effects and the serum concentrations known to produce undesirable effects. Therefore, serum concentrations should be monitored.
   (C) There is a small difference in the serum concentrations known to control migraines and the serum concentrations known to produce migraines. Therefore, serum concentrations should be monitored.
   (D) There is a small difference in the serum concentrations known to control seizures and the serum concentrations known to produce toxicities and adverse effects. Therefore, serum concentrations should be monitored.

190. Which of the following statements describes why phenytoin should NOT be administered at a rate greater than 50 mg per minute?

(A) A higher rate takes longer to achieve adequate plasma concentrations.
(B) A higher rate may lower blood pressure.
(C) A higher rate increases arthritis pain.
(D) A higher rate may cause a rash.

191. According to the passage, which of the following is NOT a common adverse reaction associated with phenytoin toxicity?

(A) Blurred vision
(B) Lethargy
(C) Dysuria
(D) Mental confusion

192. When is the therapeutic steady-state serum concentration generally achieved with an oral dosage of 300 mg daily of phenytoin?

(A) Within 5 months
(B) Within 24 hours
(C) Within 30 hours
(D) Within 1 month

STOP

End of Critical Reading section. If you have any time left, you may go over your work in this section only.

WRITING

TIME: 30 MINUTES

> **Directions:** Write a well-constructed essay addressing the statement below.

The U.S. Department of Agriculture has estimated that approximately 20 million individuals living in low-income areas have low access to healthy food options, meaning they have limited access to a grocery store or supermarket. Such limited access to healthy food may contribute to poor health and is considered a public health problem. Discuss a solution to the problem of low access to healthy food options and how addressing low access may impact population health.

BIOLOGICAL PROCESSES (1–48)

1. **A**	13. **C**	25. **C**	37. **C**
2. **B**	14. **B**	26. **A**	38. **C**
3. **C**	15. **C**	27. **C**	39. **C**
4. **D**	16. **A**	28. **D**	40. **D**
5. **A**	17. **A**	29. **C**	41. **D**
6. **B**	18. **B**	30. **A**	42. **D**
7. **D**	19. **C**	31. **B**	43. **D**
8. **A**	20. **D**	32. **C**	44. **C**
9. **C**	21. **B**	33. **A**	45. **D**
10. **B**	22. **C**	34. **A**	46. **D**
11. **C**	23. **A**	35. **C**	47. **A**
12. **B**	24. **B**	36. **B**	48. **B**

CHEMICAL PROCESSES (49–96)

49. **C**	61. **B**	73. **D**	85. **B**
50. **D**	62. **A**	74. **A**	86. **C**
51. **B**	63. **B**	75. **A**	87. **B**
52. **D**	64. **D**	76. **C**	88. **B**
53. **A**	65. **C**	77. **B**	89. **A**
54. **A**	66. **C**	78. **B**	90. **B**
55. **A**	67. **C**	79. **B**	91. **B**
56. **B**	68. **B**	80. **B**	92. **A**
57. **A**	69. **D**	81. **B**	93. **A**
58. **B**	70. **A**	82. **C**	94. **C**
59. **D**	71. **D**	83. **B**	95. **D**
60. **A**	72. **A**	84. **A**	96. **B**

QUANTITATIVE REASONING (97–144)

97. C	109. C	121. D	133. A
98. B	110. B	122. B	134. B
99. A	111. A	123. D	135. A
100. B	112. B	124. A	136. A
101. C	113. B	125. D	137. C
102. A	114. B	126. A	138. D
103. A	115. D	127. A	139. B
104. A	116. C	128. A	140. C
105. D	117. D	129. B	141. B
106. D	118. C	130. D	142. A
107. D	119. B	131. B	143. B
108. A	120. A	132. A	144. D

CRITICAL READING (145–192)

145. B	157. A	169. A	181. D
146. D	158. C	170. D	182. D
147. B	159. D	171. A	183. C
148. C	160. D	172. A	184. B
149. C	161. B	173. C	185. A
150. D	162. C	174. B	186. C
151. D	163. A	175. D	187. C
152. D	164. C	176. A	188. D
153. C	165. C	177. C	189. D
154. B	166. B	178. A	190. B
155. C	167. A	179. B	191. C
156. A	168. C	180. A	192. D

Biological Processes

1. **(A)** Peptidoglycan is made of carbon, oxygen, and hydrogen, and is considered a sugar. Polypeptides (choice B), or proteins, are made of amino acids. Peptidoglycan is not made of amino acids. Nucleic acids (choice C) contain a phosphate, a sugar, and a nitrogenous base. Peptidoglycan's structure does not match this description. Fats (choice D) contain carbons and hydrogens only.

2. **(B)** Ciprofloxacin targets DNA replication, a process which occurs during bacterial reproduction cell division and is known as bacterial fission. Penicillin (choice A) targets the process of peptidoglycan construction in the bacterial cell wall. Streptomycin (choice C) targets the process of protein production. Amphotericin B (choice D) would have no effect on bacteria as it targets ergosterol in fungal cell membranes.

3. **(C)** Streptomycin targets the ribosomes during the process of protein production. Penicillin (choice A) targets the process of peptidoglycan construction in the bacterial cell wall. Ciprofloxacin (choice B) targets DNA. Amphotericin B (choice D) would have no effect on bacteria as it targets ergosterol in fungal cell membranes.

4. **(D)** Fungi contain ergosterol in their plasma membranes. This sterol is unique to fungi and is often a target of antifungal drugs. Archaea (choice A) do not contain ergosterol in their plasma membranes. Also, archaea are not known to cause disease in humans or animals. Gram positive bacteria (choice B) and gram negative bacteria (choice C) do not contain ergosterol in their plasma membranes.

5. **(A)** The nucleolus is found inside the nucleus. The Golgi apparatus (choice B) is located to the right of the nucleus in the figure. The endoplasmic reticulum (choice C) is a series of membrane that extends from the nuclear envelope. The mitochondria (choice D) are shown as the small, kidney-shaped structures with a highly-folded inner membrane.

6. **(B)** Ribosomes, made of rRNA, are found in the cytosol and on the surface of the endoplasmic reticulum. DNA (choice A) is only found inside of the nucleus and the mitochondria in animal cells. Ribosomes, not carbohydrates (choice C), are found at the surface of the rough endoplasmic reticulum. Vesicles (choice D) are made of membrane and are larger than ribosomes.

7. **(D)** Mitochondria are similar in size and shape to prokaryotes. They also have circular DNA and ribosomes, and they undergo fission like prokaryotes. A lysosome (choice A) has no traits that are similar to a prokaryote. The Golgi apparatus (choice B) and the nucleus (choice C) also have no traits that are similar to a prokaryote.

8. **(A)** Bacteria possess a cell wall just outside of the cell membrane. The Golgi apparatus (choice B) is responsible for modifying glycolipids and glycoproteins received from the rough endoplasmic reticulum and is found inside of the cell. The smooth endoplasmic reticulum (choice C) is the location of newly synthesized lipids and is found just outside of the nucleus inside of the cell. The rough endoplasmic reticulum (choice D) is the location of newly synthesized proteins and is found just outside of the nucleus inside of the cell. Choices B, C, and D are not found in prokaryotic cells. They are only found in eukaryotic cells.

9. **(C)** DNA replication is semi-conservative. The template strand pairs with the newly synthesized strand to produce two daughter molecules that contain one parental and one newly synthesized strand. Choices A, B, and D do not describe semi-conserved DNA where one strand of DNA is from the parent and the other is new.

10. **(B)** A heterotroph is an organism that obtains its carbon, as well as energy, from organic compounds. An autotroph (choice A) is a microorganism that uses only inorganic materials as its source of nutrients. Choices C and D refer to offspring categories.

11. **(C)** The cross of "Aa" and "Aa" will result in 25% "aa" offspring.

	A	a
A	AA	Aa
a	Aa	aa

AA (homozygous), Aa (heterozygous),
and aa (homozygous)

12. **(B)** Cones (choice A) provide daylight color vision and are responsible for visual acuity, while rods (choice B) respond to dim light for black-and-white vision. The iris (choice C) surrounds the pupil and regulates its diameter. The cornea (choice D) is the anterior portion of the outer layer of the eye.

13. **(C)** Normal red blood cells (erythrocytes) have an average life span of 120 days.

14. **(B)** Adenosine triphosphate (ATP) releases energy when the last phosphate bond is broken, resulting in ADP + Pi.

15. **(C)** Glucose is a monomer. All the other choices are polymers.

16. **(A)** Kinesin and dynein move along microtubules to transport cargo like vesicles throughout the cell. These are motor proteins. Structural proteins (choice B) provide support for a cell but do not move vesicles. Storage proteins (choice C), like albumin, store molecules or ions but do not move vesicles. Receptor proteins (choice D) bind signal molecules and activate signal pathways in a cell.

17. **(A)** The order of the cell cycle is G_1 phase, S phase, G_2 phase, M phase (mitosis: prophase, metaphase, anaphase, telophase), and cytokinesis.

18. **(B)** Mesosomes (choice A) are folded sections of bacterial membranes. Plasmids (choice C) are circular pieces of DNA. Fimbriae (choice D) are bacterial extensions used for attachment.

19. **(C)** Clostridium are gram-positive, spore-forming bacilli. E. coli (choice A) is a gram-negative bacterium. Eubacterium (choice B) is not spore-forming. Lactobacillus (choice D) is a gram-positive, but not spore-forming, bacterium.

20. **(D)** Diagram D shows an autosomal recessive disease.

21. **(B)** Diagram B shows an X-linked recessive disease.

22. **(C)** Diagram C shows an autosomal dominant disease.

23. **(A)** Diagram A shows a Y-inherited disease.

24. **(B)** The Eustachian tube connects the middle ear to the throat. It is the only choice that extends into the neck. The other choices are all parts of the ear.

25. **(C)** Insulin is linked to type 2 diabetes. Glucose (choice A) is not a hormone. Cortisol (choice B) is involved with stress, and testosterone (choice D) is involved in sex development.

26. **(A)** DNA helicase (choice B) separates the two strands of DNA, while the DNA polymerases (choice C) and (choice D) work on building the new strand of DNA during DNA replication.

27. **(C)** Mycoplasmas are microorganisms that lack cell walls and do not synthesize the precursor for peptidoglycan. Photosynthetic bacteria (choice A) describes bacteria that use photons to make sugars. Archaea (choice B) have cell walls. Plasmids (choice D) are small, circular pieces of DNA found in many bacteria.

28. **(D)** The liver filters blood from the digestive tract and returns the blood to the heart via hepatic veins.

29. **(C)** The dermis (choice A) is the layer of cells below the epidermis. The hypodermis (choice B) is the thick bottom layer of skin cells. The exodermis (choice D) is not a layer of cells found in human skin tissue.

30. **(A)** Evolution refers to changes that occur in populations over time. The other choices do not describe evolution.

31. **(B)** The adrenal glands produce adrenaline and noradrenaline. The pineal gland produces melatonin and serotonin (choice A). The pancreas produces insulin and glucagon (choice C). Estrogen is produced by the ovaries in females, while testosterone is primarily produced by the testicles in males and ovaries in females (choice D).

32. **(C)** Antiport indicates that two ions are moving across a membrane in opposite directions. Uniport (choice A) indicates the movement of one ion, not two. Symport (choice B) indicates that two ions are moving across a membrane in the same direction. While sodium and potassium ions are moving in coupled transport (choice D), this term does not describe the direction of the movement of each ion.

33. **(A)** Active transport is required to move the sodium ions out of the neuron against their concentration gradient. This process uses ATP. Passive transport (choice B) indicates a movement with a concentration gradient. Sodium is moving against its concentration gradient. Simple diffusion (choice C) indicates that a molecule is moving directly through a membrane with its concentration gradient. Sodium is moving through the protein pump against its concentration gradient. Facilitated diffusion (choice D) indicates passive movement through a protein carrier. Sodium is moving actively against its concentration gradient.

34. **(A)** Active transport is required to move the potassium ions into the neuron against their concentration gradient. This process uses ATP. Passive transport (choice B) indicates a movement with a concentration gradient. Potassium is moving against its concentration gradient. Simple diffusion (choice C) indicates that a molecule is moving directly through a membrane with its concentration gradient. Potassium is moving through the protein pump, against its concentration gradient. Facilitated dif-

fusion (choice D) indicates passive movement through a protein carrier. Potassium is moving actively against its concentration gradient.

35. **(C)** The movement of ions across a cell membrane will affect the voltage of that membrane. Voltage-gated channels are sensitive to changes in membrane voltage. Ligand-gated channels (choice A) are only affected by ligands binding to active sites on the channel. Mechanical-gated channels (choice B) are only affected by physical stress placed on the channel proteins. Non-gated channel proteins (choice D) are not sensitive to changes in voltage as ions move across membranes.

36. **(B)** The Krebs cycle (choice A) and the citric acid cycle (choice D) are the same metabolic pathway and do not produce as much ATP as the electron transport chain. Electron oxidation (choice C), or a redox reaction, does not produce ATP.

37. **(C)** The other choices are part of mitosis, a phase of the cell cycle that occurs very quickly compared to interphase.

38. **(C)** Carbon dioxide is released from blood to the air in the alveoli, the site where gas exchange occurs in the lungs.

39. **(C)** Vitamin C is the only water-soluble vitamin; the other choices are fat soluble.

40. **(D)** The temporal lobe is responsible for language.

41. **(D)** The occipital lobe is involved in sight.

42. **(D)** The hippocampus is involved in memory.

43. **(D)** The cerebellum is involved in motor function.

44. **(C)** The immune response recognizes sequences in the viral proteins as foreign and makes antibodies specific for that sequence. Vaccines often contain the proteins of viruses to trigger antibody production by the immune system. In viruses, like HIV, frequent mutations change the protein sequences recognized by the immune system.

45. **(D)** Macrophages engulf and digest bacteria.

46. **(D)** Viruses may contain double-stranded DNA, single-stranded DNA, single-stranded RNA, or double-stranded RNA. Examples include the herpes simplex virus which contains double-stranded DNA, the influenza virus which contains single-stranded RNA, the rotavirus which contains double-stranded RNA, and bacteriophages which contain single-stranded DNA.

47. **(A)** Bacteriophages are viruses that infect bacteria. They are not fungi (choice B) and do not infect fungi (choice D). They can contain either DNA or RNA, so choice C is incorrect.

48. **(B)** pH affects enzymes. For example, higher or lower than normal pH levels can negatively affect the ability of an enzyme to bind its substrate. Choices A, C, and D do not affect enzyme activity.

Chemical Processes

49. **(C)** The synthesis of RNA is called transcription (choice A). The synthesis of protein is called translation (choice B). The synthesis of DNA is called replication (choice C). Translocation (choice D) means the movement of something to a new place.

50. **(D)** DNA polymerase catalyzes the synthesis of DNA using deoxyribonucleotides of adenine, guanine, cytosine, and thymine. Ribonucleotides are used by RNA polymerases to synthesize RNA (transcription). Remember that uracil in RNA is substituted with thymine in DNA, thus choice C is excluded. Both polymerases use the triphosphate forms of the nucleotides.

51. **(B)** When DNA polymerase catalyzes the addition of the next deoxynucleotide triphosphate in the synthesis of DNA, the 3′ secondary alcohol of the last nucleotide in the growing polymer adds to the phosphate at the 5′ position of the new nucleotide. Remember that with nucleotides and nucleic acids, prime numbers refer to atoms in the cyclic form of the carbohydrate ribose. Unprimed numbers would refer to atoms in the nitrogenous bases.

52. **(D)** A string of three nitrogenous bases in DNA is called a codon. The sequence is transcribed into the mRNA molecule then, during translation, a particular amino acid is incorporated into the growing protein.

53. **(A)** The sex hormones are produced from cholesterol.

54. **(A)** An arene (choice B) is a 6-membered ring with alternating single and double bonds. An alcohol is an –OH group in an organic molecule. A secondary alcohol (choice C) means that the carbon to which the –OH is attached is itself attached to two other carbons. An amide (choice D) is a carbonyl attached to a nitrogen.

55. **(A)** Hydrolysis of a nitrile (–CN) to an acid uses H_2O with H^+ or OH^-. Ketones are not oxidized under ordinary lab conditions (choice B). The hydrolysis of epoxides (choice C) yields diols, and the halogenation of an alkene (choice D) yields a dihalide.

56. **(B)** The general blocks in an infrared (IR) spectrum are: 4000 cm^{-1} to 2500 cm^{-1} for O–H, C–H, N–H; 2500 cm^{-1} to 2000 cm^{-1} for triple bonds; 2000 cm^{-1} to 1500 cm^{-1} for double bonds; and 1500 cm^{-1} to 500 cm^{-1} for all other single bonds (called the fingerprint region because the degree of complexity in the region is very high, and a match in the region conclusively identifies the molecule). Since there are not any triple bonds in atorvastatin, there would not be a band at 2100 cm^{-1}. Atorvastatin does have several O–H bonds (so choice A is expected), a couple of carbonyls and arenes (so choice C is expected), and many C–H bonds (so choice D is expected).

57. **(A)** To synthesize a compound with a nitro group and a methyl group meta to each other, you would need to first install the nitro group followed by the methyl group since nitro is a meta director but methyl is an ortho, para director. To put a nitro group on an arene ring, the reagents are nitric acid mixed with sulfuric acid (which generates the electrophile, NO_2^+).

58. **(B)** The conversion of an ester to an alcohol is a reduction and requires a hydride donor. Both choices B and C are hydride donors, but $NaBH_4$ is a much less reactive hydride donor than $LiAlH_4$. The carbonyl carbon of an ester is less reactive than the carbonyl carbon of an aldehyde or ketone; thus the more reactive $LiAlH_4$ is needed for the ester but the less reactive $NaBH_4$ would reduce a more reactive aldehyde or ketone. Choice D, hydrogen or H_2, will reduce nonpolar functional groups like alkenes and alkynes but not (usually) reduce polar functional groups like carbonyls. Choice A, potassium permanganate or $KMnO_4$, is an oxidizing agent.

59. **(D)** The functional group in the reactant in question 58 is an ester. Among the carboxylic acid derivatives, esters are near the bottom in terms of reactivity (only amides are less reactive). Thus, an ester can be made from any of the acid derivatives more reactive than esters (that would include carboxylic acid halides, carboxylic acid anhydrides, acyl phosphates, and thioesters) as well as directly from carboxylic acids. Since amides are the least reactive of the acid derivatives, none of the other acid derivatives can be made from them.

60. **(A)** Stereoisomers are molecules that have the same atom connections but different spatial arrangements. There are two classes of stereoisomers: enantiomers and diastereomers. Enantiomers are nonsuperimposable mirror images. Diastereomers are stereoisomers that are not enantiomers.

61. **(B)** The amino acids with side chains that are essentially 100% ionized at physiologic pH are glutamic acid and aspartic acid (both have a carboxylic acid in their side chain) as well as lysine (it has a primary amine in its side chain).

62. **(A)** The levels of protein structure are: primary (the amino acid sequence of the protein); secondary (localized patterns that occur by hydrogen bonding between the H of one peptide bond with the O of a different peptide bond—the two most common types are an alpha helix and a beta sheet); tertiary (the overall assembly of the entire protein, driven by the hydrophobic/hydrophilic nature of the amino acid side chains—hydrophobic side chains pull toward the interior of the folded protein while hydrophilic side chains pull toward the exterior of the folded protein where the water molecules are); and the quarternary structure (the association of multiple proteins to form an active complex—not all proteins exhibit this level of structure).

63. **(B)** See the answer explanation for question 79 for more details.

64. **(D)** Buffers are a combination of a weak acid and its conjugate base. Choices B and C can be eliminated since they are both a single entity. Choice A is a mixture of a *strong* acid and its conjugate base. The strong acids are H_2SO_4, HNO_3, HI, HBr, HCl, and $HClO_4$.

65. **(C)** Peptide bonds are amide bonds. When an amide joins two amino acids, it's called a peptide bond.

66. **(C)** First, eliminate choice D because it is a lower temperature than the starting temperature, and the question indicates that heat is absorbed by the copper, so the temperature will definitely increase. To solve this problem, it is easiest to let the units of the specific heat drive the problem set-up.

$$0.385 \text{ J/g°C} = 15.0 \text{ J}/(5.0 \text{ g} \times \text{°C temperature change})$$

Solving for the unknown, °C temperature change, you get about 8°C. The starting temperature is 25°C, so the final temperature is about 33°C.

67. **(C)** Atomic number indicates the number of protons (so choice B is eliminated) and atomic mass indicates the sum of protons and neutrons (so choice A is eliminated and choice C is found to be correct). Neither the atomic number nor the atomic mass tell you about the number of electrons. The charge on the specie is required to be able to determine the number of electrons.

68. **(B)** Isotopes of an element must have the same number of protons; otherwise they would be different elements. The number of protons (the atomic number) defines the element.

69. **(D)** To determine the molarity, you need to know the number of moles of $Cu(NO_3)_2$ and the volume of the solution (given to you in the question as 500 mL or 0.500 L). To calculate the number of moles of $Cu(NO_3)_2$, divide the mass (37.5 g) by the formula weight (187.5 g/mol) to get 0.2 moles. Now divide 0.2 mol by 0.5 L to get the answer.

70. **(A)** To determine the density of a gas, rearrange the ideal gas law.

PV = nRT can be written as PV = (mass/FW)RT, where FW is formula weight

Rearranging the equation, you get mass/V = density (in g/L) = P × FW/RT
Filling in what you know, Density = (1 × 4)/(0.082 × 308) = 0.16 g/L
Note that the temperature must be in Kelvin. 35°C + 273 = 308 K

71. **(D)** To determine partial pressure, recall that $P_{nitrogen}$ = (mole fraction of N_2) × P_{total}

Mole fraction of N_2 = moles N_2/(moles N_2 + moles He)

In this case, there are 2 moles of N_2 (56 g/28 g per mole), and there are 8 moles of He (32 g/4 g per mole), so the mole fraction of N_2 is 0.20. Multiply the mole fraction of N_2 by the total pressure to get the partial pressure of N_2.

72. **(A)** Evaporation is the conversion of a liquid into a gas; the reverse is called condensation. Since you must heat up the liquid for it to evaporate, it's an endothermic process (condensation would be an exothermic process).

73. **(D)** Increasing the temperature or the agitation (stirring) would allow the gas to escape from the liquid. Decreasing the pressure above the liquid would accomplish the same thing. Increasing the pressure of the gas above the liquid would drive it into solution.

74. **(A)** The actual yield of the reaction, 32.0 g SO_2, is given. To calculate percent yield, you must first calculate the theoretical yield, which is the maximum possible yield of the reaction, and then use the theoretical yield in the equation below to calculate percent yield.

$$\frac{\text{Actual yield}}{\text{Theoretical yield}} \times 100 = \% \text{ yield}$$

$$CS_2 + 3O_2 \rightarrow CO_2 + 2SO_2$$

$\underline{\text{g } CS_2} \rightarrow$ $\qquad$ $\underline{\text{moles } CS_2} \rightarrow$ $\qquad$ $\underline{\text{moles } SO_2} \rightarrow$

38.0 gm $\qquad\qquad$ $\dfrac{38.0 \text{ g}}{76 \text{ g/moles}}$ $\qquad$ $0.50 \text{ mole } CS_2 \times \dfrac{2 \text{ moles } SO_2}{1 \text{ mole } CS_2}$

$\qquad\qquad\qquad\qquad$ 0.50 mole $\qquad\qquad$ 1.00 mole SO_2

$\underline{\text{g } SO_2}$

$1.00 \text{ mole } SO_2 \times \dfrac{64 \text{ g } SO_2}{1 \text{ mole } SO_2} = 64 \text{ g } SO_2$ $\qquad$ $\% \text{ yield} = \dfrac{32 \text{ g}}{64 \text{ g}} \times 100 = 50\%$

75. **(A)** In a dilution problem, the number of moles of solute before dilution equals the number of moles of solute after dilution. Therefore:

Molarity × volume (before dilution) = Molarity × volume (after dilution)

$$2.0 \ \frac{\text{moles}}{\text{L}} \ (0.100 \text{ L}) = 4.0 \ \frac{\text{moles}}{\text{L}} \ (\text{volume})$$

0.05 L = volume required

Dilute 50 mL of the 4.0 M solution with water to 100 mL to prepare the 2.0 M solution.

76. **(C)** Remember that since the speed of light (c) is a constant, as the wavelength decreases, frequency increases (and vice versa). Therefore, the light with the highest frequency will be that with the lowest wavelength. A review of metric prefixes may aid in realizing that nm (nanometers) is the smallest of the units given as possible selections.

77. **(B)** A chloride ion has 8 valence electrons (a chlorine atom has 7 and when it becomes negatively charged by gaining an electron, it would have 8) and a sulfide ion also has 8 (a sulfur atom has 6 but the S^{2-} ion has 8).

78. **(B)** A basic oxide is a compound that, when it reacts with water, produces a base. Another name for a basic oxide is a basic anhydride. The oxide K_2O reacts with water to produce KOH according to the following equation:

$$K_2O + H_2O \rightarrow 2KOH$$

The other oxides, CO_2, SO_2, and P_2O_5, are all acid oxides or acid anhydrides.

$$CO_2 + H_2O \rightarrow H_2CO_3$$
$$SO_2 + H_2O \rightarrow H_2SO_3$$
$$P_2O_5 + 3H_2O \rightarrow 2 H_3PO_4$$

79. **(B)** For hydrogen bonding to exist, the hydrogen must be bonded to nitrogen, oxygen, or fluorine: H — N, H — O, H — F. Hydrogen bonding is not possible between molecules of CH_4 because the hydrogen is bonded to carbon, C. Hydrogen bonding is possible, however, between molecules of H_2O, between molecules of CH_3OH, and between molecules of NH_3.

80. **(B)** When two equilibrium reactions are added to give a third reaction, the equilibrium constant for the third reaction is calculated by multiplying the two equilibrium constants for each original reaction, $(K^1)(K^2)$. Add equations, multiply equilibrium constants.

81. **(B)** When determining the acidity of homologous compounds of members of the same family, as in HI, HBr, HCl, and HF, another concept besides electronegativity is invoked. HI is more acidic than HBr, which is more acidic than HCl, which is more acidic than HF. The larger the atom, I versus F, the more readily it can accommodate an extra electron and be stable. Therefore, I^- is more stable than F^- and consequently HI is more acidic than HF. Acidity increases as one progresses from top to bottom in a family, for example, HF < HCl < HBr < HI.

82. **(C)** Beta decay is the expulsion of a nuclear electron resulting from the conversion of a neutron to a proton (meaning the atomic number will change but the atomic mass

will not). With gamma emission (choice B) alone, neither the atomic number nor the atomic mass changes (unless some other nuclear reaction also occurs). Alpha decay (choice D) results in the change of both the atomic number and the atomic mass (the atomic mass is reduced by 4 and the atomic number is reduced by 2). Nuclear fission (choice A) is the splitting of the specie into two comparably sized nuclei.

83. **(B)** The First Law of Thermodynamics considers the conversion of energy from one form to another form without the subsequent formation or loss of any of the energy. The Second Law of Thermodynamics states that entropy, the measure of disorder, increases in spontaneous reactions and remains the same in equilibrium systems (choice C). The Third Law of Thermodynamics says that the entropy for a perfect crystal is zero at absolute zero temperature (choice A). The statement that the Gibbs Free Energy is a measure of the spontaneity of a reaction is true (choice D).

84. **(A)** Since the reactant is a tertiary alkyl halide, the substitution will occur through the SN1 mechanism. The SN1 mechanism involves a carbocation intermediate. Carbocations are planar (sp^2 hybridized) meaning that the hydrosulfide nucleophile will attack the carbocation equally from each face of the plane. Thus, both the R and the S enantiomers of the product will result, giving a racemic (or very nearly racemic) mixture, which is optically inactive.

85. **(B)** Both solutes are called acids and have pKa's, so choice C is false. The stronger the acid, the larger the Ka and the lower the pKa (since pKa = –log Ka), so choices A and D are also false. Choice B is correct because acid B is the stronger acid (larger Ka) and a solution of it would contain more hydrogen ions lowering the pH (remember pH = –log [H$^+$] so as [H$^+$] increases, pH decreases).

86. **(C)** The formula C_2H_4 is the formula for an alkene. The electrophile bromine, Br_2, adds atoms to C_2H_4 to produce the dibromide $C_2H_4Br_2$, 1,2-dibromoethane,

$$CH_2 = CH_2 + Br_2 \longrightarrow \underset{\underset{Br}{|}}{CH_2}-\underset{\underset{Br}{|}}{CH_2}$$

This is an addition reaction since two molecules add to make one.

87. **(B)** Carbohydrates, like glucose, are oxidized through glycolysis and then the citric acid cycle produces ATP and reduced cofactors (NADH and FADH$_2$). More ATP is produced when the reduced cofactors are oxidized via oxidative phosphorylation. The monomers in protein synthesis are amino acids.

88. **(B)** It is not true that all bonds in benzene are equivalent in length. All of the C–C bonds are equivalent in length but the C–H bonds are a different length from the C–C bonds. Even though the C–C bonds in benzene may be represented by alternating single and double bonds, all of these C–C bonds are the same length because of delocalization of pi electrons, that is, resonance. All of the other statements about benzene are correct.

89. **(A)** This compound is named 3-methylpentanoic acid. The carbonyl carbon is numbered 1, so the carbon atom to which the methyl group is attached is carbon 3. The

acid is named by removing the *-e* from pentane and adding *-oic acid*. The formulas for the other answers are shown below.

$$CH_3CH_2CH_2\underset{\overset{|}{CH_3}}{CH}COOH$$

$$CH_3CH_2\underset{\overset{|}{CH_3}}{CH}COOH$$

$$CH_3\underset{\overset{|}{CH_3}}{CH}CH_2COOH$$

2-methylpentanoic acid   2-methylbutanoic acid   3-methylbutanoic acid

90. **(B)** To name an alcohol, find the longest carbon chain containing the alcohol carbon, number the carbons of that chain such that the alcohol carbon has the lower number, and then identify any branches off the chain. That leads us to either choice B or choice C as the correct choice. Since there is a chiral center whose 3D arrangement has been specified in the structure, R or S can be designated. Assign priorities to the four groups attached to the chiral center based on the atomic number. Here, the OH group would be number 1, the isopropyl group would be number 2, the methyl group would be number 3, and the hydrogen group would be number 4. Orient the molecule such that priority group number 4 is away from you and look at the other three groups. If they are arranged 1, 2, 3 clockwise, it's called R, and if counterclockwise, it's S.

91. **(B)**

$$\% = \frac{\text{Part}}{\text{Whole}} \times 100$$

$$\frac{8H}{(NH_4)_2\,SO_4} \times 100 = \frac{8}{132} \times 100 = 6.06\%$$

92. **(A)** When the Br_2 adds to the alkene via anti addition, two products result: the SS and the RR stereoisomers.

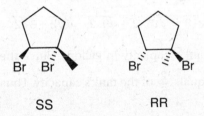

SS   RR

Since the alkene is equally accessible from either face, a 50:50 mixture of enantiomers (remember that enantiomers are opposites in absolute configuration) results. Diastereomers are stereoisomers that are not exact opposites. If the products were RR and RS, they would be diastereomers. A non-50:50 mixture of diastereomers results when the reactant contains a chiral center. A meso form would be a molecule with two chiral centers made up of the same four groups with one being R and the other being S.

93. **(A)** 2.2 mL of pentanoic acid would be 2.046 g (2.2 mL × 0.93 g/mL), which is 0.020 moles of pentanoic acid (2.046 g × 1 mol/102 g). Thus 0.020 moles of sodium hydroxide would be needed (since stoichiometry is 1:1 in the equation), which is 0.80 g (0.020 moles × 40 g/mol).

94. **(C)** Molarity is defined as moles of solute divided by liters of solution.

$$M = \frac{\text{moles of solute}}{\text{liters of solution}} = \frac{\text{g/mol. wt.}}{\text{liters of solution}}$$

Sugar, $C_6H_{12}O_6$, has a molecular weight of 180 g/mole. Substitute 18 g, 180 g/mole, and 0.5 M into the above equation to obtain the volume of the solution.

$$M = \frac{18\,g\,/\,180\,g\,/mole}{x} = 0.5\,M$$

$$x = 0.2\,L = 200\,mL$$

95. **(D)** Nuclear fission is the breakdown of a larger nucleus, usually by bombarding it with neutrons, to produce smaller atoms and more neutrons. A great deal of energy is released in this process, which is the basis for the atomic bomb. Other kinds of nuclear reactions are radioactive decay (choice A) and fusion (choice B). Radioactive decay is the spontaneous emission of nuclear particles, e.g., alpha and beta particles, as well as gamma rays, by unstable nuclei. Nuclear fusion is the combination of small nucleii to produce a larger atom with the concomitant release of a large amount of energy. Nuclear fusion occurs on the sun. The hydrogen bomb is an example of nuclear fusion. Carbon-14 dating (choice C) is a method of determining the age of an object by comparing the amount of carbon-12 and the amount of radioactive carbon-14 present in the object.

96. **(B)** Ozonolysis with reductive work up cleaves alkenes and alkynes. For alkenes, the double bond is cleaved and replaced with carbonyl groups on each carbon of the alkene. For alkynes, the triple bond is cleaved and replaced with carboxylic acid groups on each carbon of the alkyne. Acetic acid is CH_3CO_2H, so the reacting organic molecule must have been an alkyne and since two moles of acetic acid resulted, the alkyne must have had a methyl group on each alkyne carbon.

Quantitative Reasoning

97. **(C)** Note that $\sqrt{32} + \sqrt{18} = \sqrt{16 \cdot 2} + \sqrt{9 \cdot 2} = 4\sqrt{2} + 3\sqrt{2} = 7\sqrt{2}$.

98. **(B)** Let x equal the tank's capacity in gallons. Since the tank is already $\frac{3}{5}$ full, the additional 6 gallons equals $\frac{2}{5}$ of the tank's capacity. Thus,

$$6 = \frac{2}{5}x \Rightarrow 30 = 2x \Rightarrow x = 15$$

99. **(A)** We calculate the limit by first isolating the highest degree terms in the numerator and the denominator, and then reducing.

$$\lim_{x \to \infty}\left(\frac{7x^5 + 2x^3 - 5x + 50}{13x^2 - 2x^5}\right) = \lim_{x \to \infty}\left(\frac{7x^5}{-2x^5}\right) = -\frac{7}{2}$$

100. **(B)** Given the function $f(x) = \frac{x+1}{10x}$, we solve for y in the equation $x = \frac{y+1}{10y}$, that is,

$$x = \frac{y+1}{10y}$$

$$10xy = y + 1$$

$$10xy - y = 1$$

$$y(10x - 1) = 1 \Rightarrow y = \frac{1}{10x-1}$$

101. **(C)** $5^2 + 5^3 = 25 + 125 = 150$

102. **(A)** The probability that a randomly chosen piece of fruit is NOT a banana can be computed as follows:

$$\text{probability} = \frac{\text{total number of non-bananas}}{\text{total number of pieces of fruit}} = \frac{18}{26} = \frac{9}{13}$$

103. **(A)** Represent your percentage scores on the midterms by m_1 and m_2, and your percentage score on the final exam by x. Since your average on the midterms is 84%, we have

$$\frac{m_1 + m_2}{2} = 84 \Rightarrow m_1 + m_2 = 168$$

Using the respective weights for each score, we have

$$(0.24)m_1 + (0.24)m_2 + (0.52)x = \text{course average}$$
$$(0.24)(m_1 + m_2) + (0.52)x = \text{course average}$$

Now use the fact that $m_1 + m_2 = 168$.

$$(0.24)(168) + (0.52)x = \text{course average}$$

We want to find the value of x so that $(0.24)(168) + (0.52)x > 88$.

$$(0.24)(168) + (0.52)x > 88$$
$$40.32 + 0.52x > 88$$
$$0.52x > 47.68 \Rightarrow x > 91.69$$

104. **(A)** We complete the square on the given equation as follows.

$$x^2 + y^2 - 12x + 14y + 9 = 0$$
$$x^2 - 12x + 36 + y^2 + 14y + 49 = -9 + 36 + 49$$
$$(x - 6)^2 + (y + 7)^2 = 76$$
$$(x - 6)^2 + (y + 7)^2 = \left(\sqrt{76}\right)^2$$

Now use the fact that a circle with equation $(x - h)^2 + (y - k)^2 = r^2$ has center point (h, k) and a radius equal to r. In the given equation, we have $(x - 6)^2 + (y + 7)^2 = \left(\sqrt{76}\right)^2$. Thus, the radius equals $\sqrt{76}$.

105. **(D)**

$$\int_0^2 \left(12x - 6x^2\right)dx = \left[\frac{12x^2}{2} - \frac{6x^3}{3}\right]_{x=0}^{x=2} = \left[6x^2 - 2x^3\right]_{x=0}^{x=2}$$
$$= 6(2)^2 - 2(2)^3 - \left(6(0)^2 - 2(0)^3\right)$$
$$= 24 - 16 = 8$$

106. **(D)** Let $A = \{x : 1 \le x \le 500, \text{ where } 3|x\}$. Then $|A| = 166$, since $\frac{500}{3} = 166.\overline{6}$.

Let $B = \{x : 1 \le x \le 500, \text{ where } 5|x\}$. Then $|B| = 100$, since $\frac{500}{5} = 100$.

Then

$$A \cap B = \{x : 1 \le x \le 500, \text{ where } x \text{ is divisible by 3 and by 5}\}$$
$$= \{x : 1 \le x \le 500, \text{ where } x \text{ is divisible by 15}\}$$

So $|A \cap B| = 33$, since $\frac{500}{15} = 33.\overline{3}$.

We have the formula $|A \cup B| = |A| + |B| - |A \cap B|$. Therefore, we have:

$$|A \cup B| = 166 + 100 - 33 = 233$$

We want to compute the cardinality of the set $\overline{A \cup B}$, i.e.,

$$\overline{A \cup B} = \{x : 1 \le x \le 500, \text{ where } x \text{ is not divisble by 3 or by 5}\}$$

We know that $|\overline{A \cup B}| = 500 - |A \cup B| = 500 - 233 = 267$. There are 267 numbers

between 1 and 500, inclusive, that are not divisible by 3 or by 5.

107. **(D)** We use the Fundamental Theorem of Calculus as follows:

$$\int_1^2 (5x^4)\,dx = \frac{5x^5}{5}\Big]_{x=1}^{x=2} = x^5\Big]_{x=1}^{x=2} = 2^5 - 1^5 = 32 - 1 = 31$$

108. **(A)** Since the selection order matters, we are counting the number of possible permutations of length 4 that can be formed from an 8-element set. Since the balls are replaced after each selection, we have the following result. There are 8 possibilities for the first number selected, 8 possibilities for the second number selected, 8 possibilities for the third number selected, and 8 possibilities for the fourth number selected. Thus, we have a total of $8 \times 8 \times 8 \times 8 = 4{,}096$ possible four-digit numbers.

109. **(C)** We simplify the expression as follows:

$$\frac{x^2 - 11x + 24}{x - 8} = \frac{(x - 8)(x - 3)}{x - 8} = x - 3$$

110. **(B)** We use the quadratic formula.

$$x = \frac{-b \pm \sqrt{b^2 - 4ac}}{2a} = \frac{-1 \pm \sqrt{1^2 - 4 \cdot 6 \cdot 1}}{2 \cdot 6} = \frac{-1 \pm \sqrt{-23}}{12}$$

Since $\sqrt{-23}$ is not a real number, the equation has no real solutions.

111. **(A)** Each point on the graph of $y = 5f(x + 2) - 3$ is obtained by transforming the points on the graph of $y = f(x)$ as follows. Subtract 2 from each x-coordinate; multiply each y-coordinate by 5 and then subtract 3.

112. **(B)** We solve the equation for x as follows.

$$x^{\ln(x)} = e^4$$
$$\ln(x^{\ln(x)}) = \ln(e^4)$$
$$\ln(x)\ln(x) = 4$$
$$(\ln(x))^2 = 4$$
$$\ln(x) = \pm 2$$

When $\ln(x) = 2$, we have $x = e^2$. When $\ln(x) = -2$, we have $x = e^{-2}$.

113. **(B)** Note that

$$\lim_{x\to4}\left(\frac{x^2 - 10x + 24}{4 - x}\right) = \lim_{x\to4}\left(\frac{(x-4)(x-6)}{4-x}\right) = \lim_{x\to4}\left(\frac{(x-4)(x-6)}{-(x-4)}\right) = \lim_{x\to4}(-(x-6)) = -(4-6) = 2$$

114. **(B)** Add $8 + 35 + 8 + 9 + 5 + 10 + 7 + 3 + 12 = 97$. Then, divide 97 by 9, which is the total amount of numbers in the set; therefore, $97 \div 9 = 10.77$.

115. **(D)** The total rental cost is given by the daily cost plus the mileage cost. Daily cost = (\$30 per day)(7 days) = \$210. Mileage cost = (\$0.14 per mile)(x miles) = \$0.14x.

116. **(C)** The probability of heads for each independent toss is $\frac{1}{2}$. Since the coin is tossed a total of ten times, the probability of the desired outcome is

$$\frac{1}{2} \times \frac{1}{2} \times \frac{1}{2} \times \frac{1}{2} \times \frac{1}{2} \times \frac{1}{2} \times \frac{1}{2} \times \frac{1}{2} \times \frac{1}{2} \times \frac{1}{2} = \frac{1}{1024}$$

117. **(D)**

$$f'(t) = 5(4e^{4t-8}) = 20e^{4t-8} \Rightarrow f'(2) = 20e^{4(2)-8} = 20e^0 = 20$$

118. **(C)** To compute $(f + g)(x)$, add the function formulas for f and g, and then combine like terms.

$$(f + g)(x) = x^2 + 2x - 1 + 2x + 1 = x^2 + 4x$$

119. **(B)** We solve the equation as follows.

$$4(x + 3)(x - 2) = 4x^2 + x$$
$$4(x^2 + x - 6) = 4x^2 + x$$
$$4x^2 + 4x - 24 = 4x^2 + x$$
$$4x - 24 = x$$
$$3x = 24 \Rightarrow x = 8$$

120. **(A)** Each time a die is rolled, there are two possible outcomes: an even number or an odd number. Therefore, the probability that the die will land on an odd number is 50%.

121. **(D)** Note that $\frac{5}{9} - \frac{3}{10} = \frac{5 \cdot 10 - 3 \cdot 9}{9 \cdot 10} = \frac{50 - 27}{90} = \frac{23}{90}$.

122. **(B)** Let y equal the distance from home to school. This means that your sister's walking speed is $\frac{y}{30}$ and your walking speed is $\frac{y}{40}$. Let x equal the number of minutes it

takes for your sister to catch up to you. Since you have a 6-minute head start, this means that, at the moment she catches up, you have been walking for $x + 6$ minutes. Also note that, at this moment, you have both walked the same distance. Therefore, we have the following equation:

sister's distance walked = your distance walked

$$(x \text{ minutes})\left(\frac{y}{30 \text{ minutes}}\right) = (x + 6 \text{ minutes})\left(\frac{y}{40 \text{ minutes}}\right)$$

$$\frac{x \cdot y}{30} = \frac{(x+6)y}{40}$$

$$\frac{x}{30} = \frac{x+6}{40}$$

$$40x = 30x + 180$$

$$10x = 180$$

$$x = 18$$

123. **(D)** There are four ways that the sum of the numbers can equal 5, namely $1 + 4$, $4 + 1$, $2 + 3$, and $3 + 2$. Each die has six faces. This means that there are $(6)(6) = 36$ possible outcomes for tossing the two dice. Thus, the probability that the sum of the numbers equals 5 is given by $\frac{4}{36} = \frac{1}{9}$. Therefore, the probability that the sum of the numbers does NOT equal 5 is given by $1 - \frac{1}{9} = \frac{8}{9}$.

124. **(A)** We can use the Power Rule for integrals to integrate term-by-term.

$$\int (x + 2)\,dx = \int x\,dx + \int 2\,dx$$

$$= \int x\,dx + 2\int x^0\,dx$$

$$= \frac{1}{2}x^2 + 2x + C$$

125. **(D)** The highest point on the graph has a y-coordinate equal to 300.

126. **(A)** The highest point on the graph occurs when the x-coordinate equals 3.

127. **(A)** The quadratic equation $10x^2 + \pi x + q = 0$ has a double root when the discriminant equals zero. Therefore, we solve $b^2 - 4ac = \pi^2 - 4 \cdot 10 \cdot q = 0$.

$$\pi^2 - 40q = 0$$

$$\pi^2 = 40q \Rightarrow q = \frac{\pi^2}{40}$$

128. **(A)** The given function will be undefined for any x-value that causes the denominator to equal zero. Setting the denominator equal to zero yields

$$x^2 + 9x + 18 = 0$$

$$(x + 6)(x + 3) = 0$$

$$x = -6, \ x = -3$$

Thus, the domain for f must exclude $x = -6$ and $x = -3$.

129. **(B)** Note that $9^3 \cdot 9^{-1} = 9^{3-1} = 9^2 = 81$.

130. **(D)** The total number of ways to choose 3 girls and 1 boy is given by the formula:

$$\underbrace{_5C_3}_{\substack{\text{choose} \\ \text{3 girls}}} \cdot \underbrace{_3C_1}_{\substack{\text{choose} \\ \text{1 boy}}} = \frac{5!}{3!2!} \cdot \frac{3!}{1!2!} = 10 \cdot 3 = 30$$

The total number of ways to choose 4 people is given by the formula:

$$_8C_4 = \frac{8!}{4!4!} = \frac{1680}{24} = 70$$

Thus, the probability $= \frac{30}{70} = \frac{3}{7}$.

131. **(B)** A quadratic function $f(x) = ax^2 + bx + c$ will have its vertex at the point:

$$\left(-\frac{b}{2a}, f\left(-\frac{b}{2a}\right)\right)$$

$$f(x) = 9x^2 + 18x - 7 \Rightarrow = -\frac{b}{2a} = -\frac{18}{2(9)} = -\frac{18}{18} = -1$$

$$f(-1) = 9(-1)^2 + 18(-1) - 7 = 9 - 18 - 7 = -16$$

Thus, the vertex is $(-1, -16)$.

132. **(A)** We compute the derivative of $f(x) = \frac{x}{x+1}$, and then evaluate at $x = 0$ as follows. Applying the Quotient Rule for derivatives yields:

$$f'(x) = \frac{(x+1)(1) - x(1)}{(x+1)^2} = \frac{1}{(x+1)^2} \Rightarrow f'(0) = 1$$

133. **(A)** We solve the equation for x as follows:

$$\ln(p - 4x) = 2$$
$$e^{\ln(p-4x)} = e^2$$
$$p - 4x = e^2$$
$$-4x = e^2 - p \Rightarrow x = \frac{e^2 - p}{-4}$$

134. **(B)** We have the ratio $\dfrac{3 \text{ apples}}{7 \text{ oranges}} \Rightarrow \dfrac{3 \cdot 3 \text{ apples}}{7 \cdot 3 \text{ oranges}} = \dfrac{9 \text{ apples}}{21 \text{ oranges}}$.

135. **(A)** In Stage 2, the original segment is subdivided into 3 equal sub-segments, and then the middle sub-segment is removed, leaving $\frac{2}{3}$ of the original length. In Stage 3, each segment in Stage 2 is subdivided into 3 equal sub-segments, and then the middle sub-segment is removed, leaving $\frac{2}{3}$ of the length of each Stage 2 segment. Thus, the total segment length in Stage 3 equals $\left(\frac{2}{3}\right)\left(\frac{2}{3}\right) = \frac{4}{9}$ of the original segment length at Stage 1.

136. **(A)** Consider the Venn diagram.

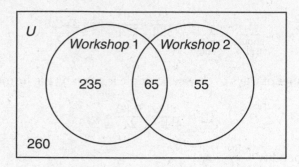

The total number of employees = 260 + 235 + 65 + 55 = 615.

137. **(C)** Note that $\lim\limits_{x \to 5.1} \left(\dfrac{f(x) - f(5.1)}{x - 5.1} \right) = f'(5.1) =$ the slope of the tangent line to the graph

when $x = 5.1$. Since the graph has a horizontal tangent line at this point, the slope equals 0 there.

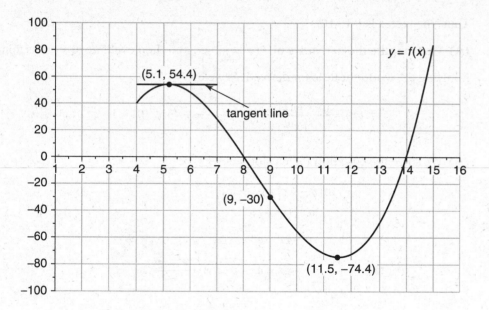

138. **(D)** A logarithmic function is undefined unless the input value is strictly greater than zero. Thus, we solve $2x - 7 > 0$ and obtain $x > 3.5$.

139. **(B)** $P(x) = 35x^2 + 420x - 50$ is a quadratic function whose graph is a parabola that opens up since the coefficient of the x^2 term is positive. This means that the function has a minimum value at the vertex of the parabola.

The minimum value occurs at the vertex, that is, when:

$$x = -\frac{b}{2a} = -\frac{420}{2(35)} = -6$$

Thus, the minimum value of the given function is:

$$P(-6) = 35(-6)^2 + 420(-6) - 50 = -1{,}310$$

140. **(C)** We simplify the expression as follows:

$$\frac{\frac{1}{x+h}-\frac{1}{x}}{h}=\frac{\frac{x}{(x+h)x}-\frac{x+h}{(x)(x+h)}}{h}=\left(\frac{x-x-h}{(x+h)x}\right)\left(\frac{1}{h}\right)=\left(\frac{-h}{(x+h)x}\right)\left(\frac{1}{h}\right)=-\frac{1}{(x+h)x}$$

141. **(B)** The Quotient Rule for logarithms states that

$$\log(M)-\log(N)=\log\left(\frac{M}{N}\right)$$

$$\log(75)-\log(3)=\log\left(\frac{75}{3}\right)$$

$$=\log(25)$$

142. **(A)** The truck must travel 48 miles in 45 minutes = 0.75 hour. We have the formula:

$$\text{speed}=\frac{\text{distance}}{\text{time}}=\frac{48\text{ miles}}{0.75\text{ hr}}=64\text{ mph}$$

143. **(B)** A circle with the equation $(x-h)^2+(y-k)^2=r^2$ has a radius equal to r. In this problem $r^2=36\Rightarrow r=6$.

144. **(D)** We solve the equation as follows:

$$\frac{2x}{x-5}+\frac{x}{x+3}=3$$

$$\frac{2x(x+3)+x(x-5)}{(x-5)(x+3)}=3$$

$$2x(x+3)+x(x-5)=3(x-5)(x+3)$$

$$2x^2+6x+x^2-5x=3x^2-6x-45$$

$$x=-6x-45\Rightarrow 7x=-45\Rightarrow x=-\frac{45}{7}$$

Critical Reading

The numbers in the margins of the reprinted passages indicate the statements in which the answer to the questions can be found.

Passage 1

145 Bronchial asthma is a common disease of children and adults. Although the clinical manifestations of asthma have been known since antiquity, it is a disease that still defies
153 precise definition. The word *asthma* is of Greek origin and means "panting." More than 2,000 years ago, Hippocrates used the word *asthma* to describe episodic shortness of breath; however, the first detailed clinical description of the asthmatic patient was made by Aretaeus in the second century. Since that time *asthma* has been used to describe any
146 disorder with episodic shortness of breath or dyspnea; thus, the terms *cardiac asthma*
152 and *bronchial asthma* have been used to delineate the etiologies of the dyspnea. These terms are now obsolete and asthma refers to a disorder of the respiratory system characterized by episodes of difficulty in breathing. An Expert Panel of the National Institutes of Health National Asthma Education Program (NAEP) has defined asthma as a lung disease characterized by (1) airway obstruction that is reversible (but not completely
147 so in some patients) either spontaneously or with treatment; (2) airway inflammation; and (3) increased airway responsiveness to a variety of stimuli. This descriptive definition for asthma is attributed to our lack of knowledge of the precise pathogenic defect that results in the clinical syndrome we recognize as asthma. The current definition
149 does allow for the important heterogeneity of the clinical presentation of asthma. New technologies have added substantially to our understanding of the interrelationships of immunology, biochemistry, and physiology to the clinical presentation of asthma, and further research may yet uncover a specific genetic defect associated with asthma. Until such time, asthma will continue to defy exact definition.

151 An estimated 10 million persons in the United States have asthma (about 5% of the population). The reported prevalence increased 29% from 1980 to 1987 to 40.1 per 1000 population. African-Americans have a 19% higher incidence of asthma than whites and are twice as likely to be hospitalized. The estimated cost of asthma in the United States in 1990 was $6.2 billion. The largest single direct medical expenditure was for inpatient hospital services (emergency care), reaching almost $1.5 billion, followed by prescription medications ($1.1 billion). The costs of medication increased 54% between 1985 and 1990. In total, 43% of the economic impact was associated with emergency room use, hospitalization, and death. Asthma accounted for 1% of all ambulatory care visits
150 according to the National Ambulatory Medical Care Survey and results in more than 450,000 hospitalizations per year.

145. **(B)** As stated in the passage, bronchial asthma is a common disease in children and adults that defies precise definition.

146. **(D)** The passage states that *cardiac asthma* and *bronchial asthma* are now two obsolete terms that delineated the etiologies of dyspnea.

147. **(B)** The passage states that the NAEP defines asthma as a lung disease characterized by: (1) airway obstruction that is reversible, but not completely so in some patients,

either spontaneously or with treatment; (2) airway inflammation; and (3) increased airway responsiveness to a variety of stimuli.

148. **(C)** The passage states that the total cost of asthma in the United States in 1990 was $6.2 billion. The cost of prescription medications accounted for $1.1 billion of the total amount. Subtracting $1.1 billion from $6.2 billion equals $5.1 billion.

149. **(C)** Wheezing and episodes of shortness of breath (choice B) and the interrelationship of immunology, biochemistry, and physiology (choice D) are already understood, and choice A is irrelevant. Researchers hope to uncover a specific genetic defect associated with asthma (choice C).

150. **(D)** Asthma results in more than 450,000 hospitalizations per year.

151. **(D)** The passage states that the estimated number of persons in the United States who have asthma is 10 million.

152. **(D)** Choices A, B, and C are incorrect choices, since "panting" (choice A) and dyspnea of cardiac (choice B) or bronchial (choice C) etiology are obsolete definitions. Choice D represents the current definition of asthma.

153. **(C)** The passage states that more than 2,000 years ago Hippocrates used the word *asthma* to describe episodic shortness of breath.

154. **(B)** The passage provides some facts about the prevalence of asthma in the United States.

Passage 2

When Italy emerged into the light of history about 700 BC, it was already inhabited by
157 various peoples of different cultures and languages. Most natives of the country lived in villages or small towns, supported themselves by agriculture or animal husbandry (Italia means "Calf Land"), and spoke an Italic dialect belonging to the Indo-European family of languages. Oscan and Umbrian were closely related Italic dialects spoken by the inhabitants of the Apennines. The other two Italic dialects, Latin and Venetic, were likewise closely related to each other and were spoken, respectively, by the Latins of Latium (a plain of west-central Italy) and the people of northeastern Italy (near modern Venice). Apulians (Iapyges) and Messapians inhabited the southeastern coast. Their language resembled the speech of the Illyrians on the other side of the Adriatic. During the fifth century BC the Po valley of northern Italy (Cisalpine Gaul) was occupied by Gallic tribes who spoke Celtic and who had migrated across the Alps from continental
160 Europe. The Etruscans were the first highly civilized people of Italy and were the only inhabitants who did not speak an Indo-European language. By 700 BC several Greek colonies were established along the southern coast. Both Greeks and Phoenicians were actively engaged in trade.

Modern historical analysis is making rapid progress in showing how Rome's early development occurred in a multicultural environment and was particularly influenced by the higher civilizations of the Etruscans to the north and the Greeks to the south.
156 Roman religion was indebted to the beliefs and practices of the Etruscans. The Romans

158 borrowed and adapted the alphabet from the Etruscans, who in turn had borrowed and adapted it from the Greek colonies of Italy. Senior officials of the Roman Republic derived their insignia from the Etruscans: curule chair, purple-bordered toga (*toga praetexta*) and bundle of rods (*fasces*). Gladiatorial combats and the military triumph were other customs adopted from the Etruscans. Rome lay 12 miles (19.3 km) inland

161 from the sea on the Tiber River, the border between Latium and Etruria. Because the site commanded a convenient river crossing and lay on a land route from the Apennines to the sea, it formed the meeting point of three distinct peoples: Latins, Etruscans, and

155 Sabines. Although Latin in speech and culture, the Roman population must have been somewhat diverse from earliest times, a circumstance that may help to account for the openness of Roman society in historical times.

155. **(C)** The Romans adopted the speech of the Latins.

156. **(A)** Roman religion was based on the beliefs of the Etruscans.

157. **(A)** Per the passage, Italy's early communities supported themselves through agriculture or animal husbandry—in other words, communities were generally agrarian (choice A) rather than trade-based (choice D). Urban (choice B) and nomadic (choice C) are incorrect because they refer to city living and moving from place to place, respectively.

158. **(C)** The correct combination is alphabet and Greek, choice C. The passage does not mention anything adapted from the Phoenecians, which eliminates choices A and D. The passage states that gladiatorial combat (choice B) was adapted from the Etruscans, but it does not state that this was originally taken from the Greeks.

159. **(D)** The first paragraph primarily focuses on the early inhabitants of Italy and their languages or dialects (choice D). Geography (choice A), migration (choice B), and economic matters (choice C) are mentioned, but are not elaborated upon to the same degree as the early inhabitants and their languages.

160. **(D)** Etruscan (choice D) is not an Indo-European language, and therefore not Italic. Latin (choice A), Oscan (choice B), and Umbrian (choice C) were all described in the passage as Italic dialects.

161. **(B)** The passage describes the site of Rome as a meeting point of three distinct peoples/cultures, which may have resulted in Rome being at least somewhat diverse from its early days. The passage does not indicate that Rome's location contributed to isolationism (in contrast, Rome is described as open), which eliminates choice A. The passage did not state that Rome was vulnerable to invasion (choice C), nor did it mention conflict between Latium and Etruria (choice D).

Passage 3

Gastroesophageal reflux disease (GERD) is a common medical disorder seen by health care practitioners of all specialties. It is generally chronic in nature, and long-term therapy may be required. While the mortality associated with GERD is very low (1 death per 100,000 patients), the quality of life experienced by the patient can be greatly diminished.

GERD refers to any symptomatic clinical condition or histologic alteration that results from episodes of gastroesophageal reflux. Gastroesophageal reflux refers to the retrograde movement of gastric contents from the stomach into the esophagus. Many people experience some degree of reflux, especially after eating, which may be considered a benign physiologic process. When the esophagus is repeatedly exposed to refluxed material for prolonged periods of time, inflammation of the esophagus (i.e., reflux esophagitis) can occur. It is important to realize that gastroesophageal reflux must precede the development of GERD or reflux esophagitis. In severe cases, reflux may lead to a multitude of serious complications including esophageal strictures, esophageal ulcers, motility disorders, perforation, hemorrhage, aspiration, and Barrett's esophagus. While mild disease is often managed with lifestyle changes and antacids, more intensive therapeutic intervention with histamine (H_2) antagonists, sucralfate, prokinetic agents, or proton pump inhibitors is generally required for patients with more severe disease. In general, response to pharmacologic intervention is dependent on the efficacy of the agent, dosage regimen employed, duration of therapy, and severity of the disease. Following discontinuation of therapy, relapse is common and long-term maintenance therapy may be required. Historically, surgical intervention has been reserved for patients in whom conventional treatment modalities fail. However, the recent development of laparoscopic antireflux surgical procedures has led to a reevaluation of the role of surgery in the long-term maintenance of GERD. Some clinicians have suggested that laparoscopic antireflux surgery may be a cost-effective alternative to long-term maintenance therapy in young patients. However, long-term comparative trials evaluating the cost effectiveness of the various treatment modalities are warranted.

The pathogenesis of gastroesophageal reflux is related to the complex balance between defense mechanisms and aggressive factors. Understanding both the normal protective mechanisms and the aggressive factors that may contribute to or promote gastroesophageal reflux helps one to design rational therapeutic treatment regimens. Gastric acid, pepsin, bile acids, and pancreatic enzymes are considered aggressive factors and may promote esophageal damage upon reflux into the esophagus. Thus, the composition (potency) and volume of the refluxate are aggressive factors that may lead to esophageal injury. Conversely, normal protective mechanisms include anatomic factors, lower esophageal sphincter pressure, esophageal clearing, mucosal resistance, and gastric emptying. Rational therapeutic regimens in the treatment of gastroesophageal reflux are designed to maximize normal defense mechanisms and/or attenuate the aggressive factors.

162. **(C)** According to the passage, the mortality rate of GERD is 1 death per 100,000 patients.

163. **(A)** One possible complication of reflux is perforation. Mucosal resistance (choice B), gastric emptying (choice C), and lower esophageal sphincter pressure (choice D) are all cited in the passage as normal protective mechanisms.

164. **(C)** The passage states that when the esophagus is repeatedly exposed to refluxed material for prolonged periods of time, inflammation of the esophagus (i.e., reflux esophagitis) can occur.

165. **(C)** The passage states that following the discontinuation of therapy, relapse is common and long-term maintenance therapy may be required.

166. **(B)** Efficacy of the agent plays a part in GERD patients' response to pharmacologic intervention.

167. **(A)** The passage states that long-term comparative trials evaluating the cost effectiveness of various treatment modalities for GERD are warranted.

168. **(C)** The passage states that laparoscopic antireflux surgery has been suggested as a possible cost-effective alternative therapy.

169. **(A)** Gastric acid and pancreatic enzymes are aggressive factors that may promote esophageal damage upon reflux into the esophagus. The factors in choice C are protective, and the factors in choice B are a combination of aggressive (bile acids) and protective (esophageal clearing). Choice D is unrelated to the passage.

Passage 4

Many people in the United States are diagnosed with diabetes mellitus. Type 2 diabetes is the most common type of diabetes and it is associated with a significant amount
170 of morbidities and mortalities. Type 2 diabetes is classified as an endocrine disorder characterized by defects in insulin secretion as well as in insulin action. In type 2 diabetes patients, a defect also exists in insulin receptor binding. These defects lead to increased serum glucose concentrations or hyperglycemia.
171   Sulfonylureas are one of the most popular classes of agents used to treat type 2 diabetes. One of the agents to treat type 2 diabetes is acarbose, an oral alpha-glucosidase inhibitor. Acarbose interferes with the hydrolysis of dietary disaccharides and complex carbohydrates, thereby delaying absorption of glucose and other monosaccharides.
172 Acarbose is available for oral administration only. To be most effective, it should be taken at the beginning of a meal. The recommended starting dose is 25 mg three
173 times daily and doses as high as 200 mg three times a day have been safely used. The most common adverse experiences associated with the use of acarbose are abdominal cramps, flatulence, diarrhea, and abdominal distension. Most of the adverse effects are due to the unabsorbed carbohydrates undergoing fermentation in the colon.
175 Acarbose has also been associated with decreased intestinal absorption of iron, thereby
176 possibly leading to anemia. The occurrence of hypoglycemia when using acarbose in
174 combination with other agents used to lower serum glucose is great. Glucose should be administered to treat hypoglycemia in patients taking acarbose because sucrose

may not be adequately hydrolyzed and absorbed. The effectiveness of this agent to lower serum glucose concentrations in patients with type 2 diabetes has been clearly demonstrated in clinical trials. Acarbose provides another option for treating type 2 diabetes.

170. **(D)** Whereas "endocrine in nature" (choice A), "hyperglycemia" (choice B), and "may be due to a defect in insulin receptor binding" (choice C) are stated in, or may be inferred from, the passage, "results in iron deficiencies" (choice D) is not listed as a characteristic of type 2 diabetes. Rather, it is mentioned as a possible adverse effect of acarbose.

171. **(A)** The passage states that a sulfonylurea agent is one of the most popular classes of agents used to treat type 2 diabetes. Glucose (choice B), sucrose (choice C), and fructose (choice D) all represent types of sugar.

172. **(A)** The passage states that to be most effective, acarbose should be taken at the beginning of a meal.

173. **(C)** Hyperglycemia (choice A) is a characteristic of type 2 diabetes. Anemia (choice B) is a possible adverse effect of acarbose, but not one of the most common side effects. Rash (choice D) is not mentioned in the passage. Gastrointestinal discomfort (choice C) is stated as the most common side effect of acarbose.

174. **(B)** The passage states that glucose is the best choice for patients taking acarbose. A sulfonylurea agent (choice A) is the most popular class of agents used to treat type 2 diabetes. Sucrose (choice C) is mentioned in the passage as a sugar that the patient may not be able to adequately hydrolyze and absorb, and fructose (choice D) is not mentioned at all.

175. **(D)** Whereas low serum glucose concentrations (choice A), gastrointestinal discomfort (choice B), and decreased iron absorption (choice C) are all described in the passage as possible adverse effects associated with the use of acarbose, obstruction of the urinary tract (choice D) is not mentioned.

176. **(A)** The passage states that sulfonylureas are one of the most popular classes of agents used to treat type 2 diabetes and that using acarbose in combination with other agents may lead to hypoglycemia. Glucose (choice B), iron (choice C), and increased caloric intake (choice D) are not described as having this effect.

177. **(C)** Since the passage does not cover the topic of diabetes in the United States, choice A cannot be the correct choice. Nor does the passage deal with all the various agents used to treat type 2 diabetes, so choice B is ruled out. Choice D is too specific; the passage does deal with some adverse effects of acarbose, but it covers much more than that. The best title for the passage is The Use of Acarbose in the Treatment of Type 2 Diabetes (choice C).

Passage 5

183 At the first session of the Confederation Congress, it was decided that nine states constituted a quorum, with two delegates necessary for a state to qualify as present. But on multiple occasions throughout the spring and summer of 1781, no official business could be done because five or more state delegations were either absent altogether or only partially represented. Part of the problem lay with the state legislatures, which

182 were slow to select their delegates; part of the problem was that the leading candidates

181 refused to serve, preferring to perform their public duties at the state level. John Witherspoon of New Jersey became the most frequent and vocal critic of this sorry

184 situation, waiting around with nothing to do because his erstwhile colleagues had failed to show up, but the attendance problem accurately reflected the political priorities of

181 the most prominent American leaders. In truth, it would be misleading to say that local and state concerns trumped the national interest, because in most minds no such thing as the national interest even existed.

A second source of systemic malfunction was the coordination of foreign policy. All business came before the full Congress, an unwieldy arrangement at best, rendered more maddeningly chaotic because the membership of state delegations kept changing. When Arthur Lee joined the Virginia delegation, for example, his inveterate suspicion of Benjamin Franklin's ties to the French Court—Lee, it soon became clear, was suspicious of everyone, especially non-Virginians—split the Virginia vote on almost every foreign policy issue, essentially negating the largest state's voice.

178. **(A)** As implied by the description provided for what constituted a quorum in the Confederation Congress, a quorum is the minimum number of individuals who must be present to make decisions (choice A). This number is set by the organization/institution/governing body involved. A quorum does not necessarily have to be a majority (choice B); indeed, as there were 13 colonies/delegations participating in the Confederation Congress, seven would have been a majority, yet the minimum number of delegations needed to constitute a quorum was set at nine. As the Congress' quorum criterion was set at less than 13, choice C is clearly incorrect. Choice D does not reflect the definition of a quorum.

179. **(B)** Although the passage mentions the issues created by Arthur Lee (choice A), it primarily describes two key barriers to conducting business in the Confederation Congress (choice B): lack of attendance, which prevented establishing a quorum, and systemic issues in addressing foreign policy. Choices C and D were not addressed in the passage.

180. **(A)** The year given for the Confederation Congress, 1781, was the year the Revolutionary War (choice A) ended. The Civil War (choice B) occurred in the 1860s. The Spanish-American War (choice C) occurred in 1898. The Great War, also known as World War I (choice D), took place in the early 1900s. Therefore, choice A is correct.

181. **(D)** Concerns at the state level took precedence in the minds of political leaders at the time of the Confederation Congress.

182. **(D)** The key obstacle faced by state legislatures when appointing delegates to the Confederation Congress was that leading candidates refused to serve.

183. **(C)** In the Confederation Congress, a quorum was established when delegations of nine states were present, with each state having at least two delegates.

184. **(B)** The passage states that John Witherspoon was frustrated that very little was getting done in the Congress due to the lack of attendance by his fellow delegates.

Passage 6

185
186 Although phenytoin may be used to treat cardiac arrhythmias, migraines, and trigeminal neuralgia, the primary use of phenytoin is to treat seizure disorders. Phenytoin, one of the most important agents used to manage seizures, works similarly to
187 other hydantoin-derivative anticonvulsants. It decreases seizure activity by stabilizing neuronal membranes and by increasing efflux or decreasing influx of sodium ions across cell membranes in the motor cortex during generation of nerve impulses. Phenytoin is commercially available as oral suspension, tablets, and capsules. It is also
188 available as an injection. The dosage of phenytoin varies according to the frequency of seizures, the type of seizures, and the patient's tolerance for phenytoin. Therefore, it is extremely important to monitor the patient for seizure activity as well as to monitor
189 phenytoin serum concentrations. Phenytoin has a narrow therapeutic window and monitoring of serum concentrations is necessary. Therapeutic serum concentrations of phenytoin are usually 10–20 mcg per mL (millimeter) and depend on the assay method
191 used. Serum concentrations above 20 mcg per mL often result in toxicity. Adverse reactions associated with dose-related toxicities include blurred vision, lethargy, rash, fever, slurred speech, nystagmus, and confusion. In some patients, seizure control is not achieved when plasma concentrations are within the therapeutic concentration range and therefore clinical response of the patient is more meaningful than plasma
192 concentrations. Generally, therapeutic steady state serum concentrations are achieved within 30 days of therapy with an oral dosage of 300 mg daily in adults. Following an intravenous administration of 1000–1500 mg, at a rate not exceeding 50 mg per minute,
190 therapeutic concentrations can be attained within 2 hours. Rapid administration of intravenous phenytoin may result in adverse effects such as decreased blood pressure and other cardiac complications. The use of phenytoin has been associated with osteomalacia, thrombocytopenia, and gastrointestinal upset.

185. **(A)** Trigeminal neuralgia is treated with phenytoin. Arthritis (choice B) is not mentioned in the passage. Osteomalacia (choice C) is mentioned as a possible adverse effect. Nystagmus (choice D) is mentioned as an adverse reaction associated with toxicity.

186. **(C)** The first sentence clearly states that phenytoin is most commonly used to treat seizure disorders. Cardiac arrhythmias (choice A) and migraines (choice B) are mentioned as other possible uses; arthritis (choice D) is not mentioned in the passage.

187. **(C)** Neither choice A nor choice B appears in the passage, and choice D states the opposite of the correct answer.

188. **(D)** Whereas phenytoin serum concentration (choice A), number of seizures experienced (choice B), and adverse events experienced (choice C) are listed as factors that affect the dosage of phenytoin, puncture sites available are not mentioned in the passage.

189. **(D)** Choice A incorrectly implies that phenytoin produces seizures. Choice B incorrectly states that there is no known difference between the serum concentrations known to produce desirable and undesirable effects. Choice C refers to migraines rather than to seizures.

190. **(B)** A higher rate of administration may lower blood pressure. Choice A is irrelevant. Choice C is inaccurate. Choice D refers to a condition (rash) that may be associated with phenytoin toxicity but not with the rapid administration of intravenous phenytoin.

191. **(C)** Blurred vision (choice A), lethargy (choice B), and mental confusion (choice D) are mentioned in the passage as adverse reactions associated with drug-related toxicities. There is no reference to dysuria (choice C).

192. **(D)** The passage states that the therapeutic steady state serum concentration may be achieved within 30 days with an oral dosage of 300 mg daily of phenytoin, which is approximately a one-month time period (choice D). Therefore, 5 months (choice A), 24 hours (choice B), and 30 hours (choice C) are all inaccurate.

10

Practice Test 2

This second sample PCAT is not a copy of an actual PCAT, but it has also been designed to closely represent the types of questions that may be included in an actual exam. Proceed with this practice exam as if you were taking the actual PCAT, adhering to the time allowed for each section in the table below.

Section	Time Allowed*
1. Chemical Processes	40 minutes
2. Biological Processes	40 minutes
3. Critical Reading	50 minutes
4. Quantitative Reasoning	45 minutes
5. Writing (Essay)	30 minutes

*Please note: The order of the subjects (test sections) may vary from test to test.

ANSWER SHEET
Practice Test 2

CHEMICAL PROCESSES (1–48)

1. Ⓐ Ⓑ Ⓒ Ⓓ
2. Ⓐ Ⓑ Ⓒ Ⓓ
3. Ⓐ Ⓑ Ⓒ Ⓓ
4. Ⓐ Ⓑ Ⓒ Ⓓ
5. Ⓐ Ⓑ Ⓒ Ⓓ
6. Ⓐ Ⓑ Ⓒ Ⓓ
7. Ⓐ Ⓑ Ⓒ Ⓓ
8. Ⓐ Ⓑ Ⓒ Ⓓ
9. Ⓐ Ⓑ Ⓒ Ⓓ
10. Ⓐ Ⓑ Ⓒ Ⓓ
11. Ⓐ Ⓑ Ⓒ Ⓓ
12. Ⓐ Ⓑ Ⓒ Ⓓ

13. Ⓐ Ⓑ Ⓒ Ⓓ
14. Ⓐ Ⓑ Ⓒ Ⓓ
15. Ⓐ Ⓑ Ⓒ Ⓓ
16. Ⓐ Ⓑ Ⓒ Ⓓ
17. Ⓐ Ⓑ Ⓒ Ⓓ
18. Ⓐ Ⓑ Ⓒ Ⓓ
19. Ⓐ Ⓑ Ⓒ Ⓓ
20. Ⓐ Ⓑ Ⓒ Ⓓ
21. Ⓐ Ⓑ Ⓒ Ⓓ
22. Ⓐ Ⓑ Ⓒ Ⓓ
23. Ⓐ Ⓑ Ⓒ Ⓓ
24. Ⓐ Ⓑ Ⓒ Ⓓ

25. Ⓐ Ⓑ Ⓒ Ⓓ
26. Ⓐ Ⓑ Ⓒ Ⓓ
27. Ⓐ Ⓑ Ⓒ Ⓓ
28. Ⓐ Ⓑ Ⓒ Ⓓ
29. Ⓐ Ⓑ Ⓒ Ⓓ
30. Ⓐ Ⓑ Ⓒ Ⓓ
31. Ⓐ Ⓑ Ⓒ Ⓓ
32. Ⓐ Ⓑ Ⓒ Ⓓ
33. Ⓐ Ⓑ Ⓒ Ⓓ
34. Ⓐ Ⓑ Ⓒ Ⓓ
35. Ⓐ Ⓑ Ⓒ Ⓓ
36. Ⓐ Ⓑ Ⓒ Ⓓ

37. Ⓐ Ⓑ Ⓒ Ⓓ
38. Ⓐ Ⓑ Ⓒ Ⓓ
39. Ⓐ Ⓑ Ⓒ Ⓓ
40. Ⓐ Ⓑ Ⓒ Ⓓ
41. Ⓐ Ⓑ Ⓒ Ⓓ
42. Ⓐ Ⓑ Ⓒ Ⓓ
43. Ⓐ Ⓑ Ⓒ Ⓓ
44. Ⓐ Ⓑ Ⓒ Ⓓ
45. Ⓐ Ⓑ Ⓒ Ⓓ
46. Ⓐ Ⓑ Ⓒ Ⓓ
47. Ⓐ Ⓑ Ⓒ Ⓓ
48. Ⓐ Ⓑ Ⓒ Ⓓ

BIOLOGICAL PROCESSES (49–96)

49. Ⓐ Ⓑ Ⓒ Ⓓ
50. Ⓐ Ⓑ Ⓒ Ⓓ
51. Ⓐ Ⓑ Ⓒ Ⓓ
52. Ⓐ Ⓑ Ⓒ Ⓓ
53. Ⓐ Ⓑ Ⓒ Ⓓ
54. Ⓐ Ⓑ Ⓒ Ⓓ
55. Ⓐ Ⓑ Ⓒ Ⓓ
56. Ⓐ Ⓑ Ⓒ Ⓓ
57. Ⓐ Ⓑ Ⓒ Ⓓ
58. Ⓐ Ⓑ Ⓒ Ⓓ
59. Ⓐ Ⓑ Ⓒ Ⓓ
60. Ⓐ Ⓑ Ⓒ Ⓓ

61. Ⓐ Ⓑ Ⓒ Ⓓ
62. Ⓐ Ⓑ Ⓒ Ⓓ
63. Ⓐ Ⓑ Ⓒ Ⓓ
64. Ⓐ Ⓑ Ⓒ Ⓓ
65. Ⓐ Ⓑ Ⓒ Ⓓ
66. Ⓐ Ⓑ Ⓒ Ⓓ
67. Ⓐ Ⓑ Ⓒ Ⓓ
68. Ⓐ Ⓑ Ⓒ Ⓓ
69. Ⓐ Ⓑ Ⓒ Ⓓ
70. Ⓐ Ⓑ Ⓒ Ⓓ
71. Ⓐ Ⓑ Ⓒ Ⓓ
72. Ⓐ Ⓑ Ⓒ Ⓓ

73. Ⓐ Ⓑ Ⓒ Ⓓ
74. Ⓐ Ⓑ Ⓒ Ⓓ
75. Ⓐ Ⓑ Ⓒ Ⓓ
76. Ⓐ Ⓑ Ⓒ Ⓓ
77. Ⓐ Ⓑ Ⓒ Ⓓ
78. Ⓐ Ⓑ Ⓒ Ⓓ
79. Ⓐ Ⓑ Ⓒ Ⓓ
80. Ⓐ Ⓑ Ⓒ Ⓓ
81. Ⓐ Ⓑ Ⓒ Ⓓ
82. Ⓐ Ⓑ Ⓒ Ⓓ
83. Ⓐ Ⓑ Ⓒ Ⓓ
84. Ⓐ Ⓑ Ⓒ Ⓓ

85. Ⓐ Ⓑ Ⓒ Ⓓ
86. Ⓐ Ⓑ Ⓒ Ⓓ
87. Ⓐ Ⓑ Ⓒ Ⓓ
88. Ⓐ Ⓑ Ⓒ Ⓓ
89. Ⓐ Ⓑ Ⓒ Ⓓ
90. Ⓐ Ⓑ Ⓒ Ⓓ
91. Ⓐ Ⓑ Ⓒ Ⓓ
92. Ⓐ Ⓑ Ⓒ Ⓓ
93. Ⓐ Ⓑ Ⓒ Ⓓ
94. Ⓐ Ⓑ Ⓒ Ⓓ
95. Ⓐ Ⓑ Ⓒ Ⓓ
96. Ⓐ Ⓑ Ⓒ Ⓓ

ANSWER SHEET
Practice Test 2

CRITICAL READING (97–144)

97. Ⓐ Ⓑ Ⓒ Ⓓ   109. Ⓐ Ⓑ Ⓒ Ⓓ   121. Ⓐ Ⓑ Ⓒ Ⓓ   133. Ⓐ Ⓑ Ⓒ Ⓓ
98. Ⓐ Ⓑ Ⓒ Ⓓ   110. Ⓐ Ⓑ Ⓒ Ⓓ   122. Ⓐ Ⓑ Ⓒ Ⓓ   134. Ⓐ Ⓑ Ⓒ Ⓓ
99. Ⓐ Ⓑ Ⓒ Ⓓ   111. Ⓐ Ⓑ Ⓒ Ⓓ   123. Ⓐ Ⓑ Ⓒ Ⓓ   135. Ⓐ Ⓑ Ⓒ Ⓓ
100. Ⓐ Ⓑ Ⓒ Ⓓ   112. Ⓐ Ⓑ Ⓒ Ⓓ   124. Ⓐ Ⓑ Ⓒ Ⓓ   136. Ⓐ Ⓑ Ⓒ Ⓓ
101. Ⓐ Ⓑ Ⓒ Ⓓ   113. Ⓐ Ⓑ Ⓒ Ⓓ   125. Ⓐ Ⓑ Ⓒ Ⓓ   137. Ⓐ Ⓑ Ⓒ Ⓓ
102. Ⓐ Ⓑ Ⓒ Ⓓ   114. Ⓐ Ⓑ Ⓒ Ⓓ   126. Ⓐ Ⓑ Ⓒ Ⓓ   138. Ⓐ Ⓑ Ⓒ Ⓓ
103. Ⓐ Ⓑ Ⓒ Ⓓ   115. Ⓐ Ⓑ Ⓒ Ⓓ   127. Ⓐ Ⓑ Ⓒ Ⓓ   139. Ⓐ Ⓑ Ⓒ Ⓓ
104. Ⓐ Ⓑ Ⓒ Ⓓ   116. Ⓐ Ⓑ Ⓒ Ⓓ   128. Ⓐ Ⓑ Ⓒ Ⓓ   140. Ⓐ Ⓑ Ⓒ Ⓓ
105. Ⓐ Ⓑ Ⓒ Ⓓ   117. Ⓐ Ⓑ Ⓒ Ⓓ   129. Ⓐ Ⓑ Ⓒ Ⓓ   141. Ⓐ Ⓑ Ⓒ Ⓓ
106. Ⓐ Ⓑ Ⓒ Ⓓ   118. Ⓐ Ⓑ Ⓒ Ⓓ   130. Ⓐ Ⓑ Ⓒ Ⓓ   142. Ⓐ Ⓑ Ⓒ Ⓓ
107. Ⓐ Ⓑ Ⓒ Ⓓ   119. Ⓐ Ⓑ Ⓒ Ⓓ   131. Ⓐ Ⓑ Ⓒ Ⓓ   143. Ⓐ Ⓑ Ⓒ Ⓓ
108. Ⓐ Ⓑ Ⓒ Ⓓ   120. Ⓐ Ⓑ Ⓒ Ⓓ   132. Ⓐ Ⓑ Ⓒ Ⓓ   144. Ⓐ Ⓑ Ⓒ Ⓓ

QUANTITATIVE REASONING (145–192)

145. Ⓐ Ⓑ Ⓒ Ⓓ   157. Ⓐ Ⓑ Ⓒ Ⓓ   169. Ⓐ Ⓑ Ⓒ Ⓓ   181. Ⓐ Ⓑ Ⓒ Ⓓ
146. Ⓐ Ⓑ Ⓒ Ⓓ   158. Ⓐ Ⓑ Ⓒ Ⓓ   170. Ⓐ Ⓑ Ⓒ Ⓓ   182. Ⓐ Ⓑ Ⓒ Ⓓ
147. Ⓐ Ⓑ Ⓒ Ⓓ   159. Ⓐ Ⓑ Ⓒ Ⓓ   171. Ⓐ Ⓑ Ⓒ Ⓓ   183. Ⓐ Ⓑ Ⓒ Ⓓ
148. Ⓐ Ⓑ Ⓒ Ⓓ   160. Ⓐ Ⓑ Ⓒ Ⓓ   172. Ⓐ Ⓑ Ⓒ Ⓓ   184. Ⓐ Ⓑ Ⓒ Ⓓ
149. Ⓐ Ⓑ Ⓒ Ⓓ   161. Ⓐ Ⓑ Ⓒ Ⓓ   173. Ⓐ Ⓑ Ⓒ Ⓓ   185. Ⓐ Ⓑ Ⓒ Ⓓ
150. Ⓐ Ⓑ Ⓒ Ⓓ   162. Ⓐ Ⓑ Ⓒ Ⓓ   174. Ⓐ Ⓑ Ⓒ Ⓓ   186. Ⓐ Ⓑ Ⓒ Ⓓ
151. Ⓐ Ⓑ Ⓒ Ⓓ   163. Ⓐ Ⓑ Ⓒ Ⓓ   175. Ⓐ Ⓑ Ⓒ Ⓓ   187. Ⓐ Ⓑ Ⓒ Ⓓ
152. Ⓐ Ⓑ Ⓒ Ⓓ   164. Ⓐ Ⓑ Ⓒ Ⓓ   176. Ⓐ Ⓑ Ⓒ Ⓓ   188. Ⓐ Ⓑ Ⓒ Ⓓ
153. Ⓐ Ⓑ Ⓒ Ⓓ   165. Ⓐ Ⓑ Ⓒ Ⓓ   177. Ⓐ Ⓑ Ⓒ Ⓓ   189. Ⓐ Ⓑ Ⓒ Ⓓ
154. Ⓐ Ⓑ Ⓒ Ⓓ   166. Ⓐ Ⓑ Ⓒ Ⓓ   178. Ⓐ Ⓑ Ⓒ Ⓓ   190. Ⓐ Ⓑ Ⓒ Ⓓ
155. Ⓐ Ⓑ Ⓒ Ⓓ   167. Ⓐ Ⓑ Ⓒ Ⓓ   179. Ⓐ Ⓑ Ⓒ Ⓓ   191. Ⓐ Ⓑ Ⓒ Ⓓ
156. Ⓐ Ⓑ Ⓒ Ⓓ   168. Ⓐ Ⓑ Ⓒ Ⓓ   180. Ⓐ Ⓑ Ⓒ Ⓓ   192. Ⓐ Ⓑ Ⓒ Ⓓ

WRITING

For the essay portion of the test, you may compose your response on page 319 or on a separate sheet of paper.

CHEMICAL PROCESSES

48 QUESTIONS (#1–#48)
TIME: 40 MINUTES

The periodic table is provided below, if needed.

H																	He
Li	Be											B	C	N	O	F	Ne
Na	Mg											Al	Si	P	S	Cl	Ar
K	Ca	Sc	Ti	V	Cr	Mn	Fe	Co	Ni	Cu	Zn	Ga	Ge	As	Se	Br	Kr
Rb	Sr	Y	Zr	Nb	Mo	Tc	Ru	Rh	Pd	Ag	Cd	In	Sn	Sb	Te	I	Xe
Cs	Ba	La	Hf	Ta	W	Re	Os	Ir	Pt	Au	Hg	Tl	Pb	Bi	Po	At	Rn
Fr	Ra	Ac	Rf	Ha	Sg	Ns	Hs	Mt									
			Ce	Pr	Nd	Pm	Sm	Eu	Gd	Tb	Dy	Ho	Er	Tm	Yb	Lu	
			Th	Pa	U	Np	Pu	Am	Cm	Bk	Cf	Es	Fm	Md	No	Lr	

Directions: Choose the best answer to each of the following questions.

QUESTIONS 1 THROUGH 4 REFER TO THE FOLLOWING PASSAGE:

Many drugs contain chiral centers. When a chiral center is synthesized in the laboratory, both forms of it (R and S) are produced. Usually one form is biologically active while the other is not since cellular molecules can discriminate between the two forms. An example of this discrimination occurs when you smell rye bread and spearmint. The molecule responsible for the characteristic aromas of the two foods is carvone—one enantiomer of carvone is in rye bread and the other enantiomer is in spearmint. Your nose does not confuse those two aromas because the receptors can easily differentiate the two stereoisomers. The same is true with drug molecules. Zyrtec (cetirizine) is an antihistamine that contains both enantiomers while only one of them is biologically active. Xyzal (levocetirizine) contains only the biologically active enantiomer of cetirizine (see the structure of levocetirizine to the right). Zyrtec is sold over the counter while Xyzal is only available by prescription.

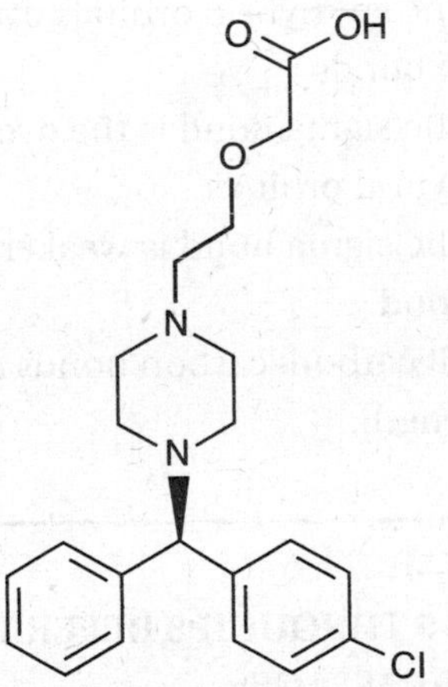

1. What is the absolute configuration of the chiral center in the structure of levocetirizine given above?

(A) R
(B) S
(C) E
(D) Z

2. Levocetirizine has an arene ring with a para chlorine. Which of the following would be used to chlorinate an arene ring?

   (A) Cl_2 and ultraviolet light
   (B) HCl
   (C) Cl_2 and $FeCl_3$
   (D) $FeCl_3$

3. Levocetirizine contains a carboxylic acid functional group. Often such groups are converted to esters to improve the side effect profile of a drug by decreasing the possibility of gastrointestinal discomfort with oral administration. Which of the following methods could be used to convert a carboxylic acid to an ester?

   (A) Add an alkene to the carboxylic acid.
   (B) Add an alcohol to the carboxylic acid.
   (C) Add an amine to the carboxylic acid.
   (D) Condense two carboxylic acids.

4. Which statement describes the carbon–carbon bonds in an arene ring?

   (A) The sp^2 hybrid orbitals overlap to form pi bonds.
   (B) The sigma bond is the overlap of sp^3 hybrid orbitals.
   (C) The sigma bond is weaker than the pi bond.
   (D) All carbon–carbon bonds are the same length.

QUESTIONS 5 THROUGH 8 REFER TO THE FOLLOWING PASSAGE:

Human immunodeficiency virus (HIV) infection is managed by several classes of drugs. One of those classes is the nucleoside reverse transcriptase inhibitors (NRTIs). These agents are nucleosides. After conversion to the corresponding triphosphate nucleotides, they inhibit reverse transcriptase, the enzyme needed by HIV to transcribe its RNA genome into DNA. The NRTIs are useful in this situation because they disrupt the production of proviral DNA. Because they are structurally similar to the nucleotides used in the synthesis of cellular nucleic acids, they may also affect DNA/RNA synthesis in uninfected cells, causing undesired side effects. Fortunately, the affinity for NRTIs of the normal cellular enzymes involved in DNA/RNA synthesis is much lower than the affinity of the viral reverse transcriptase for them. Even so, patients receiving NRTIs often experience side effects related to their impact on the synthesis of normal cellular DNA.

5. Which statement describes nucleotides?

   (A) They are polymerized to form proteins.
   (B) They contain purines and/or pyrimidines.
   (C) They contain glucose.
   (D) Their polymerization is called translation.

6. The synthesis of RNA from DNA involves

   (A) the polymerization of ribonucleotide triphosphates.
   (B) the enzyme, DNA polymerase.
   (C) ribosomes.
   (D) amino acids.

7. Which of the following statements is true regarding cellular nucleic acids?

    (A) They are found in the cytoplasm.
    (B) They contain phosphate groups.
    (C) They are synthesized from cellular protein.
    (D) They are excreted via the urea cycle.

8. The process by which protein is synthesized in the cell involves all of the following EXCEPT

    (A) mRNA.
    (B) ribosomes.
    (C) tRNA.
    (D) DNA polymerase.

QUESTIONS 9 THROUGH 12 REFER TO THE FOLLOWING PASSAGE:

Colligative properties of solutions are those that are dependent on solute concentration but not solute identity. They include freezing point depression and boiling point elevation. As a liquid changes phase from a liquid to a solid (freezes), the molecules begin to organize into a crystalline structure. The presence of a solute impedes the organization, lowering the freezing point. When a liquid changes phase from a liquid to a gas (boils), the molecules at the surface have the fewest forces "holding" them in the liquid, so they are the ones most likely to move into the gas phase. The presence of a solute means that some solute particles are at the surface, reducing the number of solvent molecules "eligible" to evaporate. Thus, the boiling point is elevated.

Antifreeze is a solution of ethylene glycol ($HOCH_2CH_2OH$) in water. The alcohol functional groups in ethylene glycol allow it to hydrogen bond with water molecules and form a homogeneous solution. The aqueous solution of ethylene glycol is used in automobile radiators to keep the water from freezing in cold weather. As is the case with other household substances, ethylene glycol is toxic to animals and should not be left out where children or animals might ingest it.

9. In addition to freezing point depression and boiling point elevation, which of the following is also a colligative property?

    (A) Viscosity
    (B) Osmotic pressure
    (C) Specific gravity
    (D) Density

10. Ethylene glycol can be synthesized by the following equation:

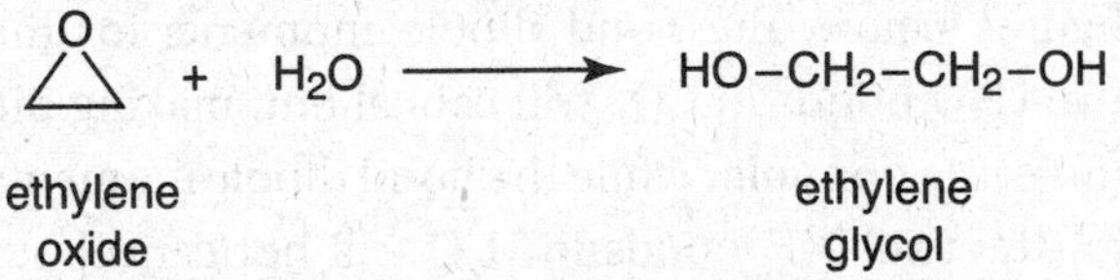

$$\text{ethylene oxide} + H_2O \longrightarrow HO-CH_2-CH_2-OH \quad (\text{ethylene glycol})$$

    What is the approximate percentage yield of ethylene glycol if the reaction of 1.0 g of ethylene oxide with 1.0 g of water yields 0.85 g of product?
    (C = 12 amu, H = 1 amu, O = 16 amu)

    (A) 85%
    (B) 61%
    (C) 40%
    (D) 25%

11. Which of the following bonds is the most polar?

    (A) C–H
    (B) C–C
    (C) C–O
    (D) O–H

12. What is the approximate molality of a solution that is 12 M ethylene glycol and has a density of 1.2 g/mL?

    (A) 10 m
    (B) 15 m
    (C) 26 m
    (D) 32 m

Molecular geometry has an impact on molecular polarity. For example, since CO_2 is a linear molecule, the polarity of each of the carbon–oxygen double bonds is "balanced," making the molecule overall nonpolar. Water, on the other hand, is not linear and is polar. Its molecular geometry is described as bent with a predicted bond angle near 109°, the tetrahedral bond angle. As noted in the figures below, the bond dipole moments for the two C=O bonds in CO_2 will cancel out, making the molecule nonpolar while the bond dipole moments for the two O-H bonds in H_2O will not cancel out because they are not "tail-to-tail." Thus, the geometry of the molecule must be determined before its molecular polarity can be predicted.

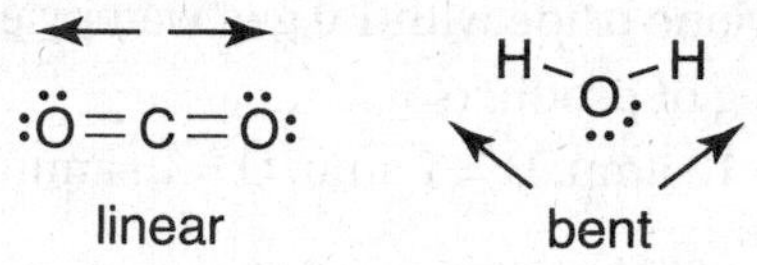

:Ö=C=Ö: H–O–H
linear   bent

Determining the molecular geometry begins with drawing the correct Lewis structure. When the Lewis structure of water is drawn, there are two unshared pairs of electrons and two shared pairs (bonds); i.e., there are 4 sets of electrons around the oxygen atom. According to the Valence Shell Electron Pair Repulsion (VSEPR) Theory, those 4 sets will spread out as far apart as possible, giving a tetrahedral geometry for the sets. The four sets of electrons are tetrahedral, but when the molecular geometry is identified, only the positions of the atoms are considered, giving a bent molecular geometry.

13. What is the molecular geometry of phosphorus trichloride, PCl_3?

(A) Triangular planar
(B) Tetrahedral
(C) Trigonal bipyramidal
(D) Trigonal pyramidal

14. How many protons are indicated in the following symbol?

$$^{37}Cl^-$$

(A) 37
(B) 36
(C) 17
(D) 20

15. What is the oxidation number of phosphorus, P, in PO_4^{-3}?

(A) –8
(B) –3
(C) +8
(D) +5

16. What is the electron configuration of the chlorine atom, Cl?

(A) $1s^2 2s^2 2p^6 3s^2$
(B) $1s^2 2s^2 2p^6$
(C) $1s^2 2s^2 2p^6 3s^2 3p^5$
(D) $1s^2 2s^2$

Car batteries are also called lead storage batteries. They contain an electrolyte solution of sulfuric acid (H_2SO_4) dissolved in water commonly called "battery acid." A solution of sulfuric acid in water is denser than pure water. As the battery discharges, the concentration of the sulfuric acid decreases, meaning the solution's specific gravity also decreases. This is the basis for using a hydrometer to measure the concentration of sulfuric acid in a battery to determine if it is time to buy a new one.

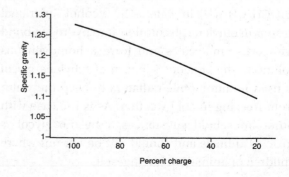

A hydrometer is a device that measures the specific gravity of a liquid. Recall that specific gravity is the ratio of the density of the liquid to the density of water at that temperature. Because it is a ratio of two densities, specific gravity is a unitless number and is easier to tabulate since units are omitted. Since the density of water is roughly 1 gm/mL, the specific gravity is approximately equal to the density of the liquid.

17. Which of the following equations represents the neutralization of sulfuric acid?

    (A) $Mg + H_2SO_4 \rightarrow MgSO_4 + H_2$
    (B) $H_2SO_4 \rightarrow 2H^+ + SO_4^{2-}$
    (C) $H_2SO_4 + 2KOH \rightarrow K_2SO_4 + 2H_2O$
    (D) $H_2SO_4 \rightarrow H_2O + SO_3$

18. How many grams of H_2SO_4 are required to produce 800 mL of 2.0 M H_2SO_4?
    (H = 1 amu, S = 32 amu, O = 16 amu)

    (A) 55 g
    (B) 80 g
    (C) 157 g
    (D) 200 g

19. How would 100 mL of a 1.5 M Na_2SO_4 solution be prepared?
    (Na = 23 amu, O = 16 amu, S = 32 amu)

    (A) Dissolve 21.3 g of Na_2SO_4 in 100 mL of water.
    (B) Dissolve 15.0 g of Na_2SO_4 in 100 mL of water.
    (C) Dissolve 21.3 g of Na_2SO_4 in enough water to make a final volume of 100 mL.
    (D) Dissolve 15.0 g of Na_2SO_4 in enough water to make a final volume of 100 mL.

20. What is the pH of battery acid if the hydrogen ion concentration equals 1×10^{-3} M?

    (A) 2
    (B) 3
    (C) 4
    (D) 5

QUESTIONS 21 THROUGH 24 REFER TO THE FOLLOWING PASSAGE:

For most substances, increasing the temperature of a solid causes it to melt, forming a liquid. Continued heating then vaporizes the liquid to a gas. Some substances, however, can undergo a phase change from a solid directly to a gas. This is called sublimation.

Probably the most common substance that sublimes is carbon dioxide. In the solid form, it is called dry ice because it is very cold (well below 0°C) but does not contain water. Grocery stores now sell dry ice, and consumers can purchase it for shipping perishable items or simply stocking the cooler without having to worry about the mess of melted ice. When dry ice sublimes, gaseous carbon dioxide is produced, meaning no soggy cooler items.

21. How many moles of carbon are present in 1.2×10^{10} atoms of carbon?
    (Avogadro's number is 6×10^{23}.)

    (A) 3×10^{-13}
    (B) 2×10^{-14}
    (C) 7×10^{-10}
    (D) 1×10^{13}

22. How many moles of carbon dioxide, CO_2, are present in 22 grams CO_2?
    (O = 16 amu, C = 12 amu)

    (A) 0.80
    (B) 0.50
    (C) 2.00
    (D) 1.30

23. If the initial pressure of CO_2 is 1.0 atm and the initial temperature is 27°C, what is the final temperature in degrees Celsius if the final pressure is 5.0 atm (assuming constant volume)?

    (A) 135°C
    (B) 1227°C
    (C) 1500°C
    (D) 2000°C

24. Which of the following statements about the behavior of gases is NOT true?

(A) Gases generally behave the same way regardless of their identity.
(B) If the volume of a gas is increased, the pressure will decrease if the temperature remains constant.
(C) If the temperature of a gas is decreased, the molecular motion of the gas particles will increase.
(D) The average kinetic energy of gas particles is directly proportional to the Kelvin temperature.

---

25. The class of biomolecules that is primarily characterized by its hydrophobicity is

(A) proteins.
(B) nucleic acids.
(C) carbohydrates.
(D) lipids.

26. Protein function is destroyed by denaturation that

(A) causes the cleavage of peptide bonds.
(B) results in the loss of secondary structure.
(C) does not affect hydrogen bonding.
(D) digests the protein.

27. To which biomolecular class does the following molecule belong?

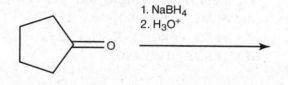

(A) Nucleic acids
(B) Proteins
(C) Lipids
(D) Carbohydrates

28. Which reagent would accomplish the following conversion?

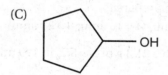

(A) H_2SO_4
(B) $K^+ {}^-OC(CH_3)_3$
(C) NH_3
(D) $LiAlH_4$

29. What is the product of the following reaction?

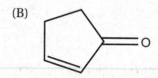

1. $NaBH_4$
2. H_3O^+

(A)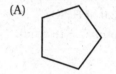

(B)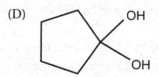

(C)

(D)

30. Which statement describes the compound, copper (II) sulfide?

(A) It is a covalent compound.
(B) The oxidation number of copper is +1.
(C) The formula is Cu_2S.
(D) It is expected to be insoluble in water.

31. Which structure for a substance with the formula $C_5H_{10}O_2$ is consistent with the following ^1H NMR data?

   δ 1.2 ppm, doublet, 6H
   δ 2.0 ppm, singlet, 3H
   δ 5.0 ppm, septet, 1H

   (A)

   (B)

   (C)

   (D)

32. Which is a resonance structure of the following ion?

   (A)

   (B)

   (C)

   (D)

33. Which of the following compounds displays hydrogen bonding?

   (A) H_2
   (B) H_2S
   (C) NH_3
   (D) CH_4

34. Lipids are involved in all of the following biological processes or structures EXCEPT

   (A) cell membrane construction.
   (B) hormones.
   (C) protein synthesis.
   (D) storage of carbon chains.

35. In an aqueous environment, proteins assume an overall conformation driven by

   (A) their nucleotide sequence.
   (B) the positioning of hydrophilic side chains toward the interior of the conformation.
   (C) a variety of forces including hydrogen bonding.
   (D) the formation of a double helix.

36. Which is expected to have the lowest boiling point?

   (A)

   (B)

   (C)

   (D)

37. The water solubility of a molecule containing a carboxylic acid functional group can be altered by converting it to an ester. Esters can be synthesized from carboxylic acids by the Fischer ester synthesis or the alcoholysis of a carboxylic acid derivative. Which of the following carboxylic acid derivatives cannot be directly converted to an ester by the addition of an alcohol?

(A) A carboxylic acid chloride
(B) A carboxylic acid anhydride
(C) An amide
(D) A nitrile

38. Which reagent(s) will accomplish the following conversion?

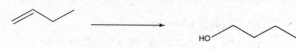

(A) 1. $Hg(OAc)_2$, H_2O
    2. $NaBH_4$
(B) 1. BH_3
    2. H_2O_2, OH^-
(C) MCPBA
(D) 1. OsO_4
    2. $NaHSO_3$

39. What is the hybridization state of the carbon, C, atom in $H_2C = CH_2$?

(A) sp
(B) sp^2
(C) sp^3
(D) sp^3d^2

40. Ascorbic acid has two pKas: 4.10 and 11.80

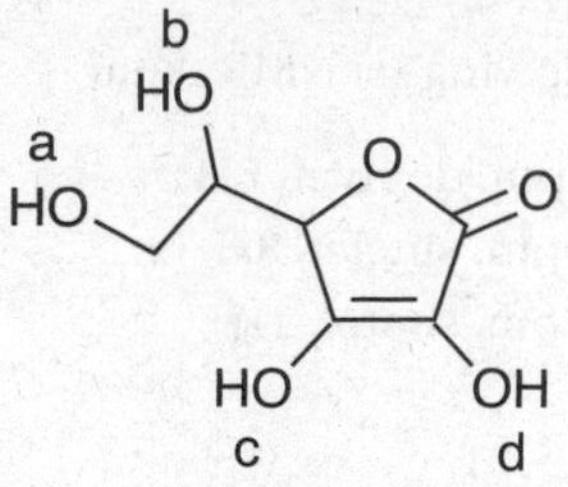

ascorbic acid

The most acidic hydrogen is the one whose removal yields the most stable conjugate base. Which proton corresponds to the more acidic pKa?

(A) a
(B) b
(C) c
(D) d

41. Which of the following solutions is a buffer solution?

(A) Hydrochloric acid and sodium chloride, $HCl + NaCl$
(B) Acetic acid and sodium acetate, $CH_3COOH + CH_3COONa$
(C) Nitric acid and sodium nitrate, $HNO_3 + NaNO_3$
(D) Sulfuric acid and sodium sulfate, $H_2SO_4 + Na_2SO_4$

42. According to the Kinetic Molecular Theory of Matter, in which of the following states of matter do atoms or molecules have the greatest freedom of motion?

(A) Solid
(B) Gas
(C) Liquid
(D) All states have the same freedom of motion.

43. Which compound could be used to react with ethyl magnesium bromide followed by protonation to form 3-pentanol?

(A)

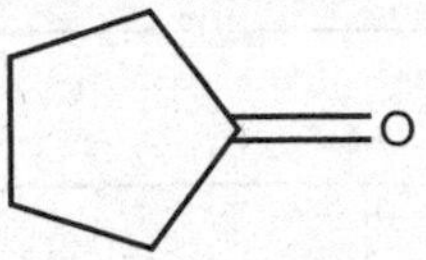

(B)

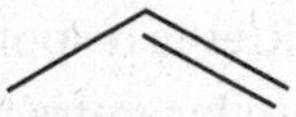

(C)

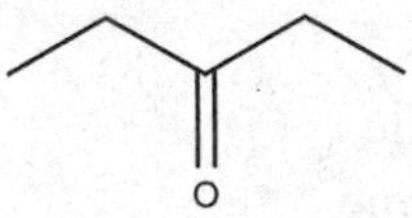

(D)

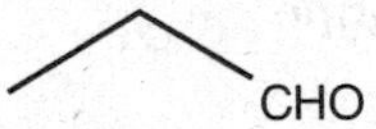

CHO

44. Which of the following is methyl 2-methylbutanoate?

(A)

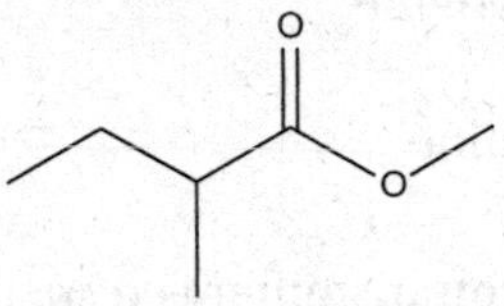

(B)

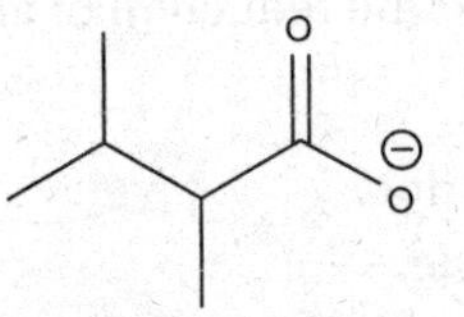

(C)

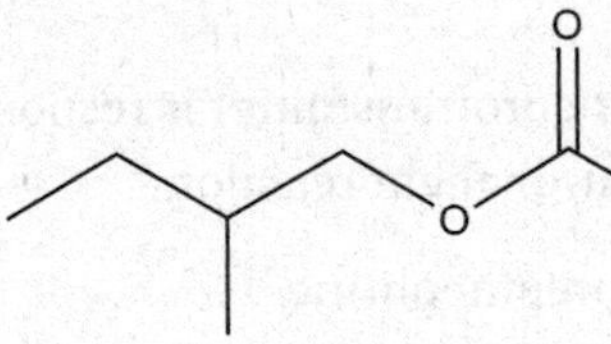

(D)

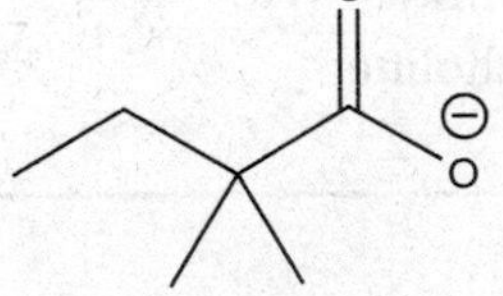

45. In the thermodynamic equation

$$\Delta G = \Delta H - T \Delta S$$

ΔG represents the change in free energy in a reaction, ΔH the change in enthalpy, and ΔS the change in entropy. The reaction is spontaneous when ΔG is

(A) +
(B) –
(C) 0
(D) The sign of ΔG has no significance.

46. Which of the following reactions shows an increase in entropy?

(A) $2KClO_3 \, (s) \rightarrow 2KCl \, (s) + 3O_2 \, (g)$
(B) $H_2O \, (g) \rightarrow H_2O \, (l)$
(C) $2H_2 \, (g) + O_2 \, (g) \rightarrow 2H_2O \, (l)$
(D) $PCl_3 \, (l) + Cl_2 \, (g) \rightarrow PCl_5 \, (s)$

47. A change in which of the following factors causes a change in the equilibrium constant of the reversible reaction shown?

$$A + B \leftrightarrow C + D \qquad K = \frac{[C][D]}{[A][B]}$$

(A) Temperature
(B) Volume
(C) Concentration
(D) Catalyst

48. Which of the following is a nuclear reaction?

(A) Beta decay
(B) Delta decay
(C) Neutralization
(D) Nuclear resonance

STOP

End of Chemical Processes section. If you have any time left, you may go over your work in this section only.

BIOLOGICAL PROCESSES

48 QUESTIONS (#49–#96)
TIME: 40 MINUTES

> **Directions:** Choose the **best** answer to each of the following questions.

49. The chromosome number is reduced from diploid to haploid by

    (A) meiosis.
    (B) mitosis.
    (C) hapnosis.
    (D) triosis.

50. In animal x, black hair (B) is dominant over white hair (b). If a homozygous black hair is crossed with a white hair, the hair color of white is expected in what percent of the offspring?

    (A) 0%
    (B) 25%
    (C) 75%
    (D) 100%

QUESTIONS 51 THROUGH 54 REFER TO THE FOLLOWING PASSAGE:

The human brain is composed of two major cell types: glial cells and neurons. Neurons are cells that receive chemical signals, form an electrical impulse, and pass a chemical signal to the next cell. The chemical signals used are called neurotransmitters. Different neurotransmitters are associated with different neuronal outcomes.

Glial cells support the neurons by providing myelin as well as maintaining a continuous supply of blood which includes glucose and oxygen. The myelin sheath surrounds the axon of the neuron and helps increase the speed of the neuronal action potential. Multiple sclerosis is linked to a depletion of the myelin sheath and an overall reduction in neuronal activity.

51. Which neurotransmitter is responsible for signaling skeletal muscle contractions?

    (A) GABA
    (B) Epinephrine
    (C) Acetylcholine
    (D) Norepinephrine

52. Which neurotransmitter is associated with alertness when awake?

    (A) Epinephrine
    (B) Acetylcholine
    (C) GABA
    (D) Dopamine

53. Which neurotransmitter is responsible for relaxation and the reduction of anxiety?

    (A) GABA
    (B) Epinephrine
    (C) Dopamine
    (D) Norepinephrine

54. Which neurotransmitter is responsible for the fight-or-flight reaction?

    (A) Norepinephrine
    (B) Serotonin
    (C) Epinephrine
    (D) Acetylcholine

55. Tetanus is associated with which type of pathogen?

    (A) Virus
    (B) Bacteria
    (C) Fungus
    (D) Protozoa

56. Which type of prokaryotic organism is found in extreme environments?

    (A) Bacteria
    (B) Archaea
    (C) Protists
    (D) Viruses

QUESTIONS 57 THROUGH 60 REFER TO THE FOLLOWING PASSAGE:

The number and size of organelles in a eukaryotic cell correlate with that cell's function. Four mammalian cell types, A–D, were evaluated for the area of the smooth and rough endoplasmic reticulum membrane (nm^2) as well as the average number of mitochondria and lysosomes present in the cell. The data were collected and ranked from largest (1) to smallest (4).

	Cell type A	Cell type B	Cell type C	Cell type D
Area of smooth endoplasmic reticulum	4	3	2	1
Area of rough endoplasmic reticulum	2	1	3	4
Average number of mitochondria per cell	1	2	4	3
Average number of lysosomes per cell	3	1	2	4

57. Based on the data shown in the table, which cell type likely secretes the largest quantity of proteins?

    (A) Cell type A
    (B) Cell type B
    (C) Cell type C
    (D) Cell type D

58. Which cell type likely produces the largest quantity of phospholipids?

    (A) Cell type A
    (B) Cell type B
    (C) Cell type C
    (D) Cell type D

59. Which cell type requires the most energy?

    (A) Cell type A
    (B) Cell type B
    (C) Cell type C
    (D) Cell type D

60. Which cell type likely requires a large amount of digestive enzymes?

    (A) Cell type A
    (B) Cell type B
    (C) Cell type C
    (D) Cell type D

---

61. Bacteria undergo cellular division in a process called

    (A) fission.
    (B) sporulation.
    (C) conjugation.
    (D) transduction.

62. During development, different embryonic cells express different sets of genes resulting in

    (A) gene mutation.
    (B) developmental abnormalities.
    (C) genetic recombination.
    (D) the formation of different cell types.

63. Bacterial chromosomes are double stranded and contain

    (A) introns and exons.
    (B) introns only.
    (C) exons only.
    (D) telomeres.

64. The valve between the right atrium and the right ventricle is the

(A) bicuspid (mitral) valve.
(B) tricuspid valve.
(C) pulmonary valve.
(D) aortic valve.

65. Given the blood vessels below:

1. aorta
2. inferior vena cava
3. pulmonary artery
4. pulmonary vein

Choose the arrangement that lists the vessels in the order a red blood cell would encounter them in going from the systemic veins back to the systemic arteries.

(A) 1, 3, 4, 2
(B) 2, 3, 4, 1
(C) 2, 4, 3, 1
(D) 3, 2, 1, 4

66. Oxygen is mostly transported in the blood

(A) in white blood cells.
(B) bound to albumin.
(C) bound to gamma globulins.
(D) bound to the heme portion of hemoglobin.

67. What cytoskeletal element supports the nuclear envelope in animal cells?

(A) Actin
(B) Microtubules
(C) Intermediate filament
(D) Cell cortex

68. Which of the following statements is true concerning vitamins?

(A) They function as coenzymes.
(B) Most can be synthesized by the body.
(C) They are normally broken down before they can be used by the body.
(D) A, D, E, and K are water-soluble vitamins.

69. Crossing over is more likely to occur between genes that are

(A) close together on the chromosome.
(B) on different chromosomes.
(C) located on the X chromosome.
(D) far apart on a chromosome.

70. In the reaction rate versus substrate concentration graph below, the curve plateaus because

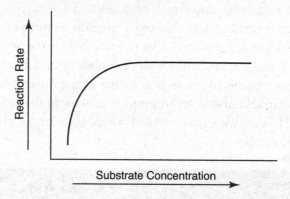

(A) a noncompetitive inhibitor is present.
(B) a competitive inhibitor is present.
(C) the active site is saturated with substrate.
(D) all the substrate has been converted to product.

QUESTIONS 71 THROUGH 74 REFER TO THE FOLLOWING PASSAGE:

The human skeleton has 206 bones. The evolution of bone, along with muscles and tendons, allowed for larger animals to move. Bones are also important for protection. The rib cage, for example, shields delicate internal organs from outside impact. The marrow tissue of bone supplies the body with new immune and blood cells.

Bone tissue is a unique mixture of protein and mineral deposits. The protein found in bone is called collagen. Collagen acts as a substrate from which to build bone. Minerals, such as calcium and phosphate, provide the strength and rigidity of bone.

71. Which of the following cells is responsible for creating the cartilage template from which bone will develop?

(A) Chondroblasts
(B) Osteoblasts
(C) Keratinocytes
(D) Osteocytes

72. Which of the following are mature cells that maintain bone?

(A) Fibroblasts
(B) Keratinocytes
(C) Osteoclasts
(D) Osteocytes

73. During development, which of the following cells creates the collagen matrix of bone?

(A) Chondroblasts
(B) Osteoblasts
(C) Osteoclasts
(D) Fibroblasts

74. During development, which of the following cells helps heal broken bones?

(A) Chondroblasts
(B) Osteoblasts
(C) Osteoclasts
(D) Osteocytes

75. Bacteria that are anaerobic heterotrophs

(A) undergo glycolysis only in the presence of oxygen.
(B) undergo glycolysis and fermentation in the presence of oxygen.
(C) undergo glycolysis only in the absence of oxygen.
(D) undergo glycolysis and fermentation in the absence of oxygen.

76. In minks, the gene for brown fur (B) is dominant to the gene for silver fur (b). Which set of genotypes represents a cross that could produce offspring with silver fur from parents that both have brown fur?

(A) Bb × Bb
(B) BB × Bb
(C) BB × bb
(D) Bb × bb

77. HIV (human immunodeficiency virus) infects mostly

(A) CT-cells.
(B) D-killer cells.
(C) T-helper cells.
(D) R-cells.

78. The sugars associated with glycolipids and glycoproteins are important in

(A) cell division.
(B) protein production.
(C) cell recognition.
(D) cell movement.

79. What are the basic nutrients the body must have?

(A) Calcium, carbohydrates, protein, fats, vitamins, minerals, water
(B) Carbohydrates, protein, fats, vitamins, minerals, water
(C) Salt, carbohydrates, protein, fats, vitamins, minerals, water
(D) Magnesium, carbohydrates, proteins, fats, vitamins, minerals, water

80. Bacteria exchange genetic material via plasmid in a process known as

(A) fission.
(B) sporulation.
(C) conjugation.
(D) transduction.

Fungal biology is of interest to many industrial organizations as these eukaryotes provide numerous benefits to mankind. For example, secondary metabolites like digestive enzymes and antibiotics that are secreted by fungi can be studied, mass produced, or synthesized for use in industry or medicine, respectively.

A liquid culture of the fission yeast *Schizosaccharomyces pombe* was exposed to high levels of UV light to introduce DNA mutations into the genomic DNA. Of the cells that were still viable, a screen was conducted to identify abnormal phenotypes. Below is a table of four selected cells and their mutant phenotype as well as a wild type control strain.

Cell type	Phenotype
Wild type	Normal growth and development
Mutant *w*	Stuck in telophase and cannot undergo cytokinesis
Mutant *x*	Cannot replicate DNA
Mutant *y*	Cannot pass metaphase checkpoint of the cell cycle
Mutant *z*	Cannot secrete digestive enzymes

81. Which cell type has a deleterious mutation in the sister chromatid protein cohesion?

   (A) Mutant *w*
   (B) Mutant *x*
   (C) Mutant *y*
   (D) Mutant *z*

82. Which cell type has a deleterious mutation in the actin gene?

   (A) Mutant *w*
   (B) Mutant *x*
   (C) Mutant *y*
   (D) Mutant *z*

83. Which cell type has a deleterious mutation in a vesicular SNARE protein?

   (A) Mutant *w*
   (B) Mutant *x*
   (C) Mutant *y*
   (D) Mutant *z*

84. Which cell type has a deleterious mutation in a subunit of DNA polymerase?

   (A) Mutant *w*
   (B) Mutant *x*
   (C) Mutant *y*
   (D) Mutant *z*

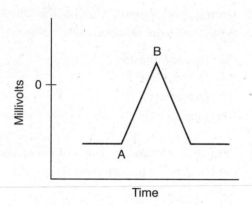

85. In the figure above, the ascending portion of the action potential observed in the cell in the graph is caused by

   (A) fluoride efflux out of the cell.
   (B) potassium influx into the cell.
   (C) sodium efflux out of the cell.
   (D) sodium influx into the cell.

Human somatic cells arise from meiosis of sex
cells. Spermatogonia give rise to sperm in males
while oogonia give rise to eggs in females. During
meiosis, the ploidy level of each cell is reduced to
23 pairs of chromosomes.

Genetic disorders may arise when a fetus receives
an abnormal number of chromosomes from either
the sperm or the egg during fertilization. This chromosomal error is a result of a nondisjunction event
that occurs among the separating chromosomes
during meiosis. The resulting fertilized egg may
have too many or too few chromosomes. Most of
these cells are unviable. A few lead to individuals
with birth defects, such as delays in physical and
mental development.

86. A nondisjunction event of the sex
chromosomes that results in two X and
one Y chromosome leads to a birth defect
known as _____.

(A) Down syndrome
(B) Turner syndrome
(C) Edwards syndrome
(D) Klinefelter syndrome

87. A nondisjunction event that results in three
copies of chromosome 21 leads to a birth
defect known as _____.

(A) Klinefelter syndrome
(B) Down syndrome
(C) Patau syndrome
(D) Edwards syndrome

88. A nondisjunction event that results in a
fetus with only one sex chromosome leads
to a birth defect known as _____.

(A) Edwards syndrome
(B) Klinefelter syndrome
(C) Patau syndrome
(D) Turner syndrome

89. A nondisjunction event that results in three
copies of chromosome 18 leads to a birth
defect known as _____.

(A) Down syndrome
(B) Turner syndrome
(C) Edwards syndrome
(D) Klinefelter syndrome

90. Which component of blood forms from
megakaryocytes?

(A) Erythrocyte
(B) Neutrophil
(C) Lymphocyte
(D) Platelet

91. The interaction of _____ and _____
cause the shortening of sacromeres during
muscle contractions.

(A) kinesin; microtubules
(B) kinesin; actin
(C) myosin; microtubules
(D) myosin; actin

92. Which form of diabetes may not require insulin injections for disease management?

(A) Type 1
(B) Type 2
(C) Type 3
(D) Type 4

93. This process occurs when double strands of a DNA segment separate and RNA nucleotides pair with DNA nucleotides.

(A) Transcription
(B) Translation
(C) Transduction
(D) Translocation

94. Apoptosis describes a process of

(A) cell specialization.
(B) cell death.
(C) cell differentiation.
(D) cell proliferation.

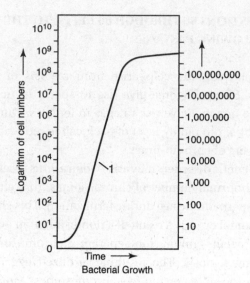

Bacterial Growth

95. In the figure above, the number 1 points to the

(A) lag phase.
(B) decline phase.
(C) stationary phase.
(D) logarithmic phase.

96. One bacterial cell is placed in a nutrient broth test tube at 12 noon. Its generation time is 30 minutes. By 2:00 P.M., the size of the population of bacteria in the test tube is

(A) 4.
(B) 8.
(C) 16.
(D) 32.

STOP

End of Biological Processes section. If you have any time left, you may go over your work in this section only.

PRACTICE TEST 2

CRITICAL READING

48 QUESTIONS (#97–#144)

TIME: 50 MINUTES

> **Directions:** Read each of the following passages, and choose the one **best** answer to each of the questions that follow each passage.

Passage 1

Bakhtin uses the term **polyphonic** to describe the novel that depicts a world in which the dialogue goes on ad infinitum without reaching a conclusion or closure. The structure is not predetermined to demonstrate the author's worldview, nor are the characters drawn to exemplify it. It is typified by the novels of Dostoyevsky, in which the reader hears many voices uttering contradictory and inconsistent statements in the context of a real-life event. Truth in Dostoyevsky's works is perceived through multiple consciousnesses and expressed in many simultaneous voices, not conceived in a single mind and spoken by a single character. There is no central voice in his novels, only multiple unfinalizable characters that talk about ideas in their distinctive, individual ways. They exist with each other and through each other as they interact in social circumstances. In addition to the characters that participate in the experience, there are the author and the reader, too, who with the characters help to create the novels' "truths," not simply one certain truth. Characters influence characters. Readers watch as they shape each other and listen as their utterances conflict with each other, all the while filtering the characters' observations through their own experiences and understanding. Bakhtin contrasts Dostoyevsky's approach with that of the nonpolyphonic monologism of Tolstoy, who reveals his own understanding of truth by expressing it through his characters' words, actions, and choices.

Another key concept in Bakhtin's theory of the novel is that of **carnival**, an idea that made its first appearance in his dissertation, "Rabelais and His World," and was further developed in *Problems of Dostoyevsky's Poetics*. His notion of carnival builds on the ancient tradition of the Saturnalia, a Roman festival that mocked and reversed the official culture, if only for a short while. For a limited period of time the powerless became the powerful, the outsider became the insider, slave and master exchanged roles.

Bakhtin judges the novel to operate with a similar social impact. Building on his study of Rabelais's novel cycle *Gargantua and Pantagruel*, the protagonists of which he sees not only as a challenge to an official culture ruled by dogmatism and deadly seriousness but also as producers of energy and vitality, he extends that analysis to consider the novel as a genre that uses laughter and parody to challenge restrictive social forces, such as the tyranny and repression of his own day. It obliterates social hierarchies and blurs distinctions between young and old, rich and poor, public and private, in short reversing the traditional systems of authority and order. In doing so, it opens the way to joyful renewal.

The polyphonic nature of the novel, in which the reader hears conflicting statements from many voices interacting and helping to shape each other, is carnivalesque. The clash of ideas destroys any notion of regular conventions, standardization, or rules, and even suggests a certain freedom of being. Each character is individually defined, and at the same time the reader witnesses how each is influenced by the other. Each one is touched by the others, and in turn shapes the character of the others. Carnival is the context in which voices are singly heard but interact together.

Excerpted from *Theory into Practice: An Introduction to Literary Criticism*, by Ann B. Dobie. Boston: Wadsworth Cengage Learning, 2012.

97. According to Bakhtin, the novel may be used to

   (A) challenge tyranny.
   (B) reinforce social hierarchies.
   (C) highlight distinctions between different segments of society.
   (D) espouse traditional systems of authority.

98. What ancient tradition is Bakhtin's concept of carnival based on?

   (A) A Roman festival that celebrated the theater
   (B) A Roman festival that celebrated the harvest
   (C) A Roman festival that celebrated the official culture
   (D) A Roman festival that mocked the official culture

99. What is the most appropriate title for the passage?

   (A) Dostoyevsky versus Tolstoy: Expressing Truth in the Novel
   (B) Interpreting Challenges to Social Change in the Works of Rabelais
   (C) Understanding Bakhtin's Theories of the Novel
   (D) Carnival and the Novel as Social Change Agent

100. According to the passage, what is missing from the novels by Dostoyevsky?

   (A) A certain truth expressed by a central voice
   (B) A protagonist who produces energy and vitality
   (C) Characters who challenge societal repression
   (D) Expression of the concept of carnival

101. In Rabelais's novel cycle, *Gargantua and Pantagruel*, what is a key characteristic of the official culture?

   (A) Violent oppression
   (B) Open-mindedness regarding social change
   (C) Humor in the face of adversity
   (D) Stubborn adherence to a belief system

102. In a polyphonic novel,

   (A) the author's worldview is expressed through the characters' words and actions.
   (B) rather than the author's singular worldview, there are multiple truths expressed through multiple characters.
   (C) the protagonists transform from adherents to the official culture into rebels who seek reform.
   (D) characters operate independently and have little influence on each other.

103. Bakhtin first introduced the concept of carnival in

   (A) *Problems of Dostoyevsky's Poetics.*
   (B) *Gargantua and Pantagruel.*
   (C) *Rabelais and His World.*
   (D) *Toward a Philosophy of the Act.*

104. According to the passage, conflicting statements and multiple voices within a novel

   (A) destroy the reader's investment in the characters and their storylines.
   (B) destroy regular conventions and suggest a certain freedom of being.
   (C) prevent the reader from understanding the overarching narrative of the novel.
   (D) prevent the author from developing connections and relationships between characters.

Passage 2

Nonadherence to medication therapy results in numerous adverse effects such as increased hospitalizations and even death. Additionally, it costs the U.S. health care system billions of dollars each year. It is important to assess patients' adherence to medications.

Improper medication adherence encompasses an assortment of behaviors. These include not having a prescription filled, forgetting or intentionally not taking a medication, consuming an incorrect amount of a medication, taking a medication at the wrong time, ceasing therapy too soon, or continuing therapy after advised to discontinue. All forms of improper medication-taking behavior may jeopardize health outcomes.

Measuring medication-taking behavior is often difficult. The ideal method of measurement should be simultaneously unobtrusive (to avoid patient sensitization and maximize cooperation), objective (to produce discrete and reproducible data for each subject), and practical (to maximize portability and minimize cost). Refill records, pill counts, electronic medication dispensers/caps, patient surveys (interviews), blood-drug level monitoring, and urine assay for drug metabolites can be used as clues to identify improper medication use.

Before altering therapy based on the assumption that a patient is taking a medication as prescribed, practitioners should ascertain the patient's medication-taking behavior. This becomes especially important when modifying dosages of medications. Due to the advantages and disadvantages of each measurement, it is important for practitioners to use a combination of methods to assess a patient's medication-usage behavior and relate these findings to the patient's clinical presentation.

105. The ideal method of medication adherence measurement should be

   (A) simultaneously functional, easy, and reliable.
   (B) simultaneously fun, personalized, and fancy-free.
   (C) simultaneously practical, objective, and unobtrusive.
   (D) simultaneously advantageous, creative, and unpretentious.

106. According to the passage, current techniques for assessing a patient's medication usage include

   (A) blood-drug level monitoring, pill counts, refill records, and half-life tables.
   (B) refill records, patient interviews, electronic medication dispensers, and nucleic acid levels.
   (C) pill counts, electronic medication dispensers, patient interviews, X-rays, and refill records.
   (D) blood-drug level monitoring, refill records, electronic medication dispensers, and urine assays for drug metabolites.

107. Improper medication adherence

   (A) encompasses taking a medication too soon, not taking enough of the drug, and forgetting to take the medication.
   (B) results in few adverse effects.
   (C) results in little cost to the U.S. health care system.
   (D) is easily measured.

108. Before altering therapy based on the assumption that the medication is being taken as prescribed, practitioners should

(A) assess the patient's behavior concerning taking his/her medication.
(B) check the patient's blood glucose levels and ask about his/her dietary intake.
(C) discern the patient's refill rate and whether he/she was on schedule.
(D) decide if the patient is in the maintenance phase of adherence.

109. The most appropriate title for this passage would be

(A) Factors Impacting U.S. Health Care Costs
(B) Interventions to Ameliorate Medication Nonadherence
(C) Prevention of Medication Nonadherence
(D) Defining and Measuring Medication Nonadherence

110. It is important to assess patients' adherence to medication because

(A) if they are not adherent then their medication will not work.
(B) it can result in adverse effects such as increased hospitalizations and perhaps death.
(C) it costs the U.S. government trillions in lawsuits each year.
(D) maintenance of adherence contributes to an increase in suicides.

Passage 3

As many as 50 million Americans have high blood pressure, defined as a systolic blood pressure ≥ 140 mm Hg and a diastolic blood pressure ≥ 90 mm Hg. Although blood pressure generally increases with age, the onset of hypertension most often occurs in the third, fourth, or fifth decade of life. The prevalence of hypertension in the elderly population (age ≥ 65 years) is approximately 63% in whites and 76% in blacks. In younger generations (35 to 45 years of age), the prevalence is markedly different with 44% among black men, 37% among black women, 26% among white men, and 17% among white women.

A specific cause of sustained hypertension cannot be found in the vast majority of individuals with high blood pressure. Genetic factors have been suggested to play a role in essential hypertension due to the fact that high blood pressure may be hereditary. Evidence that a single gene may account for specific subtypes of hypertension has also been suggested. Genetic traits include high angiotensin levels, increased aldosterone and other adrenal steroids, and high sodium-lithium counter-transport. More direct approaches for preventing or treating hypertension could be achieved by identifying individuals with these traits. Factors such as sodium excretion and transport rates, blood pressure response to plasma volume expansion, electrolyte homeostasis, and glomerular filtration rate help explain the predisposition for a person to develop hypertension.

Antihypertensive drug therapy should be individualized according to various patient characteristics and fundamental pathophysiologic circumstances. Dietary intake has been shown to be similar in all races but blacks ingest less potassium and calcium than whites. Supplemental potassium and calcium has been shown to cause a modest reduction in blood pressure in some studies. Therefore, it would seem reasonable to ascertain the effects of increasing the amount of potassium and calcium in the diet as part of the nonpharmacologic regulation of hypertension. The initial treatment for hypertension is lifestyle changes unless target-organ damage is present. These changes include sodium restriction, weight reduction, increased physical activity, and ethanol reduction or abstinence. In terms of target-organ damage, diuretics and beta-blockers are first-line therapy. Control of blood pressure and prevention of cardiovascular morbidity and mortality are the goals of antihypertensive therapy. By maintaining arterial blood pressure below 140 mm Hg systolic and 90 mm Hg diastolic and by controlling other risk factors such as smoking, hyperlipidemia, and diabetes, morbidity and mortality may be averted.

111. The onset of hypertension most often occurs in which decades?

(A) Third and fifth
(B) Third, fourth, and fifth
(C) Fourth, fifth, and sixth
(D) Fifth, sixth, and seventh

112. Based on the information presented in the first paragraph, one may conclude that

(A) hypertension is a rarely diagnosed disease state.
(B) hypertension is more prevalent among white individuals compared with their black counterparts in both the elderly and younger populations.
(C) hypertension is more prevalent among black individuals compared with their white counterparts in both the elderly and younger populations.
(D) hypertension rarely occurs prior to the sixth decade of life.

113. According to the passage, initial treatment for hypertension is lifestyle changes which include

(A) smoking cessation, weight reduction, decreased physical activity, and ethanol restriction.
(B) sodium restriction, weight reduction, increased physical activity, and ethanol reduction or abstinence.
(C) ethanol reduction or abstinence, sodium restriction, reduced mental activity or stress, and gaining weight.
(D) weight reduction, increased sodium intake, ethanol reduction, and increased stress.

114. Two of the factors that help provide an explanation of hypertensive development are centered around

(A) diuretic usage and abstinence.
(B) electrolyte homeostasis and sodium excretion.
(C) increased calcium intake and proper medication adherence.
(D) decreased medication therapy costs and decreased steroid usage.

115. Genetic factors have been suggested to play a role in essential hypertension based on the fact that

(A) parents can get it from their children.
(B) if ancestors have high angiotensin levels they have a higher rate of morbidity.
(C) geneticists know which gene causes hypertension.
(D) high blood pressure may be hereditary.

116. Antihypertensive therapy should be individualized according to

(A) patient characteristics and fundamental pathophysiologic circumstances.
(B) number of offspring and dietary habits stemming from care of those offspring.
(C) features found in the patient's family tree.
(D) the climate of the state where the patient lives.

117. Morbidity and mortality associated with hypertension may be averted if an individual can maintain an arterial blood pressure of

(A) 155 mm Hg systolic and 77 mm Hg diastolic.
(B) 136 mm Hg systolic and 99 mm Hg diastolic.
(C) 160 mm Hg systolic and 98 mm Hg diastolic.
(D) 135 mm Hg systolic and 85 mm Hg diastolic.

118. How many Americans currently suffer from high blood pressure?

(A) As many as 60 billion

(B) As many as 50 billion

(C) As many as 50 million

(D) As many as 40 million

Passage 4

We humans sense old age through feeling those creaky joints or observing those graying hairs but, according to Apfeld and Kenyon reporting in a recent issue of Nature, the nematode worm senses its age by smelling and tasting the environment. These investigators show that worms with defective olfactory organs (that would normally detect odor molecules in the environment) live longer than their comrades with a keener sense of smell. By comparing these worms with other mutant nematodes that live an unusually long time, the researchers found clues to how a reduced ability to "smell the roses" might lengthen life span.

The worm's olfactory sense organs—amphids on the head and plasmids on the tail—are composed of a cluster of nerve cells, the ends of which are modified into cilia. The cilia are encircled by a sheath and a socket cell that form a pore in the worm's skin through which the tips of the cilia protrude. Odor molecules and soluble compounds bind to G protein-coupled receptors (similar to the olfactory and taste receptors of mammals) located at the tip of each cilium. Worms with a poor sense of smell—because their olfactory organs have defective or absent cilia, blocked pores, or damaged sheaths—live much longer, yet are otherwise normal (for example, their feeding and reproductive behaviors are unchanged). Mutations in TAX-4—a channel regulated by cyclic GMP that sits under the G protein-coupled receptor and transduces the sensory signals into electrical impulses—also imbue the worm with a longer life.

But mutations in the worm's olfactory machinery are not the only defects that extend its life span. In an earlier study, Kenyon's group found that defects in the reproductive system could prolong life by decreasing the activity of DAF-2 (a receptor for an insulin-like molecule) and increasing the activity of DAF-16 (a transcription factor). By looking at worms defective in both sensory perception and reproduction, Apfeld and Kenyon worked out a putative pathway through which smell might influence a worm's longevity.

An environmental signal, perhaps produced by bacteria (the worm's favorite food), binds to G protein-coupled olfactory receptors on sensory cilia activating TAX-4, which then incites electrical activity in the sensory neurons. This activity triggers secretory vesicles in the neurons to release insulin-like molecules, which bind to DAF-2 and activate the insulin-like signaling pathway. This then switches on genes that will ensure the worm dies at the usual age of 2 weeks. A reduced ability to sense olfactory cues would result in a decrease in DAF-2 activation and an increase in life span.

This chain of events is not proven, but insulin-like molecules that might bind to DAF-2 have been identified in the nematode. Such a pathway would also make physiological sense. After all, if food is scarce it may behoove the worm to live longer to ensure that it has the chance to produce its full quota of offspring. A scarcity of food also promotes longevity in rodents and primates. But so far it seems that in these more complicated creatures a poor sense of smell is not a harbinger of a ripe old age.

Excerpted from "Nota Bene: Sensing Old Age" by Orda Smith, *Science*, Vol. 287, January 2000. Page 54. Reprinted with permission from AAAS.

119. A worm usually lives to the "old age" of

   (A) 3 weeks.
   (B) 5 weeks.
   (C) 1 week.
   (D) 2 weeks.

120. TAX-4 is

   (A) a channel regulated by cyclic GMP
        which sits beneath the G protein-
        coupled receptor and transduces the
        sensory signals into electrical impulses.
   (B) a cyclic regulated AMP which lies
        above the G protein-coupled receptor
        and transduces the neurological signals
        into electrical impulses.
   (C) a liability where the nematode has to
        deal with four times the amount of
        cyclic GMP next to the G protein-
        coupled receptor.
   (D) a receptor for an insulin-like molecule
        which activates the insulin-like
        pathway.

121. A nematode worm detects its age by

   (A) a biological stopwatch which notes
        sunrise and sunset.
   (B) burrowing through the soil at speeds
        up to 0.01 mph.
   (C) whether it has had the chance to pro-
        duce its full quota of offspring.
   (D) smelling and tasting the environment.

122. The worm's olfactory sense organs are
     composed of

   (A) a cluster of nervous tissue surrounded
        by a sheath which protects it.
   (B) socket cells that are embedded in the
        head and tail of the worm.
   (C) a cluster of nerve cells of which the
        ends are modified into cilia.
   (D) its individual mouth and nose which
        are covered with cilia.

123. What other traits in the worm extend its life
     span?

   (A) Defects in the circulatory system
   (B) Mutations in the excretory system
   (C) Alterations in the lymphatic system
   (D) Aberrations in the reproductive system

124. DAF-2 is

   (A) a receptor for an insulin-like molecule.
   (B) a transcription factor.
   (C) a transduction factor.
   (D) a binding site for a glucose molecule.

125. A logical pathway by which smell might
     influence a worm's longevity was achieved
     by studying

   (A) worms flawed in both circulatory and
        sensory perception.
   (B) worms defective in both reproduction
        and sensory perception.
   (C) worms deficient in only the reproduc-
        tive system.
   (D) worms impaired in the nervous and
        circulatory systems.

126. Secretory vesicles in the neurons are
     stimulated by what to release insulin-like
     molecules?

   (A) TAX-4 incites electrical activity.
   (B) DAF-2 activates the insulin-like
        pathway.
   (C) DAF-16 regulates the electrical activity.
   (D) TAX-2 initiates the secretory vesicles.

127. A scarcity of food is known to promote
     longevity in

   (A) nematodes.
   (B) nematodes and rodents.
   (C) nonprimates and nematodes.
   (D) rodents and primates.

128. The reduced ability to sense olfactory cues results in

(A) a decrease in life span and an increase in DAF-2 activation.
(B) a decrease in DAF-2 activation and an increase in life span.
(C) a decrease in TAX-4, which incites electrical activity.
(D) a decrease in DAF-16, which creates more gene activity.

Passage 5

The most prevalent theme of the Group Member involves some loss of individuality within the group. Multiple lines of work in social psychology have explored the consequences of immersing oneself in the group to varying degrees. Usually these consequences are seen as bad. The Group Member can become deindividuated, may engage in group-think, and might even participate in mob violence. These negative effects reveal the group aspect of the Foolish Decision Maker . . . (If they were foolish to start with, they become even more so.) Indeed, the assumption that people degenerate into inferior creatures by virtue of belonging to groups has crept into many other lines of research in social psychology, including social loafing, crowding, social facilitation, and diffusion of responsibility in bystander intervention.

The Group Member need not be a bad person, however. After all, interactions in groups is an almost inevitable part of human social life, especially if we include families as groups (which they most certainly are).

The motivations of the Group Members differ somewhat depending on which of two approaches is taken. One approach considers processes within the group. The Group Member must find ways to be accepted and liked by the other members, which often requires determining how the member is similar to them and can fit in with them (getting along). The Group Member must also seek to rise through the group hierarchy (getting ahead), which may require finding ways to stand out among the group. More recent characterizations of the Group Member involve the cognitive work that is involved in the various steps of entering the group, becoming socialized into full membership, finding a niche or rising through the ranks, exerting leadership, and exiting the group.

The other approach is to look at processes between groups. Intergroup processes have become a dominant focus of social psychology in Europe and Australia and have also been studied elsewhere. The emphasis is on how the individual identifies with the group and relates to members of other groups. The Group Member is thus committed and loyal to his or her group and is competitive with and often prejudiced or even hostile toward other groups.

Excerpted from "Social Psychologists and Thinking about People" in *Advanced Social Psychology: The State of the Science*, by Roy F. Baumeister and Eli J. Finkel. New York: Oxford University Press, 2010.

129. Cognitive work of the Group Member involves

(A) becoming socialized and finding a niche.
(B) challenging the leader for dominance.
(C) demonstrating his/her hostility to rival groups.
(D) diffusing responsibility to bystanders.

130. What would be the most appropriate title for this passage?

(A) Social Psychology Perspectives on Understanding the Group Member
(B) Social Psychology Perspectives on Maintaining Individuality within a Group
(C) Social Psychology Perspectives on the Motivations of the Group Member
(D) Social Psychology Perspectives on Consequences of Group Membership

131. What does the passage identify as the most prevalent theme of the Group Member?

    (A) Group loyalty
    (B) Enhancement of individuality
    (C) Groupthink
    (D) Loss of individuality

132. In the context of this passage, "getting along" and "getting ahead" refer to

    (A) establishing respectful communication between groups and advancing within the governing body created by the groups.
    (B) establishing a fit within the group and advancing within the group hierarchy.
    (C) establishing a friendship with a Group Member as an entry point to immersing oneself in a group, and advancing within the group hierarchy.
    (D) establishing a relationship with a Group Member as an outsider to the group, and using that relationship to advance within the social hierarchy.

133. Which of the following topics has become of significant interest to social psychologists in Europe and Australia?

    (A) Group differentiation
    (B) Intergroup conflict
    (C) Intergroup processes
    (D) Group leadership

134. Commitment to a group may result in

    (A) efforts to recruit members from other groups.
    (B) isolation from family.
    (C) competition with other groups.
    (D) increased interaction with family.

135. According to the passage, how does group membership affect individuals who are considered Foolish Decision Makers?

    (A) They become more foolish.
    (B) They become less foolish.
    (C) No effect is indicated.
    (D) Foolish Decision Makers are generally refused group membership.

136. Other areas of social psychology research that address the negative aspects of group membership include which of the following?

    (A) Exerting leadership
    (B) Social loafing
    (C) Getting along
    (D) Social withdrawal

Passage 6

Drug interactions, a common type of drug-related problem, are categorized as pharmacokinetic, pharmacodynamic, or a combination of both. Pharmacokinetic drug interactions include changes in absorption, distribution, excretion, and metabolism, whereas pharmacodynamic drug interactions may lead to antagonistic or synergistic effects. Not all drug interactions are undesirable; in fact, many drug interactions are used to produce desirable effects. Patients who take drugs with narrow therapeutic indices and drugs that interfere with the pharmacokinetic properties of other drugs are at increased risk of experiencing a drug interaction. Also, patients who take multiple medications per day or take multiple doses of medications per day are at increased risk. Because renal transplant patients take immunosuppressive agents that have narrow therapeutic indices and are subjected to multiple medications per day, they are vulnerable to experiencing adverse drug events. To prevent adverse drug interactions, an alternative therapy should be considered when possible or the dose or schedule of the drugs should be adjusted to reduce the occurrence of an adverse experience. Additionally, adequate monitoring to prevent and detect adverse effects is an essential part of patient care.

A common pharmacokinetic interaction involves drugs that interfere with the absorption of other medications. Drugs that bind and decrease the gastrointestinal absorption of another drug, such as cholestyramine decreasing the absorption of tacrolimus, typically can be prevented by administering the agents two to three hours apart from each other. Prokinetic agents interfere with the rate of absorption. Since many transplant patients take prokinetic agents, such as metochlopromide, this may increase the bioavailability of other medications. This is of significant importance since immunosuppressive agents have narrow therapeutic indices and toxicity may result from this interaction. If the prokinetic agent cannot be avoided, careful monitoring (e.g., serum drug levels, clinical presentation of the patient) and adjustments should be made to prevent immunosuppressant toxicity.

137. The passage indicates that prokinetic agents

(A) interfere with the rate of metabolism.
(B) affect all interactions in the gastrointestinal tract.
(C) interfere with the rate of absorption.
(D) should be monitored and adjusted.

138. Drug interactions are characterized as

(A) pharmacokinetic only.
(B) pharmacokinetic, pharmacodynamic, or a combination of both.
(C) pharmacodynamic only.
(D) pharmacosynthetic only.

139. Toxicity can result from a prokinetic agent being administered with an immunosuppressive agent because

(A) cholestyramine has a narrow therapeutic index.
(B) patients have to take immunosuppressive agents multiple times per day.
(C) the prokinetic agent may increase the bioavailability of the immunosuppressive agent.
(D) all drug interactions are undesirable.

140. Pharmacokinetic drug interactions include

(A) changes in allocation, circulation, and dispersion.
(B) changes in absorption, distribution, excretion, and metabolism.
(C) reactions which affect the composition of other medications.
(D) cumulative and additive effects.

141. Patients who are at an increased risk of experiencing a drug interaction include

(A) patients who take multiple medications per day or take multiple doses of medications per day.
(B) patients who take drugs with wide therapeutic indices.
(C) patients who take drugs that do not interfere with the pharmacokinetic properties of other drugs.
(D) patients who are taking medications for a brief time period.

142. In this passage, an example of a drug that binds and decreases the gastrointestinal absorption of another drug is

(A) tacrolimus.
(B) metochlopromide.
(C) sirolimus.
(D) cholestyramine.

143. To prevent adverse drug reactions,

   (A) consult neighbors regularly.
   (B) consider an alternate therapy or alter the dose or schedule of the drugs.
   (C) time medication regimens with meals.
   (D) increase water intake.

144. If the prokinetic agent cannot be avoided, to prevent immunosuppressant toxicity,

   (A) carefully arrange the patient's medication consumption schedule.
   (B) monitor compliance to see if the prokinetic factor is really necessary.
   (C) monitor the serum levels and the clinical presentation of the patient, and make appropriate adjustments.
   (D) do not educate the patient on the types of adverse drug reactions which may occur.

STOP

End of Critical Reading section. If you have any time left, you may go over your work in this section only.

Directions: Choose the **best** answer to each of the following questions.

---

145. Evaluate the integral $\int_{2}^{3}(10x^4)\,dx$.

    (A) 550
    (B) 760
    (C) 650
    (D) 422

146. Find the total number of 7-letter anagrams, using letters from the set {P, Q, R}, that contain exactly three Rs, but no two Rs consecutively.

    (A) 320
    (B) 240
    (C) 160
    (D) 120

147. Eighty-six degrees Fahrenheit =

    (A) 30 degrees Celsius
    (B) 15 degrees Celsius
    (C) 20 degrees Celsius
    (D) 25 degrees Celsius

148. Given that $\ln(a) = 12$ and $\ln(b) = 3$,
    $\ln\left(\dfrac{a}{b}\right) =$

    (A) 9
    (B) 4
    (C) ln(9)
    (D) ln(4)

149. A patient takes 20 mL of medicine 3 times daily. How many teaspoons are needed for a 10-day supply of medicine?
    (One teaspoon = 5 mL)

    (A) 120
    (B) 80
    (C) 140
    (D) 100

150. What is the mean value for the sequence {4, 5, 11, 18, 20, 22, 34, 35, 38}?

    (A) 20.77
    (B) 25.77
    (C) 30.77
    (D) 35.77

151. A box contains 8 balls, numbered 1 through 8. Four balls are removed at random from the box, one after another, and are not replaced. The numbers on the balls removed from the box are written down in the order in which they are removed, forming a four-digit number. How many different four-digit numbers can be obtained in this way?

    (A) 4,096
    (B) 1,680
    (C) 5,040
    (D) 3,360

152. A square plot of land 210 feet on one side contains 1 acre. Approximately how many square feet are in 3 acres of land?

    (A) 132,300
    (B) 44,100
    (C) 88,200
    (D) 66,150

153. Given the function $f(x) = \dfrac{5x}{x^3+1}$, compute $\dfrac{dy}{dx}$.

(A) $\dfrac{10x^3-5}{\left(x^3+1\right)^2}$

(B) $\dfrac{5-10x^3}{\left(x^3+1\right)^2}$

(C) $\dfrac{5+10x^3}{\left(x^3+1\right)^2}$

(D) $\dfrac{-10x^3-5}{\left(x^3+1\right)^2}$

154. $10^2 + 9^2 =$

(A) 90^4

(B) 19^4

(C) 1.81×10^2

(D) 1^4

155. Suppose point P is on the x-axis such that P is 7 units away from the point $(5, -3)$. Determine all possible coordinates of point P.

(A) $(5 + 2\sqrt{10}, 0)$ and $(5 - 2\sqrt{10}, 0)$

(B) $(5 + 4\sqrt{10}, 0)$ and $(5 - 4\sqrt{10}, 0)$

(C) $(2\sqrt{6}, 0)$ and $(-2\sqrt{6}, 0)$

(D) $(4\sqrt{6}, 0)$ and $(-4\sqrt{6}, 0)$

156. John has $6.60 in quarters and dimes. He has twice as many quarters as dimes. How many quarters does he have?

(A) 11

(B) 20

(C) 18

(D) 22

157. Simplify the expression $\dfrac{3}{x} - \dfrac{2}{y}$.

(A) $\dfrac{3y-2x}{xy}$

(B) $\dfrac{1}{xy}$

(C) $\dfrac{1}{x-y}$

(D) $\dfrac{xy}{x-y}$

158. Given the function $f(x) = 3x - 1$, determine the formula for $f^{-1}(x)$.

(A) $f^{-1}(x) = \dfrac{1}{3x-1}$

(B) $f^{-1}(x) = \dfrac{x+1}{3}$

(C) $f^{-1}(x) = \dfrac{x-1}{3}$

(D) $f^{-1}(x) = \dfrac{1}{3x+1}$

QUESTIONS 159 THROUGH 161 ARE BASED ON THE GRAPH BELOW OF THE FUNCTION $y = f(x)$:

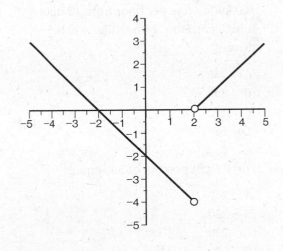

159. $\displaystyle\lim_{x \to 2^+} f(x) =$

(A) 0 and -4

(B) Does not exist

(C) 0 or -4

(D) 0

160. $\lim\limits_{x\to 2^-} f(x) =$

    (A) −4
    (B) Does not exist
    (C) 0 or −4
    (D) 0 and −4

161. $\lim\limits_{x\to 2} f(x) =$

    (A) −4
    (B) Does not exist
    (C) 0
    (D) 0 and −4

---

162. $\log(mn) =$

    (A) $\log(m) - \log(n)$
    (B) $\log(m) + \log(n)$
    (C) $\log\left(\dfrac{m}{n}\right)$
    (D) $\dfrac{\log(m)}{\log(n)}$

163. A truck travels at a steady speed of 100 kilometers per hour from 12 noon until 6 P.M. How many miles will be driven?

    (A) 968
    (B) 600
    (C) 372
    (D) 106

164. Forty-eight percent of 500 equals

    (A) 240
    (B) 250
    (C) 260
    (D) 220

165. $\displaystyle\int_{e}^{e^2}\left(\dfrac{6}{x}\right)dx =$

    (A) 6
    (B) $\dfrac{6}{e^2} - \dfrac{6}{e}$
    (C) 18
    (D) $\dfrac{6}{e^2} + \dfrac{6}{e}$

166. Determine the derivative for the function $p(x) = e^{-x} \cdot \cos(3x)$.

    (A) $e^{-x}\cos(3x) + 3e^{-x}\sin(3x)$
    (B) $-e^{-x}\cos(3x) - 3e^{-x}\sin(3x)$
    (C) $-e^{-x}\cos(3x) + 3e^{-x}\sin(3x)$
    (D) $e^{-x}\cos(3x) - 3e^{-x}\sin(3x)$

167. $\lim\limits_{x\to\infty}\left(\dfrac{8x^6 + 4x^2 - 10x + 5}{7x^6 + 12x^3}\right) =$

    (A) ∞
    (B) Undefined
    (C) 1
    (D) $\dfrac{8}{7}$

168. A man is tossing a coin. The first three tosses have been heads. What are the chances that heads will occur on the fourth toss?

    (A) 50%
    (B) 25%
    (C) 12.5%
    (D) 6.25%

169. The height, h, of a projectile is given by $h(x) = -0.004x^2 + 16x$, where x is the horizontal distance the projectile travels. The projectile hits the ground after it has traveled a horizontal distance of

    (A) 200 feet
    (B) 2,000 feet
    (C) 400 feet
    (D) 4,000 feet

170. A student determines that the mean of six measurements of the boiling point of an unknown chemical solution is 210°C. The mean of the first five measurements is 208°C. Determine the value of the sixth measurement.

(A) 220°C
(B) 212°C
(C) 216°C
(D) 218°C

171. Event A has a probability of $\frac{5}{9}$. What is the probability that event A does NOT occur?

(A) $\frac{4}{9}$

(B) $-\frac{5}{9}$

(C) $\frac{9}{5}$

(D) Not enough information

172. Calculate the value of x in the expression $4x = \frac{1}{2}$.

(A) $\frac{1}{42}$

(B) $\frac{1}{24}$

(C) $\frac{1}{16}$

(D) $\frac{1}{8}$

QUESTIONS 173 AND 174 ARE BASED ON THE DATA SHOWN IN THE TABLE BELOW:

Drug Prescribed	# of Patients
Drug A	680
Drug B	200
Drug C	42
Drug D	350
Other	20

173. What percentage of patients received prescriptions for Drug B or Drug C?

(A) 0.1873%
(B) 10.99%
(C) 0.1099%
(D) 18.73%

174. What percentage of patients did NOT receive a prescription for Drug A?

(A) 0.4737%
(B) 37.73%
(C) 0.3773%
(D) 47.37%

175. Digoxin injection is supplied in ampules of 500 micrograms per 2 mL. What quantity must a nurse administer to deliver a dose of 0.75 milligrams?

(A) 2.25 mL
(B) 1.75 mL
(C) 2.0 mL
(D) 3.0 mL

176. Determine the slope of the line passing through the points (10, 3) and (4, –6).

(A) $\frac{3}{2}$

(B) $-\frac{3}{2}$

(C) $\frac{2}{3}$

(D) $-\frac{2}{3}$

QUESTION 177 IS BASED ON THE GRAPH BELOW OF THE FUNCTION $y = f(x)$**:**

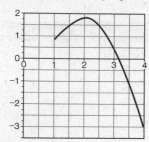

177. Identify the graph of the function $y = f(x-3)$.

(A)

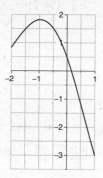

(B)

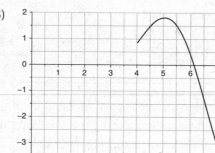

(C)

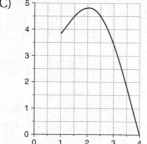

(D)

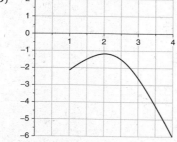

178. A patient's creatine clearance rate (CrCl) can be calculated by using the following formula:

$$CrCl = \frac{140 - \text{age in years}}{72 \cdot SCr} \cdot (\text{ideal body weight in kilograms})$$

What is the approximate CrCl for a 58-year-old patient who has a SCr of 2.6 and an ideal body weight of 76 kg?

(A) 23
(B) 33
(C) 30
(D) 37

179. The range of the function f is given by $(-\infty, 6)$. Determine the domain for f^{-1}.

(A) $(-\infty, 6)$
(B) $(6, \infty)$
(C) $\left(\frac{1}{6}, \infty\right)$
(D) $\left(-\infty, \frac{1}{6}\right)$

QUESTIONS 180 THROUGH 183 ARE BASED ON THE GRAPH BELOW OF THE FUNCTION $y = f(x)$:

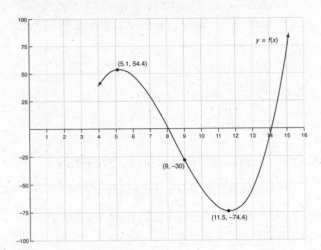

180. Choose an interval for which $f'(x) > 0$.

    (A) $x > 11.5$

    (B) $4 < x < 8$

    (C) $x > -74.4$

    (D) $0 < x < 40$

181. Identify the x-value(s) for which $f''(x) < 0$.

    (A) $9 > x > \infty$

    (B) $-\infty < x < 9$

    (C) $9 < x < \infty$

    (D) $-\infty > x > 9$

182. Identify the relative maxima (if any) for f.

    (A) $(5.1, 54.4)$

    (B) $(9, -30)$

    (C) None

    (D) $(11.5, -74.4)$

183. $\lim\limits_{x \to 8}\left(\dfrac{f(x) - f(8)}{x - 8}\right) =$

    (A) 0

    (B) A positive number

    (C) A negative number

    (D) Not enough information

184. Determine the average rate of change of the function $f(x) = x^3$ on the interval $2 \le x \le 4$.

    (A) 28

    (B) 56

    (C) 36

    (D) 38

185. Portions of the interior of an equilateral triangle are removed in stages according to the following pattern. At each stage, the midpoints of the sides of each shaded triangle form a triangle to be removed.

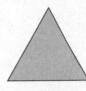 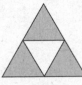 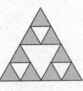

Stage 1   Stage 2   Stage 3

The shaded area that remains at Stage 3 is what fraction of the original shaded area at Stage 1?

    (A) $\dfrac{9}{16}$

    (B) $\dfrac{7}{16}$

    (C) $\dfrac{3}{4}$

    (D) $\dfrac{1}{4}$

186. What is the slope of the line shown in the graph below?

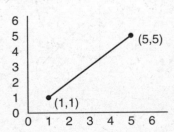

    (A) 1

    (B) 2

    (C) 4

    (D) 10

187. What is the median of the following values:

   10, 12, 9, 10, 11, 9, 9, 10, 8, 12?

   (A) 2
   (B) 9.5
   (C) 10
   (D) 12

188. How many three-letter codes can be formed from the set {A, B, C, D, E}? Repeated letters are allowed.

   (A) 60
   (B) 120
   (C) 80
   (D) 125

189. Determine the x-coordinate of the points, if any, where the graph of $f(x) = \dfrac{x}{x+2}$ has a horizontal tangent line.

   (A) When $x = -2$
   (B) When $x = 0$
   (C) When $x = 2$
   (D) Never

190. Find the sum of the y-coordinates of points P and Q shown in the diagram.

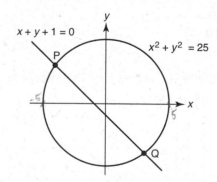

   (A) 1
   (B) 2
   (C) –2
   (D) –1

191. Event A has a probability of 0.35. Event B has a probability of 0.22. The probability that events A and B both occur is 0.09. What is the probability that either event A or event B occurs?

   (A) 0.57
   (B) 0.52
   (C) 0.48
   (D) 0.66

192. Find the exact value of the shaded area bounded above by the graph of $f(x) = \dfrac{3}{x}$ and below by the x-axis from $x = 1$ to $x = \sqrt{e}$.

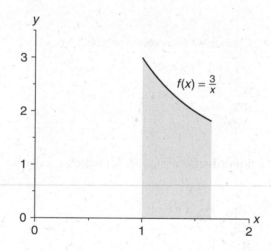

   (A) $\ln(1.5)$
   (B) $\dfrac{2}{3}$
   (C) 1.5
   (D) $\ln\left(\dfrac{2}{3}\right)$

STOP

End of Quantitative Reasoning section. If you have any time left, you may go over your work in this section only.

WRITING

TIME: 30 MINUTES

Directions: Write a well-constructed essay addressing the statement below.

In recent years, the U.S. Congress has had difficulty reaching a consensus regarding legislation to address the issue of illegal immigration and the more than 11 million illegal immigrants residing in the United States. Discuss a solution to the problem of illegal immigration in the United States.

ANSWER KEY
Practice Test 2

CHEMICAL PROCESSES (1–48)

1.	A	13.	D	25.	D	37.	C
2.	C	14.	C	26.	B	38.	B
3.	B	15.	D	27.	D	39.	B
4.	D	16.	C	28.	B	40.	C
5.	B	17.	C	29.	C	41.	B
6.	A	18.	C	30.	D	42.	B
7.	B	19.	C	31.	D	43.	D
8.	D	20.	B	32.	A	44.	A
9.	B	21.	B	33.	C	45.	B
10.	B	22.	B	34.	C	46.	A
11.	D	23.	B	35.	C	47.	A
12.	C	24.	C	36.	C	48.	A

BIOLOGICAL PROCESSES (49–96)

49.	A	61.	A	73.	B	85.	D
50.	A	62.	D	74.	C	86.	D
51.	C	63.	C	75.	D	87.	B
52.	A	64.	B	76.	A	88.	D
53.	A	65.	B	77.	C	89.	C
54.	A	66.	D	78.	C	90.	D
55.	B	67.	C	79.	B	91.	D
56.	B	68.	A	80.	C	92.	B
57.	B	69.	D	81.	C	93.	A
58.	D	70.	C	82.	A	94.	B
59.	A	71.	A	83.	D	95.	D
60.	B	72.	D	84.	B	96.	C

ANSWER KEY
Practice Test 2

CRITICAL READING (97–144)

97.	A	109.	D	121.	D	133.	C
98.	D	110.	B	122.	C	134.	C
99.	C	111.	B	123.	D	135.	A
100.	A	112.	C	124.	A	136.	B
101.	D	113.	B	125.	B	137.	C
102.	B	114.	B	126.	A	138.	B
103.	C	115.	D	127.	D	139.	C
104.	B	116.	A	128.	B	140.	B
105.	C	117.	D	129.	A	141.	A
106.	D	118.	C	130.	A	142.	D
107.	A	119.	D	131.	D	143.	B
108.	A	120.	A	132.	B	144.	C

QUANTITATIVE REASONING (145–192)

145.	D	157.	A	169.	D	181.	B
146.	C	158.	B	170.	A	182.	A
147.	A	159.	D	171.	A	183.	C
148.	A	160.	A	172.	D	184.	A
149.	A	161.	B	173.	D	185.	A
150.	A	162.	B	174.	D	186.	A
151.	B	163.	C	175.	D	187.	C
152.	A	164.	A	176.	A	188.	D
153.	B	165.	A	177.	B	189.	D
154.	C	166.	B	178.	B	190.	D
155.	A	167.	D	179.	A	191.	C
156.	D	168.	A	180.	A	192.	C

ANSWERS EXPLAINED

Chemical Processes

1. **(A)** The chiral center is the carbon with the wedged bond to nitrogen. The absolute configuration will be either R or S. (E and Z refer to the configuration of alkenes, not chiral centers. Both the E/Z and R/S systems use the Cahn-Ingold-Prelog System of assigning priorities.) To assign R or S to the chiral center, prioritize each of the four groups attached to the chiral carbon. The nitrogen will be priority #1 (priority is based on atomic number), and #4 is the implied hydrogen (it is behind the plane of the paper—remember that for tetrahedral carbons, at most, two bonds can be in the plane, the third is above the plane and wedged, and the fourth is behind the plane and dotted, if expressed). The arene with the chlorine will be priority #2, and the other arene is #3. Since the hydrogen is already positioned away from us, we can read the absolute configuration by the direction of the other three. Here, 1-2-3 goes clockwise so the configuration is R.

2. **(C)** Chlorine (in the presence of ultraviolet light) chlorinates alkanes by a free radical substitution reaction. HCl would chlorinate an alkene or an alkyne by electrophilic addition. Chlorine and iron (III) chloride chlorinate an arene ring by electrophilic aromatic substitution. The iron (III) chloride acts as a Lewis acid to polarize the Cl–Cl bond, making one end of the chlorine molecule sufficiently partial positive to act as an electrophile toward the pi electrons of the arene ring.

3. **(B)** To make esters, you can add an alcohol to a carboxylic acid, a carboxylic acid halide, a carboxylic acid anhydride, an acyl phosphate, or a thioester. Condensing two carboxylic acids makes a carboxylic acid anhydride. An amine and a carboxylic acid undergo an acid-base reaction with the acid being converted to the carboxylate and the amine protonated.

4. **(D)** Even though an arene ring is drawn with double and single bonds, because of resonance, the bonds are actually identical and are between a double and a single bond. The carbons are sp^2 hybridized, and the sigma bonds are the overlap of sp^2 hybrid orbitals while the pi bonds are the overlap of unhybridized p orbitals. Sigma bonds are stronger than pi bonds.

5. **(B)** Nucleotides are polymerized to form nucleic acids, DNA, and RNA. Nucleotides are composed of an aromatic nitrogenous base (the purines: adenine and guanine; the pyrimidines: cytosine, uracil, and thymine), a ribose/deoxyribose carbohydrate, and at least one phosphate. The polymerization of the nucleotides is called transcription for the synthesis of RNA and replication for the synthesis of DNA.

6. **(A)** The synthesis of RNA requires ribonucleotide triphosphates and RNA polymerase.

7. **(B)** As mentioned in question 5, nucleotides contain at least one phosphate. When they are polymerized, one phosphate remains and links the carbohydrate of one nucleotide to the carbohydrate of the next one. RNA is found in the cytoplasm but DNA is found only in the nucleus of animal cells. The urea cycle is the series of reactions whereby amine groups (from amino acids) and carbon dioxide are converted to urea (H_2NCONH_2) for excretion in the urine.

8. **(D)** DNA polymerase is the enzyme catalyzing the synthesis of DNA.

9. **(B)** There is a fourth colligative property, vapor pressure depression.

10. **(B)** According to the equation, the reaction between ethylene oxide and water is 1:1. To determine the percent yield, we need to know the theoretical yield. There is 1.0 g of ethylene oxide (formula weight 44), so there are 1.0 g/(44 g/mole) = 0.023 moles of ethylene oxide. There is also 1.0 g of water (formula weight 18), so there are 1.0 g/(18 g/mole) = 0.056 moles of water. Ethylene oxide is the limiting reactant, so the theoretical yield of ethylene glycol (formula weight 62) is 0.023 moles × (62 g/mole) = 1.4 g. The percent yield is (0.85 g/1.4 g) × 100 = 61%.

11. **(D)** Polarity of covalent bonds is related to the difference in electronegativities of the two atoms involved. The farther two atoms are from each other on the periodic table, the more different their electronegativities will be. Thus, the O–H bond is the most polar of those listed.

12. **(C)** Molality is defined as the number of moles of solute per kilogram of solvent. Molarity is defined as the number of moles of solute per liter of solution. Notice that one is defined in terms of the solvent, and the other is defined in terms of the solution. That is the big challenge here. The solution is 12 M ethylene glycol meaning there are 12 moles of ethylene glycol per liter of solution. Since the density of the solution is given, we can determine the mass of 1 L of solution.

$$1000 \text{ mL} \times 1.2 \text{ g/mL} = 1200 \text{ g of solution}$$

Of that 1200 g, some is ethylene glycol (12 moles in fact) and the rest is the solvent. The mass of ethylene glycol is 12 moles × 62 g/mole = 744 g ethylene glycol. The mass of the solvent is 1200 g – 744 g or 456 g (0.456 kg). The molality of the solution is 12 moles solute/0.456 kg solvent = 26.3 m ≈ 26 m.

13. **(D)** To determine molecular geometry, you must first draw the Lewis structure. With one phosphorus atom and three chlorines, there are 26 valence electrons total. Place the phosphorus in the middle and the chlorines around it, connecting each chlorine to the central phosphorus atom with a pair of electrons. Complete the octets of the peripheral chlorine atoms (that commits 24 of the valence electrons), leaving two electrons to go on the phosphorus. All atoms have an octet so no multiple bonds are needed. To determine the molecular geometry, look at the four sets of electrons on the phosphorus atom (three sets are the bonds to chlorines and the fourth set is the unshared pair)—they will spread out as far as possible (according to the Valence Shell Electron Pair Repulsion Theory), assuming a geometry of a tetrahedral (choice B). When the name of the molecular geometry is given, however, the name refers only to the three-dimensional location of the atoms. Here, the phosphorus is inside the tetrahedron, and the three chlorines are directed toward three of the four corners of the tetrahedron (with the unshared pair directed toward the fourth corner), giving the atoms a geometry called trigonal pyramidal (choice D). A triangular planar (choice A) geometry is one for three sets of electrons, and a trigonal bipyramidal (choice C) geometry is for five sets of electrons.

14. **(C)** All chlorine atoms or ions will have 17 protons because the atomic number of Cl is 17. If the number of protons is anything other than 17, the symbol will not be Cl. The superscript number (37) gives the atomic mass, which is the sum of the protons and neutrons. The charge (–1) gives information about the number of electrons. Since

there are 17 protons (17 positive charges) and the ion has a –1 charge, there must be 18 electrons.

15. **(D)** To determine the oxidation number of an element in a formula, it is necessary to assign oxidation numbers to all the other elements in the formula. For example, in PO_4^{-3}, oxygen has an oxidation number of –2. There are four atoms of oxygen in the formula, so the total oxidation value of oxygen is $4(-2) = -8$. Since the ion has a charge of –3, the oxidation number of phosphorus should be such that when it is combined with –8, a charge of –3 remains. Therefore, the oxidation number of phosphorus is $-3 = -8 + ?$. The value of +5 = ?. Oxygen is assigned an oxidation number of –2, except when it is present in a peroxide, e.g., H_2O_2, when the oxidation number is –1.

16. **(C)** The electron configuration can be read from the periodic table. The first two columns of the periodic table represent the filling of s orbitals, the last six columns represent the filling of p orbitals, and the middle ten columns represent the filling of d orbitals. The shell number for the s and p orbitals is the same as the row number, while the shell number for the d orbitals is one less than the row number. Find Cl in the third row, then read off the orbitals starting at the upper left corner until you reach Cl. Starting at the top left, $1s^2 2s^2 2p^6 3s^2 3p^5$.

17. **(C)** A neutralization reaction is a reaction between an acid and a base. The most common bases are ionic compounds of hydroxide ion. Choice A is an oxidation–reduction reaction. The easiest way to see that is to notice that on the left magnesium is neutral, while on the right it is paired with sulfate ions, so it must be Mg^{+2} (meaning it has lost electrons to become an ion). Notice that choices B and D involve only one reactant, so they cannot possibly be a reaction between an acid and a base (two things).

18. **(C)** A 2.0 M H_2SO_4 solution contains 2 moles of H_2SO_4 per liter. We need 800 mL or 0.800 L. Multiplying 0.8 L by 2.0 gives 1.6 moles H_2SO_4. The formula weight of H_2SO_4 is 98, so 1.6 moles is 157 g H_2SO_4.

19. **(C)** To make 100 mL of a 1.5 M Na_2SO_4 solution, you first need to know what mass of Na_2SO_4 is needed. A 1.5 M solution contains 1.5 moles of Na_2SO_4 per liter, so in 100 mL (0.100 L) there would be 0.15 moles of Na_2SO_4. Since the formula weight of Na_2SO_4 is 142, 0.15 moles would be 21.3 g of Na_2SO_4 (0.15 moles $\times$ 142 g/mole = 21.3 g). Choices A and C have the correct mass of Na_2SO_4. The difference is in how much solvent is added. In choice A, the instructions say to add 100 mL of water while in choice C the instructions say to add water to make a final volume of 100 mL. Choice C is correct because the solution's volume is 100 mL (according to the definition of molarity). Adding 100 mL of solvent does not mean the volume of the solution will be 100 mL.

20. **(B)** The pH of a solution is the negative log of the hydrogen ion concentration. Logs refer to the power of ten required for the number given. The log of 10 is 1 ($10^1 = 10$). The log of 100 is 2 ($10^2 = 100$). The log is the exponent that 10 must be raised to in order to get the number you have been asked about. In this question, you have been asked what power of 10 (log) must you raise 10 to in order to get 1×10^{-3}. The answer is –3. Then, since the pH is the negative of that number, the pH equals 3.

21. **(B)** To calculate the number of moles, recall that one mole contains 6×10^{23} items.

$$1.2 \times 10^{10} \text{ atoms} \times (1 \text{ mole}/6 \times 10^{23} \text{ atoms}) = 2 \times 10^{-14} \text{ moles}$$

Recall that 1.2×10^{10} equals 12×10^9. Then, you have $(12 \times 10^9)/(6 \times 10^{23})$.

$\dfrac{12}{6} = 2$ and $\dfrac{10^9}{10^{23}} = 10^{-14}$.

22. **(B)** Moles may be defined as grams/molar mass.

$$\text{moles} = \frac{\text{grams}}{\text{molar mass}}$$

The molar mass of carbon dioxide, CO_2, is

$$1 \text{ C} = 1(12) = 12$$
$$2 \text{ O} = 2(16) = 32$$
$$12 + 32 = 44 \ \frac{\text{grams}}{\text{mole}}$$

Dividing 22 grams by $44 \ \dfrac{\text{grams}}{\text{mole}}$ gives 0.50 mole.

23. **(B)** From the ideal gas law ($PV = nRT$), you can get $\dfrac{P}{T} = nRV$. Thus, $\dfrac{P}{T}$ is a constant. Remember to change the temperature to Kelvin ($273 + 27 = 300$ K).

$$\frac{1 \text{ atm}}{300 \text{ K}} = \frac{5 \text{ atm}}{\text{new temperature}}$$

Solving for the new temperature, you get 1500 K, which is 1227°C.

24. **(C)** The reason why there are "gas laws" or equations that describe the behavior of gases in general is because gases behave similarly. One of the gas laws is Boyle's law which states that as the volume of a gas is increased, its pressure will decrease (or $P_1V_1 = P_2V_2$). The Kinetic Molecular Theory of gases (the theory that summarizes our understanding of gases as a result of the observations of the gas laws) states that the kinetic energy of gas particles increases with increased Kelvin temperature (i.e., they are directly proportional).

25. **(D)** Of the major classes of biomolecules, the lipids are characterized by their hydrophobicity (or lipophilicity) due to their structural nonpolarity. The other biomolecular classes (proteins, carbohydrates, and nucleic acids) have more polar features (like carbon–oxygen bonds, carbon–nitrogen bonds, oxygen–hydrogen bonds, and nitrogen–hydrogen bonds) and are therefore more hydrophilic (lipophobic).

26. **(B)** Denaturation involves the disruption of noncovalent intermolecular forces (in particular, hydrogen bonding, dipole–dipole interactions). Peptide bonds are covalent, and digestion involves the cleavage of these.

27. **(D)** The major biomolecular classes are carbohydrates (which have multiple alcohol groups), nucleic acids (which have phosphates, carbohydrates, and aromatic heterocycles), proteins (which have amide/peptide bonds), and lipids (which have long carbon chains).

28. **(B)** When an alkyl halide is converted to an alkene, a base is used. If the halide is primary or secondary, a strong base is required to accomplish an E2 elimination. NH_3 is a weak base but potassium t-butoxide is a strong base.

29. **(C)** $NaBH_4$ is a hydride-reducing agent that reduces aldehydes and ketones to alcohols.

30. **(D)** Copper (II) sulfide is an ionic compound because it is composed of a metal and a nonmetal. The Roman numeral II indicates that it is in the +2 oxidation state (i.e., +2 charge); thus, its formula will be CuS. According to the solubility rules, sulfides are generally insoluble in water.

31. **(D)** ^1H NMR gives information about the hydrogens in a molecule. Since there are three signals, there are three kinds of hydrogen in the molecule. Choice A can be excluded since this molecule has only four kinds of hydrogen, and choice C can be excluded since this molecule has five kinds of hydrogen. After comparing the number of signals in the spectrum to the number of different kinds of hydrogen in the molecule, look at the splitting pattern and integration information. Simple splitting patterns follow the n + 1 rule, meaning that the splitting pattern for a group of hydrogens will be equal to the number of neighboring hydrogens (those on an adjacent carbon) plus one. A doublet indicates that the hydrogens represented by that signal have one neighboring hydrogen, a singlet indicates that the hydrogens represented by that signal have no neighboring hydrogens, and a septet indicates that the hydrogens represented by that signal have six neighboring hydrogens. Both remaining choices B and D are consistent with the observed splitting pattern. The next level of comparison should be the chemical shifts of the signals. Since the septet is farthest downfield, the hydrogen represented by the signal must be the most deshielded in the molecule. In choice B, the signal for the methyl hydrogens (represented by the singlet since there are no neighboring hydrogens) would be farthest downfield (due to the adjacent oxygen)—the singlet is not the signal farthest downfield so choice B can be excluded. That leaves choice D as the correct answer, and indeed the hydrogen represented by the septet (since it has six neighboring hydrogens) is expected to be the signal farthest downfield.

32. **(A)** Resonance structures do not have atoms in different places, only pi and unshared electrons. The only structure for which this is true is choice A.

33. **(C)** Hydrogen bonding, the strongest intermolecular force, is the attraction between a partial negative atom of one molecule and a *very* partial positive hydrogen of another molecule. In order for the hydrogen to be of sufficient partial positive charge to be termed hydrogen bonding, the hydrogen must be covalently bonded to N, O, or halogen. It is only when hydrogen is covalently bonded to one of these atoms that the hydrogen will be partial positive enough to participate in hydrogen bonding.

34. **(C)** Cell membranes contain phospholipids, steroid hormones are lipids, and triglycerides in adipose tissue are lipids that store carbon chains for later oxidation through beta oxidation.

35. **(C)** The conformation of a protein is driven by its amino acid sequence that determines the kinds of amino acid side chains present. The hydrophilic side chains will be oriented toward the exterior of the conformation (where the polar water molecules

are) and the hydrophobic side chains oriented toward the interior of the conformation (where water is excluded).

36. **(C)** Boiling point is based on molecular weight (the heavier the molecule, the higher the boiling point) and the strength of intermolecular attractions. For the options available, choices A and C have the lowest molecular weight. For those two, the only intermolecular force possible is Van der Waals force (also known as London force). The more extended molecule in choice A would have more available sites for this type of force, but the more compact molecule in choice C would have fewer available sites (less surface area) so the intermolecular forces among molecules of choice C would be less extensive, and it would boil at a lower temperature.

37. **(C)** Amides are carboxylic acid derivatives, but they are less reactive than esters due to the significant electron donation to the carbonyl carbon by nitrogen through resonance. Carboxylic acid derivatives can only be made directly from other more reactive carboxylic acid derivatives; thus, an ester cannot be made directly from an amide. Nitriles (choice D) are not carboxylic acid derivatives. They must be hydrolyzed to a carboxylic acid and then converted to a carboxylic acid derivative prior to alcoholysis (the conversion of a carboxylic acid derivative to an ester by the addition of alcohol). Carboxylic acid halides and carboxylic acid anhydrides (choice B) are carboxylic acid derivatives and are more reactive than esters, so they can be directly converted to esters by alcoholysis.

38. **(B)** To hydrate an alkene, there are two major options: oxymercuration–demercuration (the reagents in choice A) and hydroboration–oxidation (the reagents in choice B). Oxymercuration–demercuration yields the Markovnikov alcohol (the new H goes on the least highly substituted carbon of the alkene and the OH goes on the more highly substituted carbon of the alkene) and hydroboration–oxidation yields the anti-Markovnikov alcohol (the reverse orientation).

39. **(B)** Each carbon atom in $H_2C = CH_2$ is bonded to three other atoms, bonded by two single bonds to two hydrogen atoms and bonded by a double bond to the other carbon atom. To determine the shape of the molecule, the double bond is considered to be one set of electrons. Therefore, each carbon is assumed to have three electron sets around itself and the shape of the molecule around each carbon atom is trigonal planar with a 120° bond angle. The hybridization of the trigonal planar carbon atom is sp^2.

40. **(C)** Deprotonation of alcohols a or b yields alkoxides that cannot be resonance-stabilized. Deprotonation of c yields an enolate that is resonance-stabilized through two additional resonance structures (since it is beta to the ketone). Deprotonation of d yields an enolate that is resonance-stabilized through only one additional resonance structure. Greater resonance stabilization (i.e., more resonance structures) corresponds to greater stability. The greater the stability of a conjugate base, the more acidic the acid.

41. **(B)** A buffer solution is one in which the pH remains constant even when small amounts of acid or base are added to the solution. A buffer solution consists of a weak acid and its conjugate base, or a weak base and its conjugate acid. Acetic acid, CH_3COOH, is the only weak acid present, along with its salt sodium acetate, CH_3COONa. The other acids, HCl, HNO_3, and H_2SO_4, are all strong acids.

42. **(B)** According to the Kinetic Molecular Theory of Matter, the molecules in a solid (choice A) are close together, the molecules of a liquid (choice C) are farther apart, and the molecules of a gas (choice B) are farthest apart. The farther apart molecules are, the more freely they can move.

43. **(D)** Grignard reagents attack carbonyl carbons. The reaction of ethyl Grignard with the ketone in choice A would give ethyl cyclopentanol whereas its reaction with choice C would give 3-ethyl-3-pentanol. The reaction of ethyl Grignard with the aldehyde in choice D gives 3-pentanol.

44. **(A)** To name esters, name the alkyl group attached to the oxygen first (in this case, methyl) and then name the rest of the molecule as if it is a carboxylate. Choice B is not even an ester (it would be named 2,3-dimethylbutanoate). Choice C is named 2-methylbutyl ethanoate. Choice D is also not an ester (it would be named 2,2-dimethylbutanoate).

45. **(B)** The change in free energy, ΔG, represents the energy which can be used to do work in a reaction. The change in free energy may be used to determine whether a reaction will take place as written or not.

    If $\Delta G < 0$, the reaction occurs spontaneously in the direction written.

    If $\Delta G > 0$, the reaction does not occur spontaneously in the direction written, but does occur spontaneously in the opposite direction.

    If $\Delta G = 0$, the reaction is at equilibrium and no change occurs.

46. **(A)** Entropy is a measure of the amount of disorder in a reaction system. More freedom of movement, or disorder, of molecules is possible in a gas than in a liquid than in a solid. In equation A, a solid is converted to a solid and a gas. More disorder can be present in the reaction system in the products, where a gas is produced, than in the reactants, where a solid is used. Disorder increases. In equation B, a gas is converted to a liquid. Disorder decreases. In equation C, two different gases are converted to a liquid. Disorder decreases. In equation D, a liquid and a gas are converted to a solid. Disorder decreases.

47. **(A)** Only a change in temperature can cause a change in the equilibrium constant of a reaction. Changes in either the volume (choice B) or concentration (choice C) of one of the components in the reaction system will cause a corresponding change in the volume or concentration of another component in the system to maintain a constant equilibrium. A catalyst (choice D) will cause a change in the mechanism and the activation energy of a reaction but has no effect upon the equilibrium constant.

48. **(A)** Beta decay is the loss of a nuclear electron (beta particle), resulting in the conversion of a neutron to a proton. Delta decay (choice B) is nonsense. Neutralization (choice C) is the reaction between an acid and a base. Nuclear resonance (choice D) is what some nuclei do when subjected to radio waves while in a magnetic field (what is going on in NMR or MRI).

Biological Processes

49. **(A)** Meiosis is a process comprised of two nuclear divisions in rapid succession that result in four gametocytes, each containing half the number of chromosomes found in somatic cells. When the two gametes unite in fertilization, the fusion reconstitutes the diploid number of chromosomes. Mitosis (choice B) leads to a new cell with the same number of chromosomes as the parent cell. Choices C and D are not real terms.

50. **(A)** 0% will have white hair color.

	B	B
b	Bb	Bb
b	Bb	Bb

51. **(C)** Acetylcholine is used to trigger a contraction in skeletal muscles. GABA (choice A) is associated with lowering anxiety. Epinephrine (choice B) regulates heart rate and blood pressure. Norepinephrine (choice D) stimulates the fight-or-flight reaction.

52. **(A)** Epinephrine levels are highest when we are awake and alert. Acetylcholine (choice B) is used to trigger a contraction in skeletal muscles. GABA (choice C) is associated with lowering anxiety. Dopamine (choice D) is involved in cognition and mood.

53. **(A)** GABA is associated with lowering anxiety. Epinephrine (choice B) regulates heart rate and blood pressure. Dopamine (choice C) is involved in cognition and mood. Norepinephrine (choice D) stimulates the fight-or-flight reaction.

54. **(A)** Norepinephrine stimulates the fight-or-flight reaction. Serotonin (choice B) is associated with balance and mood. Epinephrine (choice C) regulates heart rate and blood pressure. Acetylcholine (choice D) is used to trigger a contraction in skeletal muscles.

55. **(B)** Tetanus is caused by a neurotoxin secreted by a bacterium.

56. **(B)** Archaea are prokaryotic cells that live in extreme environments, while prokaryotic bacteria (choice A) do not live in extreme environments. Protists (choice C) are eukaryotic and do not live in extreme environments. Viruses (choice D) are not cellular.

57. **(B)** Proteins that exit the cell are created in the rough endoplasmic reticulum; cell type B has the largest area of rough endoplasmic reticulum membrane. Cell type A (choice A) has the second largest area of rough endoplasmic reticulum membrane. Cell type C (choice C) has the second smallest area of rough endoplasmic reticulum membrane. Cell type D (choice D) has the smallest area of rough endoplasmic reticulum membrane.

58. **(D)** New phospholipids are placed in the smooth endoplasmic reticulum; cell type D has the largest area of smooth endoplasmic reticulum membrane and therefore is likely to produce the largest amount of phospholipids. Cell type A (choice A) has the smallest area of smooth endoplasmic reticulum membrane. Cell type B (choice B) has the second smallest area of smooth endoplasmic reticulum membrane. Cell type C (choice C) has the second largest area of smooth endoplasmic reticulum membrane.

59. **(A)** Cells with large numbers of mitochondria require more ATP or energy to function; cell type A has the largest number of mitochondria of the cell types listed. Cell type B (choice B) has the second largest number of mitochondria of the cell types listed. Cell type C (choice C) has the smallest number of mitochondria of the cell types listed. Cell type D (choice D) has the second smallest number of mitochondria of the cell types listed.

60. **(B)** Digestive enzymes are localized to the lysosomes in a cell; cell type B has the largest number of lysosomes. Cell type A (choice A) has the second smallest number of lysosomes. Cell type C (choice C) has the second largest number of lysosomes. Cell type D (choice D) has the smallest number of lysosomes.

61. **(A)** Bacteria undergo cell division called binary fission. Bacteria may produce spores (choice B), such as endospores for protection, but they are not used in cell division. Bacteria exchange plasmid DNA via conjugation (choice C). Transduction (choice D) is when bacteria receive new genetic material via bacteriophage.

62. **(D)** Each cell contains a complete set of genes. The differentiation status of a cell is determined by the subset of the gene expressed in that cell.

63. **(C)** Bacterial chromosomes are circular and have only exons.

64. **(B)** The tricuspid valve is the valve closing the orifice between the right atrium and the right ventricle of the heart. The bicuspid valve (choice A) is the valve closing the orifice between the left atrium and the left ventricle of the heart. The pulmonary valve (choice C) connects the right ventricle and the pulmonary artery. The aortic valve (choice D) connects the left ventricle with the left atrium.

65. **(B)** The red blood cell would enter the right atrium through the inferior vena cava and pass into the right ventricle. The red blood cell would exit the right ventricle through the pulmonary trunk, pass through the lungs, and return to the left atrium through the pulmonary vein. From the left atrium, the red blood cell would enter the left ventricle and leave the heart through the aorta.

66. **(D)** About 97% of the oxygen transported in blood is bound to the heme portion of hemoglobin inside erythrocytes. About 3% is dissolved in plasma.

67. **(C)** The nuclear lamina is made of a type of cytoskeletal element called intermediate filaments. They support the nuclear envelope in animal cells. Choices A, B, and D all refer to cytosolic cytoskeletal elements.

68. **(A)** Vitamins function as coenzymes, parts of coenzymes, or parts of enzymes. Most vitamins cannot be synthesized by the body (choice B), and they are not broken down before use (choice C). Vitamins A, D, E, and K are fat-soluble vitamins (choice D).

69. **(D)** The probability is that crossing over increases for genes far apart on a chromosome.

70. **(C)** A reaction in which the enzyme is the catalyst may be written as follows:

Enzyme + Substrate – Enzyme-Substrate Complex – Enzyme + Product

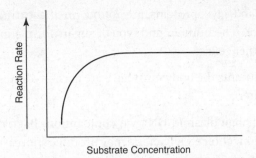

Substrate Concentration

The substrate binds to a specific site on the surface of the enzyme, known as the active site, after which the product and enzyme are released. The enzyme is then available to bind to another substrate. At low substrate concentration, the reaction rate increases sharply with increasing substrate concentration because there are abundant free enzyme molecules available to bind to an added substrate. At high substrate concentration, the reaction rate reaches a plateau as the enzyme active sites become saturated with substrate. The enzyme-substrate complex and no free enzymes are available to bind to the added substrate.

71. **(A)** Chondroblasts maintain cartilage. Osteoblasts (choice B) are involved in bone creation, creating the collagen needed in bone. They also regulate calcium ions. Keratinocytes (choice C) are found in the skin and produce keratin. Osteocytes (choice D) are mature bone cells that maintain bone mineral levels.

72. **(D)** Osteocytes are mature bone cells that maintain bone mineral levels. Fibroblasts (choice A) are associated with connective tissue, not bone. Keratinocytes (choice B) are found in the skin and produce keratin. Osteoclasts (choice C) are involved in bone healing.

73. **(B)** Osteoblasts are involved in bone creation, creating the collagen needed in bone. They also regulate calcium ions. Chondroblasts (choice A) maintain cartilage. Osteoclasts (choice C) are involved in bone healing. Fibroblasts (choice D) are associated with connective tissue, not bone.

74. **(C)** Osteoclasts are involved in bone healing. Chondroblasts (choice A) maintain cartilage. Osteoblasts (choice B) are involved in bone creation, creating the collagen needed in bone. Osteocytes (choice D) are mature bone cells that maintain bone mineral levels.

75. **(D)** Anaerobic heterotrophs undergo glycolysis and fermentation in the absence of oxygen to make energy. Choices A and B are incorrect because anaerobic indicates that oxygen is not needed. Choice C is incorrect because anaerobic heterotrophs undergo both glycolysis and fermentation in the absence of oxygen.

76. **(A)** One-fourth of their offspring, on average, will have silver fur. Choices C and D are not possibilities because none of the parents have silver fur.

	B	b
B	BB	Bb
b	Bb	bb

77. **(C)** The T-helper cells (T_4) are the most infected.

78. **(C)** Glycolipids and glycoproteins are found on the extracellular side of the cell plasma membrane. The number and type of sugars form a unique pattern that helps cells recognize other cells.

79. **(B)** The basic nutrients the body must have are carbohydrates, protein, fats, vitamins, minerals, and water.

80. **(C)** Bacteria exchange plasmid DNA via conjugation. Bacteria undergo cell division called binary fission (choice A). Bacteria may produce spores (choice B), such as endo-spores for protection. These are not used for genetic exchange. Transduction (choice D) is when bacteria receive new genetic material via bacteriophage.

81. **(C)** Cohesion keeps sister chromatids together until anaphase. Without cohesion, the mitosis checkpoint cannot sense tension.

82. **(A)** Actin forms a ring that constricts or pinches the cell membrane during cyto-kinesis.

83. **(D)** SNAREs initiate vesicular fusion to a target membrane. Digestive enzymes are carried to the cell's membrane via vesicles and are secreted via exocytosis.

84. **(B)** DNA polymerase is the enzyme responsible for DNA replication.

85. **(D)** A large sodium (Na^+) influx into the cell results in the resting potential of a neuron becoming more positive. An action potential is produced when the charge difference across the plasma membrane reverses and then returns to the resting condition which requires the movement of sodium (Na^+) ions into the cell. There is generally a higher concentration of potassium (K^+) ions inside the cell than outside, and conversely a higher concentration of sodium (Na^+) ions outside the cell than inside. Following the action potential, the sodium-potassium exchange pump restores ion concentrations by moving sodium (Na^+) ions out of the cell and potassium (K^+) ions into the cell.

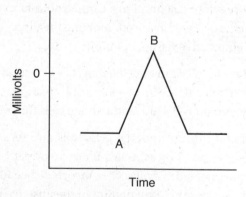

86. **(D)** Klinefelter syndrome is an abnormal number of sex chromosomes. Down syndrome (choice A) is also known as Trisomy 21. Turner syndrome (choice B) is the absence of a second sex chromosome. Edwards syndrome (choice C) is also known as Trisomy 18.

87. **(B)** Down syndrome is also known as Trisomy 21. Klinefelter syndrome (choice A) is an abnormal number of sex chromosomes. Patau syndrome (choice C) is known as Trisomy 13. Edwards syndrome (choice D) is also known as Trisomy 18.

88. **(D)** Turner syndrome is the absence of a second sex chromosome. Edwards syndrome (choice A) is also known as Trisomy 18. Klinefelter syndrome (choice B) is an abnormal number of sex chromosomes. Patau syndrome (choice C) is known as Trisomy 13.

89. **(C)** Edwards syndrome is also known as Trisomy 18. Down syndrome (choice A) is also known as Trisomy 21. Turner syndrome (choice B) is the absence of a second sex chromosome. Klinefelter syndrome (choice D) is an abnormal number of sex chromosomes.

90. **(D)** Platelets form from the breakdown of megakaryocytes in the blood stream. Erythrocytes, red blood cells (choice A), neutrophils (choice B), and lymphocytes (choice C), are all formed in bone marrow and do not arise from megakaryocytes.

91. **(D)** Myosin binds to actin to shrink sarcomeres during muscle contractions. Kinesin (choices A and B) is a motor protein involved in vesicular transport in cells. Myosin does not interact with microtubules (choice C).

92. **(B)** Type 2 diabetes may not require insulin injections for disease management. Choices C and D are not real conditions. Type 1 diabetes (choice A) is a result of the body not producing any insulin; therefore, insulin must be given as a treatment.

93. **(A)** Translation (choice B) involves the building of proteins, one amino acid at a time, from an mRNA template. Transduction (choice C) is the process in which bacteria receive new DNA from a bacteriophage. Translocation (choice D) is the movement of a large molecule, like a protein, across a membrane.

94. **(B)** Cell death is another term for apoptosis. Cell specialization (choice A) and differentiation (choice C) refer to stem cells that have changed to specific cell types. Cell proliferation (choice D) indicates cells that are undergoing the cell cycle often.

95. **(D)** The log (logarithmic) phase is the upward growth of bacteria in culture.

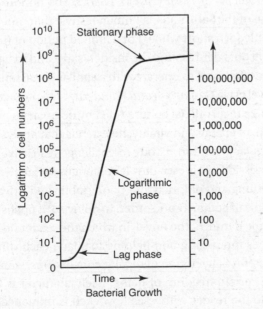

Bacterial Growth

96. **(C)** Since bacterium multiplies by binary fission at a generation time of 30 minutes, the population within 2 hours (12 noon–2:00 P.M.) is 2 at 12:30 P.M., 4 at 1 P.M., 8 at 1:30 P.M., and 16 at 2:00 P.M.

Critical Reading

The numbers in the margins of the reprinted passages indicate the statements in which the answer to the questions can be found.

Passage 1

Bakhtin uses the term **polyphonic** to describe the novel that depicts a world in which the dialogue goes on ad infinitum without reaching a conclusion or closure. The structure is not predetermined to demonstrate the author's worldview, nor are the characters drawn to exemplify it. It is typified by the novels of Dostoyevsky, in which the reader hears many voices uttering contradictory and inconsistent statements in the context of a real-life event. Truth in Dostoyevsky's works is perceived through multiple consciousnesses and expressed in many simultaneous voices, not conceived in a single

100 mind and spoken by a single character. There is no central voice in his novels, only multiple unfinalizable characters that talk about ideas in their distinctive, individual ways. They exist with each other and through each other as they interact in social circumstances. In addition to the characters that participate in the experience, there are the author and the reader, too, who with the characters help to create the novels' "truths," not simply one certain truth. Characters influence characters. Readers watch as they shape each other and listen as their utterances conflict with each other, all the while filtering the characters' observations through their own experiences and understanding. Bakhtin contrasts Dostoyevsky's approach with that of the nonpolyphonic monologism of Tolstoy, who reveals his own understanding of truth by expressing it through his characters' words, actions, and choices.

103   Another key concept in Bakhtin's theory of the novel is that of **carnival**, an idea that made its first appearance in his dissertation, "Rabelais and His World," and was further

98 developed in *Problems of Dostoyevsky's Poetics*. His notion of carnival builds on the ancient tradition of the Saturnalia, a Roman festival that mocked and reversed the official culture, if only for a short while. For a limited period of time the powerless became the powerful, the outsider became the insider, slave and master exchanged roles.

Bakhtin judges the novel to operate with a similar social impact. Building on his study of Rabelais's novel cycle *Gargantua and Pantagruel*, the protagonists of which he sees not

101 only as a challenge to an official culture ruled by dogmatism and deadly seriousness but

97 also as producers of energy and vitality, he extends that analysis to consider the novel as a genre that uses laughter and parody to challenge restrictive social forces, such as the tyranny and repression of his own day. It obliterates social hierarchies and blurs distinctions between young and old, rich and poor, public and private, in short reversing the traditional systems of authority and order. In doing so, it opens the way to joyful renewal.

The polyphonic nature of the novel, in which the reader hears conflicting statements

104 from many voices interacting and helping to shape each other, is carnivalesque. The clash of ideas destroys any notion of regular conventions, standardization, or rules, and even suggests a certain freedom of being. Each character is individually defined, and at the same time the reader witnesses how each is influenced by the other. Each one is touched by the others, and in turn shapes the character of the others. Carnival is the context in which voices are singly heard but interact together.

97. **(A)** As per the third paragraph of the passage, Bakhtin believed that the novel may be used to challenge tyranny and repression.

98. **(D)** According to the passage, Bakhtin's concept of carnival was based on Saturnalia, a Roman festival that mocked and reversed the official culture.

99. **(C)** Since the passage discusses two key theories of the novel set forth by Bakhtin, the most appropriate title would be "Understanding Bakhtin's Theories of the Novel" (choice C). Only the first paragraph briefly discusses expressions of truth in the works of Dostoyevsky and Tolstoy (choice A), while choices B and C fail to address Bakhtin's theory of the polyphonic novel.

100. **(A)** As per the first paragraph, there is no central voice in the novels by Dostoyevsky.

101. **(D)** The passage characterizes the official culture of *Gargantua and Pantagruel* as "ruled by dogmatism and deadly seriousness." Dogmatism is defined as stubborn adherence to a belief system.

102. **(B)** As explained in the first paragraph, in a polyphonic novel there are multiple characters who express multiple points of view or truths (choice B) while interacting and influencing each other. The characters are not used to express the singular truth or viewpoint of the author (choice A), nor do they operate independently and have little influence on each other (choice D). Choice C is not stated in the passage.

103. **(C)** Bakhtin first introduced the concept of carnival in his dissertation, *Rabelais and His World*.

104. **(B)** As stated in the last paragraph, the clash of ideas from conflicting statements and multiple voices destroys regular conventions and suggests a certain freedom of being.

Passage 2

110 Nonadherence to medication therapy results in numerous adverse effects such as increased hospitalizations and even death. Additionally, it costs the U.S. health care system billions of dollars each year. It is important to assess patients' adherence to medications.

107 Improper medication adherence encompasses an assortment of behaviors. These include not having a prescription filled, forgetting or intentionally not taking a medication, consuming an incorrect amount of a medication, taking a medication at the wrong time, ceasing therapy too soon, or continuing therapy after advised to discontinue. All forms of improper medication-taking behavior may jeopardize health outcomes.

105 Measuring medication-taking behavior is often difficult. The ideal method of measurement should be simultaneously unobtrusive (to avoid patient sensitization and maximize cooperation), objective (to produce discrete and reproducible data for each subject), and practical (to maximize portability and minimize cost). Refill records, pill

106 counts, electronic medication dispensers/caps, patient surveys (interviews), blood-drug level monitoring, and urine assay for drug metabolites can be used as clues to identify improper medication use.

108 Before altering therapy based on the assumption that a patient is taking a medication as prescribed, practitioners should ascertain the patient's medication-taking behavior.

This becomes especially important when modifying dosages of medications. Due to the advantages and disadvantages of each measurement, it is important for practitioners to use a combination of methods to assess a patient's medication-usage behavior and relate these findings to the patient's clinical presentation.

105. **(C)** The passage specifically states that the ideal method of measurement should be simultaneously unobtrusive (to avoid patient sensitization and maximize cooperation), objective (to produce discrete and reproducible data for each subject), and practical (to maximize portability and minimize cost).

106. **(D)** According to the passage, half-life tables, nucleic acid levels, and X-rays are not techniques for assessing a patient's medication usage. Choice D lists techniques used to assess medication usage.

107. **(A)** According to the passage, improper medication adherence includes those items listed in choice A. Choices B, C, and D are not true.

108. **(A)** Before altering therapy based on the assumption that the medication is being taken as prescribed, practitioners should assess the patient's behavior concerning taking his/her medication.

109. **(D)** Since the content of the passage primarily discusses the behaviors that encompass medication nonadherence, as well as methods used to measure medication-taking behaviors, choice D represents the most appropriate proposed title. The passage does not address other factors impacting U.S. health care costs, nor does it discuss the prevention of or interventions to treat medication nonadherence.

110. **(B)** Medications may still work even if the patient does not take it as advised, therefore ruling out choice A. Choice C is not the answer because the passage specifically stated billions, not trillions, and no mention of lawsuits was made. Also, no mention of suicides (choice D) was made. The first sentence of the passage discussed that nonadherence to medication therapy results in numerous adverse effects such as increased hospitalizations and even death. Therefore, the answer is choice B.

Passage 3

118 As many as 50 million Americans have high blood pressure, defined as a systolic blood pressure ≥140 mm Hg and a diastolic blood pressure ≥90 mm Hg. Although blood
111 pressure generally increases with age, the onset of hypertension most often occurs in
112 the third, fourth, or fifth decade of life. The prevalence of hypertension in the elderly population (age ≥65 years) is approximately 63% in whites and 76% in blacks. In younger generations (35 to 45 years of age), the prevalence is markedly different with 44% among black men, 37% among black women, 26% among white men, and 17% among white women.

A specific cause of sustained hypertension cannot be found in the vast majority of
115 individuals with high blood pressure. Genetic factors have been suggested to play a role in essential hypertension due to the fact that high blood pressure may be hereditary. Evidence that a single gene may account for specific subtypes of hypertension has also

been suggested. Genetic traits include high angiotensin levels, increased aldosterone and other adrenal steroids, and high sodium-lithium counter-transport. More direct approaches for preventing or treating hypertension could be achieved by identifying

114 individuals with these traits. Factors such as sodium excretion and transport rates, blood pressure response to plasma volume expansion, electrolyte homeostasis, and glomerular filtration rate help explain the predisposition for a person to develop hypertension.

116   Antihypertensive drug therapy should be individualized according to various patient characteristics and fundamental pathophysiologic circumstances. Dietary intake has been shown to be similar in all races but blacks ingest less potassium and calcium than whites. Supplemental potassium and calcium has been shown to cause a modest reduction in blood pressure in some studies. Therefore, it would seem reasonable to ascertain the effects of increasing the amount of potassium and calcium in the diet as part of the nonpharmacologic regulation of hypertension. The initial treatment for

113 hypertension is lifestyle changes, unless target-organ damage is present. These changes include sodium reduction, weight reduction, increased physical activity, and ethanol reduction or abstinence. In terms of target-organ damage, diuretics and beta-blockers are first-line therapy. Control of blood pressure and prevention of cardiovascular mor-

117 bidity and mortality are the goals of antihypertensive therapy. By maintaining arterial blood pressure below 140 mm Hg systolic and 90 mm Hg diastolic and by controlling other risk factors such as smoking, hyperlipidemia, and diabetes, morbidity and mortality may be averted.

111. **(B)** The onset of hypertension most often occurs in the third, fourth, and fifth decades.

112. **(C)** The passage states that, in both the younger and elderly generations, respectively, the prevalence of hypertension in black individuals is greater than in white individuals.

113. **(B)** Although all the choices may represent lifestyle changes, according to the passage, lifestyle changes that are suggested to lower blood pressure include sodium restriction, weight reduction, increased physical activity, and ethanol reduction or abstinence. Weight gain and increased stress may increase blood pressure.

114. **(B)** Two of the factors that help provide an explanation of hypertensive development are centered around electrolyte homeostasis and sodium excretion.

115. **(D)** Genetic factors have been suggested to play a role in essential hypertension based on the fact that high blood pressure may be hereditary.

116. **(A)** Antihypertensive therapy should be individualized according to patient characteristics and fundamental pathophysiologic circumstances.

117. **(D)** The passage states that by maintaining arterial blood pressure below 140 mm Hg systolic and 90 mm Hg diastolic and by controlling other risk factors, morbidity and mortality may be averted.

118. **(C)** As many as 50 million Americans suffer from high blood pressure, as per the passage.

Passage 4

121 We humans sense old age through feeling those creaky joints or observing those gray-ing hairs but, according to Apfeld and Kenyon reporting in a recent issue of Nature, <u>the nematode worm senses its age by smelling and tasting the environment</u>. These investigators show that worms with defective olfactory organs (that would normally detect odor molecules in the environment) live longer than their comrades with a keener sense of smell. By comparing these worms with other mutant nematodes that live an unusually long time, the researchers found clues to how a reduced ability to "smell the roses" might lengthen life span.

122 The worm's <u>olfactory sense organs—amphids on the head and plasmids on the tail—are composed of a cluster of nerve cells, the ends of which are modified into cilia.</u> The cilia are encircled by a sheath and a socket cell that form a pore in the worm's skin through which the tips of the cilia protrude. Odor molecules and soluble compounds bind to G protein-coupled receptors (similar to the olfactory and taste receptors of mammals) located at the tip of each cilium. Worms with a poor sense of smell—because their olfactory organs have defective or absent cilia, blocked pores, or damaged sheaths—live much longer, yet are otherwise normal (for example, their feeding and 120 reproductive behaviors are unchanged). <u>Mutations in TAX-4—a channel regulated by cyclic GMP that sits under the G protein-coupled receptor and transduces the sensory signals into electrical impulses</u>—also imbue the worm with a longer life.

123 But mutations in the worm's olfactory machinery are not the only defects that extend 124 its life span. In an earlier study, Kenyon's group found that <u>defects in the reproductive 125 system could prolong life by decreasing the activity of DAF-2 (a receptor for an insulin-like molecule) and increasing the activity of DAF-16 (a transcription factor). By looking at worms defective in both sensory perception and reproduction, Apfeld and Kenyon worked out a putative pathway through which smell might influence a worm's longevity.</u>

126 An environmental signal, perhaps produced by bacteria (the worm's favorite food), binds to G protein-coupled olfactory receptors on sensory cilia <u>activating TAX-4, which then incites electrical activity in the sensory neurons.</u> This activity triggers secretory vesicles in the neurons to release insulin-like molecules, which bind to DAF-2 and acti-119 vate the insulin-like signaling pathway. <u>This then switches on genes that will ensure the 128 worm dies at the usual age of 2 weeks. A reduced ability to sense olfactory cues would result in a decrease in DAF-2 activation and an increase in life span.</u>

This chain of events is not proven, but insulin-like molecules that might bind to DAF-2 have been identified in the nematode. Such a pathway would also make physiological sense. After all, if food is scarce it may behoove the worm to live longer to 127 ensure that it has the chance to produce its full quota of offspring. <u>A scarcity of food also promotes longevity in rodents and primates).</u> But so far it seems that in these more complicated creatures a poor sense of smell is not a harbinger of a ripe old age.

119. **(D)** A worm usually lives 2 weeks.

120. **(A)** TAX-4 is a channel regulated by cyclic GMP which sits beneath the G protein-coupled receptor and transduces the sensory signals into electrical impulses.

121. **(D)** A nematode worm detects its age by smelling and tasting the environment.

122. **(C)** The worm's olfactory sense organs are composed of a cluster of nerve cells of which the ends are modified into cilia.

123. **(D)** Aberrations in the reproductive system extend the life span of the worm.

124. **(A)** DAF-2 is a receptor for an insulin-like molecule.

125. **(B)** A logical pathway by which smell might influence a worm's longevity was achieved by studying worms defective in both reproduction and sensory perception.

126. **(A)** Sensory vesicles in the neurons are stimulated by TAX-4 to release insulin-like molecules.

127. **(D)** A scarcity of food is known to promote longevity in rodents and primates.

128. **(B)** The reduced ability to sense olfactory cues results in a decrease in DAF-2 activation and an increase in life span.

Passage 5

131 The most prevalent theme of the Group Member involves some loss of individuality within the group. Multiple lines of work in social psychology have explored the consequences of immersing oneself in the group to varying degrees. Usually these consequences are seen as bad. The Group Member can become deindividuated, may

135 engage in groupthink, and might even participate in mob violence. These negative effects reveal the group aspect of the Foolish Decision Maker . . . (If they were foolish to start with, they become even more so.) Indeed, the assumption that people degenerate

136 into inferior creatures by virtue of belonging to groups has crept into many other lines of research in social psychology, including social loafing, crowding, social facilitation, and diffusion of responsibility in bystander intervention.

The Group Member need not be a bad person, however. After all, interactions in groups is an almost inevitable part of human social life, especially if we include families as groups (which they most certainly are).

The motivations of the Group Members differ somewhat depending on which of two approaches is taken. One approach considers processes within the group. The Group Member must find ways to be accepted and liked by the other members, which

132 often requires determining how the member is similar to them and can fit in with them (getting along). The Group Member must also seek to rise through the group hierarchy (getting ahead), which may require finding ways to stand out among the group. More recent characterizations of the Group Member involve the cognitive work

129 that is involved in the various steps of entering the group, becoming socialized into full membership, finding a niche or rising through the ranks, exerting leadership, and exiting the group.

133 The other approach is to look at processes between groups. Intergroup processes have become a dominant focus of social psychology in Europe and Australia and have also been studied elsewhere. The emphasis is on how the individual identifies with the

134 group and relates to members of other groups. The Group Member is thus committed and loyal to his or her group and is competitive with and often prejudiced or even hostile toward other groups.

129. **(A)** As stated in the third paragraph, cognitive work of the Group Member involves becoming socialized into full membership and finding a niche.

130. **(A)** The passage describes both the motivations of group members (choice C) and the consequences of group membership (choice D). Therefore, the more general "Social Psychology Perspectives on Understanding the Group Member" (choice A) is a better choice as a title because it encompasses the multiple topics addressed in the passage. Choice B is not addressed in the passage.

131. **(D)** As per the passage, the most prevalent theme of the Group Member is loss of individuality.

132. **(B)** "Getting along" refers to establishing a fit within the group, and "getting ahead" is defined as advancing within the group hierarchy.

133. **(C)** The topic of intergroup processes has become of significant interest to social psychologists in Europe and Australia.

134. **(C)** As stated in the last paragraph, commitment to the group may result in competition with other groups.

135. **(A)** According to the passage, Foolish Decision Makers become *more* foolish as a result of group membership.

136. **(B)** Other areas of social psychology research that address the negative aspects of group membership include social loafing.

Passage 6

138   Drug interactions, a common type of drug-related problem, are categorized as pharma-
140 cokinetic, pharmacodynamic, or a combination of both. Pharmacokinetic drug interactions include changes in absorption, distribution, excretion, and metabolism, whereas pharmacodynamic drug interactions may lead to antagonistic or synergistic effects. Not all drug interactions are undesirable; in fact, many drug interactions are used to produce desirable effects. Patients who take drugs with narrow therapeutic indices and drugs that interfere with the pharmacokinetic properties of other drugs are at increased
141 risk of experiencing a drug interaction. Also, patients who take multiple medications per day or take multiple doses of medications per day are at increased risk. Because renal transplant patients take immunosuppressive agents that have narrow therapeutic indices and are subjected to multiple medications per day, they are vulnerable to expe-
143 riencing adverse drug events. To prevent adverse drug interactions, an alternative therapy should be considered when possible or the dose or schedule of the drugs should be adjusted to reduce the occurrence of an adverse experience. Additionally, adequate monitoring to prevent and detect adverse effects is an essential part of patient care.

     A common pharmacokinetic interaction involves drugs that interfere with the
142 absorption of other medications. Drugs that bind and decrease the gastrointestinal absorption of another drug, such as cholestyramine decreasing the absorption of tacrolimus, typically can be prevented by administering the agents two to three hours apart
137 from each other. Prokinetic agents interfere with the rate of absorption. Since many
139 transplant patients take prokinetic agents, such as metochlopromide, this may increase

the bioavailability of other medications. This is of significant importance since immunosuppressive agents have narrow therapeutic indices and toxicity may result from this interaction. If the prokinetic agent cannot be avoided, careful monitoring (e.g., serum drug levels, clinical presentation of the patient) and adjustments should be made to prevent immunosuppressant toxicity.

144

137. **(C)** The passage indicates that prokinetic agents interfere with the rate of absorption.

138. **(B)** The passage states that drug interactions are characterized as (1) pharmacokinetic, (2) pharmacodynamic, or (3) a combination of both.

139. **(C)** Toxicity can result from a prokinetic agent being administered with an immunosuppressive agent because the prokinetic agent may increase the bioavailability of the immunosuppressive agent.

140. **(B)** Pharmacokinetic drug interactions include changes in absorption, distribution, excretion, and metabolism.

141. **(A)** Patients who are at an increased risk of experiencing a drug interaction include those who take multiple medications per day or take multiple doses of medications per day.

142. **(D)** Cholestyramine is an example of a drug that binds and decreases the gastrointestinal absorption of another drug.

143. **(B)** To prevent adverse drug reactions, consider an alternate therapy or alter the dose or schedule of the drugs.

144. **(C)** If the prokinetic agent cannot be avoided, to prevent immunosuppressant toxicity, monitor the serum levels and the clinical presentation of the patient, and make appropriate adjustments.

Quantitative Reasoning

145. **(D)** We use the Fundamental Theorem of Calculus for integrals.

$$\int_2^3 \left(10x^4\right) dx = \frac{10x^5}{5}\bigg|_2^3 = 2x^5\bigg|_2^3 = \left(2\cdot(3)^5\right)-\left(2\cdot(2)^5\right) = 486-64 = 422$$

146. **(C)** First consider the four "non-R" letters. We have 2 choices for each of the 4 spaces, which gives $2^4 = 16$ possibilities. We now have the string _ * _ * _ * _ * _ , where the *s represents the "non-R" choices. Note we have 5 possible places to put the 3 Rs so that no 2 Rs are consecutive. Therefore, we have $_5C_3 = \frac{5!}{3!2!} = 10$ ways to place the Rs.

Thus, we have $\underbrace{2^4}_{\substack{\text{place the} \\ \text{non-}R\text{s}}} \cdot \underbrace{10}_{\substack{\text{place} \\ \text{the }R\text{s}}} = (16)(10) = 160$ possibilities

147. **(A)** Use the conversion formula:

$$\text{Celsius Temp} = \frac{5}{9} \cdot (\text{Fahrenheit Temp} - 32) = \frac{5}{9} \cdot (86 - 32) = \frac{5}{9} \cdot (54) = 30$$

148. **(A)** We use the Quotient Rule for logarithms.

$$\ln\left(\frac{a}{b}\right) = \ln(a) - \ln(b) = 12 - 3 = 9$$

149. **(A)** Since 1 teaspoon = 5 mL, 4 teaspoons = (4)(5) = 20 mL, taken 3 times daily. This means the patient takes (4)(3) = 12 teaspoons per day. Thus, a 10-day supply requires (12)(10) = 120 teaspoons.

150. **(A)** We compute $\dfrac{4+5+11+18+20+22+34+35+38}{9} = \dfrac{187}{9} \approx 20.77$.

151. **(B)** Since the selection order matters, we are counting the number of possible permutations of a length of 4 that can be formed from an 8-element set. The balls are chosen without replacement, so we have the following result:

There are 8 possibilities for the first number selected, 7 possibilities for the second number selected, 6 possibilities for the third number selected, and 5 possibilities for the fourth number selected. Thus, we have a total of $8 \cdot 7 \cdot 6 \cdot 5 = 1{,}680$ possible four-digit numbers.

152. **(A)** The total area of the given square plot = (210)(210) = 44,100 square feet. Since the given plot contains 1 acre, we have the equation

$$44{,}100 \text{ square feet} = 1 \text{ acre}$$

Multiplying the square feet by 3 yields:

$$(3)(44{,}100) \text{ square feet} = 3 \text{ acres}$$
$$132{,}300 \text{ square feet} = 3 \text{ acres}$$

153. **(B)** We use the Quotient Rule for derivatives.

$$\frac{d}{dx}\left(\frac{f(x)}{g(x)}\right) = \frac{g(x)f'(x) - f(x)g'(x)}{(g(x))^2} = \frac{(x^3+1)(5) - (5x)(3x^2)}{(x^3+1)^2}$$
$$= \frac{5x^3 + 5 - 15x^3}{(x^3+1)^2} = \frac{5 - 10x^3}{(x^3+1)^2}$$

154. **(C)** Calculate each number separately such that $10^2 = 100$ and $9^2 = 81$. Added together they equal 181. 181 can also be expressed as 1.81×10^2.

155. **(A)** Since point P is on the x-axis, P must have coordinates given by $(x, 0)$. The length of the segment with endpoints (x_1, y_1) and (x_2, y_2) is given by:

$$\text{length} = \sqrt{(x_2 - x_1)^2 + (y_2 - y_1)^2}$$

Applying the formula with length = 7, $(x_1, y_1) = (x, 0)$ and $(x_2, y_2) = (5, -3)$ yields:

$$7 = \sqrt{(5-x)^2 + (-3-0)^2}$$
$$7 = \sqrt{(5-x)^2 + (-3)^2}$$
$$7 = \sqrt{(5-x)^2 + 9}$$

Now square both sides.

$$(7)^2 = \left(\sqrt{(5-x)^2 + 9}\right)^2$$

$$49 = (5-x)^2 + 9$$

$$40 = (5-x)^2$$

$$\pm\sqrt{40} = 5-x$$

$$\pm 2\sqrt{10} = 5-x \Rightarrow x = 5 \pm 2\sqrt{10}$$

156. **(D)** Let x = the number of dimes, and $2x$ = the number of quarters. This yields the equation $10 \cdot x + 25 \cdot 2x$ = total money in cents. Therefore, we solve the equation:

$$10 \cdot x + 25 \cdot 2x = 660$$

$$60x = 660 \Rightarrow x = \frac{660}{60} = 11$$

Thus, John has 11 dimes, so $11 \cdot 2 = 22$, which means he has 22 quarters.

157. **(A)** We combine the terms by finding a common denominator.

$$\frac{3}{x} - \frac{2}{y} = \left(\frac{3}{x}\right)\left(\frac{y}{y}\right) - \left(\frac{2}{y}\right)\left(\frac{x}{x}\right)$$

$$= \left(\frac{3y}{xy}\right) - \left(\frac{2x}{yx}\right)\left(\frac{3y-2x}{xy}\right)$$

158. **(B)** Given the function $f(x) = 3x - 1$, we solve for y in the equation $x = 3y - 1$.

$$x = 3y - 1$$

$$x + 1 = 3y \Rightarrow y = \frac{x+1}{3}$$

159. **(D)** As x approaches 2 from the right-hand side, the values of $f(x)$ approach 0.

160. **(A)** As x approaches 2 from the left-hand side, the values of $f(x)$ approach –4.

161. **(B)** The left-hand and right-hand limits are not equal.

162. **(B)** The Product Rule for logarithms states that

$$\log(m) + \log(n) = \log(m \cdot n)$$

163. **(C)** From 12 noon to 6 P.M. is 6 hours. At a speed of 100 kilometers (km) per hour, the truck will travel 600 kilometers. Several conversions can be used to change kilometers to miles. One mile = 1.6 kilometers; one kilometer = 0.62 miles. For this problem 600 km $\cdot$ 0.62 miles per km = 372 miles.

164. **(A)** We need to solve the equation $\frac{48}{100} = \frac{x}{500}$. Multiplying both sides by 500 yields:

$$\left(\frac{48}{100}\right)(500) = \left(\frac{x}{500}\right)(500)$$

$$240 = x$$

165. **(A)** We use the integration rule.

$$\int_{e}^{e^2}\left(\frac{6}{x}\right)dx = 6\ln(x)\Big]_{e}^{e^2} = 6\ln(e^2) - 6\ln(e) = 6 \cdot 2 - 6 \cdot 1 = 6$$

166. **(B)** Use the Product Rule for derivatives:

$$\frac{d}{dx}\left(f(x) \cdot g(x)\right) = f'(x) \cdot g(x) + f(x) \cdot g'(x)$$

In this problem, we let $f(x) = e^{-x}$ and $g(x) = \cos(3x)$. Also note that $\frac{d}{dx} e^{-x} = -e^{-x}$ and $\frac{d}{dx}\cos(3x) = -3\sin(3x)$. Therefore, we have:

$$p'(x) = (-e^{-x}) \cdot \cos(3x) + e^{-x} \cdot (-3\sin(3x))$$
$$= (-e^{-x})\cos(3x) - 3e^{-x}\sin(3x)$$

167. **(D)** Since x approaches positive infinity, the numerator and the denominator are each dominated by their highest-powered terms; that is,

$$\lim_{x \to \infty}\left(\frac{8x^6 + 4x^2 - 10x + 5}{7x^6 + 12x^3}\right) \to \frac{8x^6}{7x^6} = \frac{8}{7}$$

168. **(A)** When a coin is tossed, only two outcomes are possible, heads or tails. No matter how many times a coin has been tossed, the probability on any one toss is 50 : 50 or 1 chance out of 2 for either heads or tails. Thus, there is a 50% chance for heads (or tails) on this toss.

169. **(D)** The projectile hits the ground when the height equals zero. We solve the equation $-0.004x^2 + 16x = 0$.

$$-0.004x^2 + 16x = 0$$
$$x(-0.004x + 16) = 0 \Rightarrow x = 0 \quad \text{or} \quad -0.004x + 16 = 0$$
$$16 = 0.004x$$
$$\frac{16}{0.004} = x$$
$$x = 4{,}000$$

170. **(A)** Represent the first five measurements by m_1, m_2, m_3, m_4, and m_5. Since the mean of the first five measurements is 208°C, we have the equation:

$$\frac{m_1 + m_2 + m_3 + m_4 + m_5}{5} = 208$$

Thus, $m_1 + m_2 + m_3 + m_4 + m_5 = (5)(208) = 1{,}040$. Now represent the sixth measurement by m_6. Since the mean of the six measurements is 210°C, we have the equation:

$$\frac{m_1 + m_2 + m_3 + m_4 + m_5 + m_6}{6} = 210$$

Since $m_1 + m_2 + m_3 + m_4 + m_5 = 1{,}040$, we have:

$$\frac{1{,}040 + m_6}{6} = 210$$

$$1{,}040 + m_6 = (6)(210) \Rightarrow m_6 = 220$$

171. **(A)** The probability that event A does not occur is given by the formula:

Probability that event A does not occur = 1 − probability of event A = $1 - \frac{5}{9} = \frac{4}{9}$

172. **(D)** The expression $4x = \frac{1}{2}$ can be solved by dividing both sides of the equation by four to provide the new equation $x = \frac{1}{2} \div 4$. The four can become $\frac{4}{1}$. Now the equation is $x = \frac{1}{2} \div \frac{4}{1}$. This rearranges, for the purpose of division, to become $x = \frac{1}{2} \times \frac{1}{4}$. Solving yields $x = \frac{1}{8}$.

173. **(D)** We need to compute the following:

% of patients who received Drug B + % of patients who received Drug C

$$= \frac{\text{# of patients who received Drug B}}{\text{total # of patients}} + \frac{\text{# of patients who received Drug C}}{\text{total # of patients}}$$

$$= \frac{200}{1,292} + \frac{42}{1,292} = \frac{242}{1,292} \approx 0.1873 = 18.73\%$$

174. **(D)** We need to compute the following:

% of patients who did NOT receive Drug A $= 1 -$ % of patients who received Drug A

$$= 1 - \frac{\text{# of patients who received Drug A}}{\text{total # of patients}}$$

$$= 1 - \frac{680}{1,292} \approx 0.4737 = 47.37\%$$

175. **(D)** Note that 1 milligram (mg) = 1,000 micrograms (mcg). Thus, a dose of 0.75 mg = (0.75)(1000) = 750 mcg. We are given the ratio $\frac{2}{500 \text{ mcg}}$. Therefore, the desired dose is given by:

$$\left(\frac{2}{500 \text{ mcg}}\right)(750 \text{ mcg}) = 3$$

176. **(A)** We calculate the slope using the formula $\frac{\Delta y}{\Delta x} = \frac{-6-3}{4-10} = \frac{-9}{-6} = \frac{3}{2}$.

177. **(B)** Given the function $y = f(x)$, if k is a positive number, then $y = f(x - k)$ shifts the graph of f to the right by k units. Thus, $y = f(x - 3)$ shifts the original graph 3 units to the right.

178. **(B)** We plug into the given formula:

$$\text{CrCl} = \left(\frac{(140-58)}{(72 \cdot 2.6)}\right) \cdot (76) = \left(\frac{82}{187}\right) \cdot (76) \approx 33$$

179. **(A)** Since f^{-1} represents the inverse function for f, the domain of f^{-1} corresponds to the range of f.

180. **(A)** The derivative of f is positive when the graph of f has a positive slope. Of the possible choices, the only valid interval is $x > 11.5$.

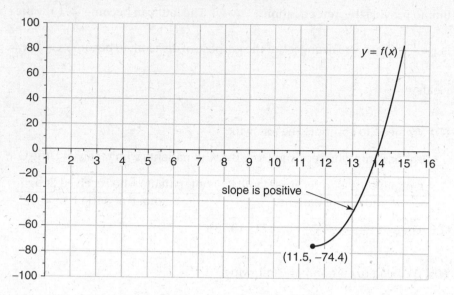

181. **(B)** The graph is concave down when $-\infty < x < 9$.

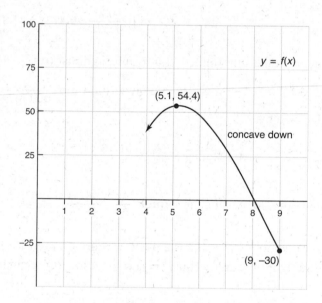

182. **(A)** A relative maximum corresponds to a "peak" on the graph.

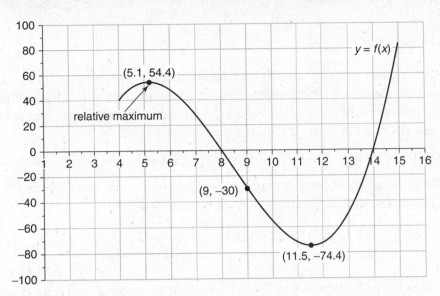

183. **(C)** Note that $\lim\limits_{x \to 8}\left(\dfrac{f(x) - f(8)}{x - 8} \right) = f'(8)$ is the slope of the graph when $x = 8$.

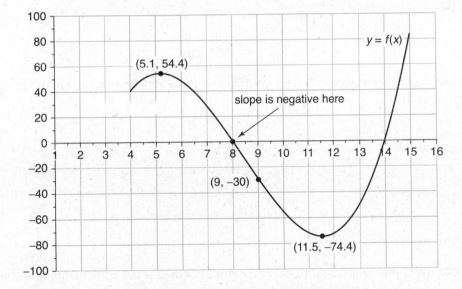

184. **(A)** We compute $\dfrac{f(4) - f(2)}{4 - 2} = \dfrac{64 - 8}{2} = 28$.

185. **(A)** In Stage 2, the original shaded area is subdivided into 4 equal triangles, and then one triangle is removed, leaving $\dfrac{3}{4}$ of the original shaded area. In Stage 3, each shaded triangle in Stage 2 is subdivided into 4 equal triangles, and then one triangle is removed, leaving $\dfrac{3}{4}$ of the Stage 2 shaded area. Thus, the shaded area in Stage 3 equals $\left(\dfrac{3}{4}\right)\left(\dfrac{3}{4}\right) = \dfrac{9}{16}$ of the original shaded area at Stage 1.

186. **(A)** The formula for slope (m) of a line is $m = \dfrac{y_2 - y_1}{x_2 - x_1}$. Substituting the values into the formula yields $m = \dfrac{5-1}{5-1} = 1$.

187. **(C)** Arrange the values in order from least to highest: 8, 9, 9, 9, <u>10</u>, <u>10</u>, 10, 11, 12, 12. Because there are an even number of values, you will need to find the average of the two values that fall in the middle of the list (10 and 10 as underlined). Add $10 + 10 = 20$. Then, divide 20 by 2, $20 \div 2 = 10$. The median value is 10.

188. **(D)** There are 5 options for each of the 3 letters. Total $= 5^3 = 125$.

189. **(D)** If the graph of f has a horizontal tangent line at the point where $x = a$, then $f'(a) = 0$. Applying the Quotient Rule for derivatives yields:

$$f'(x) = \frac{(x+2)(1)-(x)(1)}{(x+2)^2} = \frac{x+2-x}{(x+2)^2} = \frac{2}{(x+2)^2}$$

Setting $f'(x) = 0$ yields $\dfrac{2}{(x+2)^2} = 0 \Rightarrow 2 = 0$. Thus, the graph of f never has a horizontal tangent line.

190. **(D)** The coordinates of points P and Q must solve the system of equations:

$$x^2 + y^2 = 25$$
$$x + y + 1 = 0$$

Solving the second equation for x yields $x = -y - 1$. Substituting for x in the first equation yields:

$$(-y-1)^2 + y^2 = 25$$
$$y^2 + 2y + 1 + y^2 = 25$$
$$2y^2 + 2y - 24 = 0$$
$$y^2 + y - 12 = 0$$
$$(y+4)(y-3) = 0 \Rightarrow y = -4 \text{ or } y = 3$$

The sum of these values is $-4 + 3 = -1$.

191. **(C)** With the understanding that the symbol $\cup$ means the set of elements either in A or B or in both, and the symbol $\cap$ means the set that contains all those elements that A and B have in common, we use the formula:

$$P(A \cup B) = P(A) + P(B) - P(A \cap B) = 0.35 + 0.22 - 0.09 = 0.48$$

192. **(C)** The exact area of the shaded region is given by the definite integral $\displaystyle\int_{1}^{\sqrt{e}} \frac{3}{x}\, dx$.

Using the Fundamental Theorem of Calculus yields:

$$\int_{1}^{\sqrt{e}} \frac{3}{x}\, dx = 3\ln|x|\Big]_{1}^{\sqrt{e}} = \left(3\ln(\sqrt{e}) - 3\ln(1)\right) = 3 \cdot \left(\frac{1}{2}\right) - 0 = 1.5$$

Appendix: Weights, Measures, and Conversions

LENGTH

1 inch (in)		= 2.54 cm
1 foot (ft)	= 12 in	= 0.3048 m
1 yard (yd)	= 3 ft	= 0.9144 m
1 mile (mi)	= 1,760 yd	= 1.6093 km
1 millimeter (mm)		= 0.0394 in
1 centimeter (cm)	= 10 mm	= 0.3937 in
1 meter (m)	= 1,000 mm	= 1.0936 yd
1 kilometer (km)	= 1,000 m	= 0.6214 mi

AREA

1 square inch (in^2)		= 6.4516 cm^2
1 square foot (ft^2)	= 144 in^2	= 0.093 m^2
1 square yard (yd^2)	= 9 ft^2	= 0.8361 m^2
1 acre	= 4,840 yd^2	= 4,046.86 m^2
1 square mile (mi^2)	= 640 acres	= 2.59 km^2
1 square centimeter (cm^2)	= 100 mm^2	= 0.155 in^2
1 square meter (m^2)	= 10,000 cm^2	= 1.196 yd^2
1 hectare (ha)	= 10,000 m^2	= 2.4711 acres
1 square kilometer (km^2)	= 100 ha	= 0.3861 mi^2

WEIGHT

1 ounce (oz)	= 437.5 grains	= 28.35 g
1 pound (lb)	= 16 oz	= 0.4536 kg
1 kilogram (kg)	= 1,000 g	= 2.2 lb
1 short ton	= 2,000 lb	= 0.9072 metric ton
1 long ton	= 2,240 lb	= 1.0161 metric ton
1 milligram (mg)		= 0.0154 grain
1 gram (g)	= 1,000 mg	= 0.0353 oz
1 tonne	= 1,000 kg	= 1.1023 short tons
1 tonne		= 0.9842 long ton

VOLUME

1 cubic inch (in³)		= 16.387 cm³
1 cubic foot (ft³)	= 1,728 in³	= 0.028 m³
1 cubic yard (yd³)	= 27 ft³	= 0.7646 m³
1 cubic centimeter (cm³)		= 0.061 in³
1 cubic decimeter (dm³)	= 1,000 cm³	= 0.0353 ft³
1 cubic meter (m³)	= 1,000 dm³	= 1.3079 yd³
1 liter (L)	= 1 dm³	= 0.2642 gal
1 hectoliter (hL)	= 100 L	= 2.8378 bushel (bu)
1 fluid ounce (fl oz)		= 29.573 mL
1 liquid pint (pt)	= 16 fl oz	= 0.4732 L
1 liquid quart (qt)	= 2 pt	= 0.946 L
1 gallon (gal)	= 4 qt	= 3.7854 L

TEMPERATURE

$$\text{Celsius}° = \frac{5}{9}(\text{F}° - 32°)$$

$$\text{Fahrenheit}° = \frac{9}{5}(\text{C}°) + 32$$

$$\text{Kelvin} = 273.15 + \text{C}°$$

NOTES

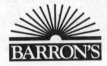
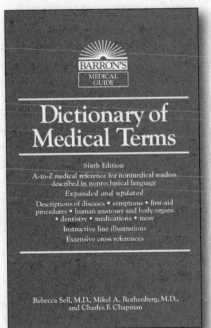

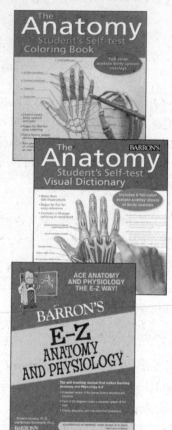
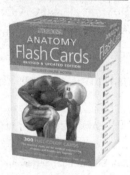

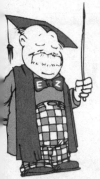
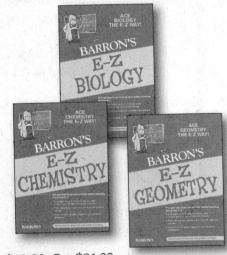
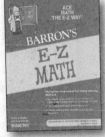
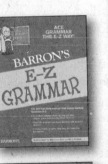
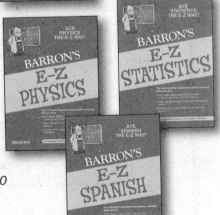
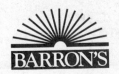

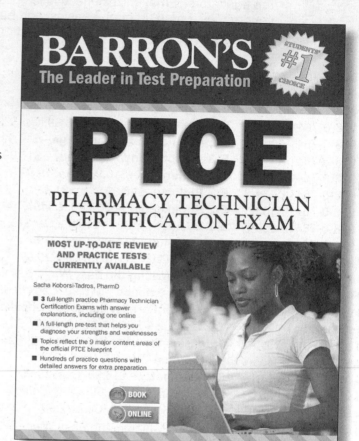